Lecture Notes
Psychiatry

Paul Harrison

DM, FRCPsych
Professor of Psychiatry
University of Oxford

John Geddes

MD, FRCPsych
Professor of Epidemiological Psychiatry
University of Oxford

Michael Sharpe

MD, FRCP, FRCPsych
Professor of Psychological Medicine
University of Edinburgh

Ninth Edition

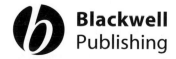

Blackwell
Publishing

© 2005 P.J. Harrison, J.R. Geddes and M. Sharpe
© 1964, 1968, 1972, 1974, 1979, 1984, 1989, 1998 by Blackwell Science Ltd
Published by Blackwell Publishing Ltd
Blackwell Publishing, Inc., 350 Main Street, Malden, Massachusetts 02148-5020, USA
Blackwell Publishing Ltd, 9600 Garsington Road, Oxford OX4 2DQ, UK
Blackwell Publishing Asia Pty Ltd, 550 Swanston Street, Carlton, Victoria 3053, Australia

First published 1964
Reprinted 1966
Second edition 1968
Reprinted 1970
Third edition 1972
Fourth edition 1974
Reprinted 1976
Fifth edition 1979
Portuguese edition 1980
Sixth edition 1984
Seventh edition 1989
Reprinted 1991, 1993
Eighth edition 1998
Reprinted 1999, 2001, 2002, 2003, 2004
Ninth edition 2005

Library of Congress Cataloging-in-Publication Data
Harrison, P. J. (Paul J.), 1960–
    Lecture notes. Psychiatry.—9th ed. / Paul Harrison, John Geddes, Michael Sharpe.
        p.   ;   cm.
    Rev. ed. of: Lecture notes on psychiatry. 8th ed. c1998.
    Includes bibliographical references and index.
    ISBN-13: 978-1-4051-1869-9 (alk. paper)
    ISBN-10: 1-4051-1869-5 (alk. paper)

    1. Psychiatry—Outlines, syllabi, etc.   2. Psychiatry—Examinations, questions, etc.
    [DNLM: 1. Psychiatry—Examination Questions.   2. Psychiatry—Handbooks.   WM 34 H321L 2005]   I. Title:
Psychiatry.   II. Geddes, John, MD.   III. Sharpe, Michael.   IV. Harrison, P. J. (Paul J.), 1960- Lecture notes on
psychiatry.   V. Title.

    RC457.2.H375 2005
    616.89—dc22

                                                                                                    2004024194

ISBN-13: 978-1-4051-1869-5
ISBN-10: 1-4051-1869-5

A catalogue record for this title is available from the British Library

Set in 8/12 Stone Serif by SNP Best-set Typesetter Ltd., Hong Kong
Printed and bound in India by Replika Press Pvt. Ltd.

Commissioning Editor: Vicki Noyes
Development Editors: Nic Ulyatt/Karen Moore
Production Controller: Kate Charman

For further information on Blackwell Publishing, visit our website:
http://www.blackwellpublishing.com

Contents

Preface vi

1 Getting started 1
2 The core psychiatric assessment 6
3 Psychiatric assessment modules 16
4 Risk: harm, self-harm and suicide 36
5 Completing and communicating the assessment 41
6 Aetiology 49
7 Treatment 57
8 Psychiatric services 80
9 Mood disorders 87
10 Neurotic, stress-related and somatoform disorders 101
11 Eating, sleep and sexual disorders 113
12 Schizophrenia 122

13 Organic psychiatric disorders 136
14 Substance misuse 150
15 Personality disorders 160
16 Childhood disorders 168
17 Learning disability (mental retardation) 181
18 Psychiatry in other settings 188

Multiple choice questions 194
Answers to multiple choice questions 198
Appendix 1: ICD-10 classification of psychiatric disorders 201
Appendix 2: Keeping up-to-date and evidence-based 202
Further reading 203
Index 207

Preface

Four percent of medical students end up as psychiatrists. This book is aimed equally at the other 96%, because the skills, attitudes and knowledge you will learn by studying psychiatry are relevant to all doctors—and other health professionals.

After providing what we hope and believe are convincing reasons why psychiatry is worth studying and how to start (Chapter 1), we take a practical approach to 'doing' psychiatry. Our guide to assessment comprises a relatively brief core (Chapter 2), followed by more detailed modules to be used as required (Chapter 3), and a guide to risk assessment (Chapter 4). Chapter 5 describes how to draw everything together and communicate the information to others.

The middle chapters cover the principles of aetiology (Chapter 6), treatment (Chapter 7) and services (Chapter 8). We have tried to be evidence-based in our treatment recommendations. Useful sources of evidence and ways of keeping up to date are provided in Appendix 2.

The main psychiatric disorders of adults are covered in Chapter 9–15, followed by childhood disorders (Chapter 16) and learning disability (Chapter 17). Last but not least, Chapter 18 discusses the psychiatric assessment and treatment in non–psychiatric medical settings—the place where most psychiatry actually happens.

In writing the book we have tried to make psychiatry both logical and enjoyable. Naturally, it is also intended to help you to pass the end-of-course exam, so we've highlighted important facts in each chapter and have included some multiple choice questions, and suggestions for other sources of information.

We are grateful to Marian Perkins and Tim Andrews for expert advice on child psychiatry and learning disability respectively, and to the many other colleagues who have generously shared their expertise with us.

The book is dedicated to Sandra, Rosie, Charlotte and Grace; Jane and Caitlin; Liz, Joe and Anna.

PJH, JRG and MCS
December 2004

Chapter 1

Getting started

Psychiatry can seem disconcertingly different from other specialties, especially if your first experience is on a psychiatric in-patient unit. How do I approach a patient? What am I trying to achieve? Is he dangerous? Does it have anything to do with the rest of medicine? This chapter is meant to help orientate anyone facing the same situation. Like the rest of the book, it is based on three principles:

- Psychiatry is part of medicine.
- Psychiatric knowledge, skills and attitudes are relevant to all doctors.
- Psychiatry should be as effective, pragmatic and evidence-based as every other medical specialty.

What is psychiatry?

'Psychiatry is . . . weird doctors in Victorian asylums using bizarre therapies on people who are either untreatably mad or who are not really ill at all.' Although remnants of such ill-informed stereotypes persist, the reality of modern psychiatry is very different and rather more mundane! Psychiatry is, in fact, fundamentally similar to the rest of medicine: it is based upon making reliable diagnoses and applying evidence-based treatments that have success rates comparable to those used in other specialties. Most patients with psychiatric illness are not mad and most are treated in primary care. Nor are psychiatric patients a breed apart—psychiatric diagnoses are common in medical pa-

tients. And psychiatrists are no stranger than other doctors, probably.

Psychiatric disorders may be defined as illnesses that are conventionally treated with treatments used by psychiatrists, just as surgical conditions are those thought best treated by surgery. The specialty designation does not indicate a profound difference in the illness or type of patient. In fact it can change as new treatments are developed; peptic ulcer moved from being a predominantly surgical to a medical condition once effective drug treatments were developed. Similarly, conditions such as dementia may move between psychiatry and neurology.

The conditions in which psychiatrists have developed expertise have tended to be those that either manifest with disordered psychological functioning (emotion, perception, thinking and memory) or those which have no clearly established biological basis. However, scientific developments are showing us that these so-called psychological disorders are associated with abnormalities of the brain, just as so-called medical disorders are profoundly affected by psychological factors. Consequently, the delineation between psychiatry and the rest of medicine can increasingly be seen as only a matter of convenience and convention.

However, traditional assumptions continue to influence both service organization (with psychiatric services usually being planned and often

1

situated separate from other medical services) and terminology (see below).

Where is psychiatry going?

Psychiatry is evolving rapidly and three themes permeate this book:
- *Psychiatry, like the rest of medicine, is becoming less hospital-based.* Most psychiatric problems are seen and treated in primary care, with many others handled in the general hospital. Only a minority are managed by specialist psychiatric services. So psychiatry should be learned and practised in these other settings too.
- *Psychiatry is becoming more evidence-based.* Diagnostic, prognostic and therapeutic decisions should, of course, be based on the best available evidence. It may come as a surprise to discover that current psychiatric interventions are as evidence-based (and sometimes more so) as in other specialties.
- *Psychiatry is becoming more neuroscience-based.* Developments in brain imaging and molecular genetics are beginning to make real progress in the neurobiological understanding of psychiatric disorders. These developments are expanding the knowledge base and range of skills which the next generation of doctors will need.

Why study psychiatry?

Studying psychiatry is worthwhile for all trainee doctors, and other health practitioners, because its *knowledge*, *skills* and *attitudes* are applicable to every branch of medicine. Specifically, studying psychiatry will give you:
- A basic knowledge of specialist psychiatric disorders.
- A working knowledge of common psychiatric problems encountered in all medical settings.
- The ability to assess effectively someone with a 'psychiatric problem'.
- Skills in the assessment of psychological aspects of medical conditions.
- A holistic or 'biopsychosocial' perspective from which to understand all illness.

Useful knowledge

Formerly, patients with severe psychiatric disorders were often institutionalized and their management was exclusively the domain of psychiatrists. The advent of community care (Chapter 8) means that other doctors, especially GPs, encounter and participate in their management, so all doctors need basic information about these 'specialist' psychiatric disorders. Equally, all doctors need to recognize and treat the more common psychiatric illnesses, such as anxiety and depressive disorders. These are extremely prevalent in all medical settings, including primary care and general hospitals (Chapter 18).

Useful skills

Most psychiatric disorders are diagnosed from the history, and many treatments are based on listening and talking. So, psychiatrists have had to retain particular expertise in interviewing patients, in assessing their state of mind, and in establishing a therapeutic doctor–patient relationship. These skills remain important in all medical practice. For example, all doctors should be able to:
- Make the patient feel comfortable enough to express their symptoms and feelings clearly.
- Use basic psychotherapeutic skills. For example, knowing how to help a distressed patient and how best to communicate bad news.
- Discuss and prescribe antidepressants and other common psychotropic drugs with confidence.

Without these 'soft' skills, the 'hard' skills of technological, evidence-based medicine cannot be fully effective. For example, an impatient, non-empathic doctor is less likely to elicit the symptoms needed to make the correct diagnosis, and her patient is less likely to adhere to the treatment plan she prescribes.

Useful attitudes

Psychiatric diagnoses are still associated with stigma and misunderstanding. These stem largely from the misconception that illnesses that do not have established 'physical pathology are 'mental' and that such 'mental' illness is not real, represents personal inadequacy and is the person's own fault. Studying psychiatry will help you to challenge these attitudes. You will see many patients with severe symptoms in whom no 'organic' pathology has been established, but who have real symptoms and disability. You will be repeatedly reminded of the stigma which patients with psychiatric problems experience from the public and (sadly) some health professionals. Finally, you will be confronted with the reality of human frailty. Recognizing these issues and dealing with them appropriately — by developing positive, educated and effective attitudes — is another important consequence of studying psychiatry. You might conclude, as we have done that:

● Suffering is real even when there is no 'test' to prove it.

● Psychological and social factors are relevant to all illnesses and can be scientifically studied.

● Much harm is done by negative attitudes towards patients with psychiatric diagnoses.

● Your own experience and personality will influence your relationship with patients — your positive attributes as well as your vulnerabilities and prejudices.

How to start psychiatry

The psychiatric interview

The first, key skill to learn is how to listen to and talk with (in that order) patients. The *psychiatric interview* has two functions:

● It forms the main part of the psychiatric assessment by which diagnoses are made.

● It can be used therapeutically — in the psychotherapies, the communication between patient and therapist is the currency of treatment (Chapter 7).

Psychiatric assessment

Because of its central importance, the principles of psychiatric assessment are outlined here. The prac-

ticalities are described in the next two chapters. Psychiatric assessment has three goals:

● To elicit the information needed to make a diagnosis, since a diagnosis provides the best available framework for making clinical decisions. This may seem obvious, but it hasn't always been so.

● To understand the causes and context of the disorder.

● To form a therapeutic relationship with the patient.

Though these goals are the same in all of medicine, the balance of psychiatric assessment differs:

● The interview provides a greater proportion of diagnostic information. Physical examination and laboratory investigations play a lesser, though occasionally crucial, role.

● The interview includes a detailed examination of the patient's current thoughts, feelings, experiences and behaviour (the *mental state examination*) in addition to the standard questioning about the presenting complaint and past history (the *psychiatric history*).

● A greater wealth of background information about the person is collected (the *context*).

Psychiatric assessments have a reputation for being excessively long. We take a pragmatic approach to the *process* of assessment. A *core assessment* is used to collect the essential diagnostic and contextual information (Chapter 2). Then, more detailed *modules* are used if anything has led you to hypothesize that the patient has a particular disorder (Chapter 3).

● This two-stage approach considerably shortens most assessments — to 30–45 minutes or less. It also happens to be what psychiatrists actually do — as opposed to what they tell their students to do.

Diagnostic categories

Solving a problem is always easier when you know the range of possible answers. Similarly, before embarking on your first assessment, it helps to know the major psychiatric diagnoses and their cardinal features. Table 1.1 is a simplified guide. As you gain experience, aim for more specific diagnoses which correspond to those listed in the International

Table 1.1 A basic guide to psychiatric classification.

Category	Examples of disorders	Basic characteristics	Common presentations
Organic disorder	Dementia, delirium	Defined by 'organic' cause	Forgetfulness, confusion
Psychosis	Schizophrenia, bipolar disorder	Delusions, hallucinations	Bizarre ideas, odd behaviour
Neurosis	Anxiety disorders	Emotional disturbance	Worried, tired, stressed
Somatoform disorders	Somatization disorder	Unexplained physical symptoms	Chronic pain, fear of disease
Mood disorders	Depression	Low mood	Tearful, fed up, somatic complaints
Substance misuse	Opiate dependence	Effects of the drug	Addiction, withdrawal, depression
Personality disorder	Dissocial, histrionic	Dysfunctional personality traits	Exacerbation of traits when stressed
Learning disability	Down's syndrome, autism	Congenitally low IQ	Developmental delay, physical appearance

Classification of Diseases, 10th revision (ICD-10) which are used in this book.

- There is an American alternative to ICD-10, called the Diagnostic and Statistical Manual of Mental Disorders (DSM-IV), widely used in research. The two systems are broadly similar.
- Whatever the classification, remember the underused category of 'no psychiatric disorder'.
- A term like 'nervous breakdown' has no useful psychiatric meaning—it may describe almost any of the categories in Table 1.1.

Psychiatric classification

The classification of psychiatric disorders has several problems that you should be aware of before you start:

- *Most diagnoses are syndromes, defined by combinations of symptoms, but some are based on aetiology or pathology.* For example, depression can be caused by a brain tumour (diagnosis: organic mood disorder) or after bereavement (diagnosis: abnormal grief reaction), or without clear cause (diagnosis: depressive disorder). This combination of different sorts of category leads to some difficulties, which will become apparent later.
- *Comorbidity: many patients suffer from more than one psychiatric disorder* (or a psychiatric disorder and a medical disorder). The comorbid disorders may or may not be causally related, and may or may not both require treatment. As a rule, comorbidity complicates management and worsens prognosis.
- *Hierarchy: not all diagnoses carry equal weight.* Traditionally, organic disorder trumps everything (i.e. if it is present, coexisting disorders are not diagnosed), and psychosis trumps neurosis. This principle is no longer applied consistently, partly because it is hard to reconcile with the frequency and clinical importance of comorbidity.
- *Psychiatric classification is not an exact science.* All classifications have drawbacks, and psychiatry has more than its share. Despite the imperfections, rational clinical practice requires a degree of order to be created. Most of the diagnostic categories have good reliability and utility in predicting treatment response and prognosis.

After the assessment: summarizing and communicating the information

Completion of the psychiatric assessment is followed by several steps:

- *Make a differential diagnosis*, using your knowledge of the key features of each psychiatric disorder.

• *Attempt to understand how and why the disorder has arisen* (Chapter 6).

• *Develop a management plan*, based on an awareness of the best available treatment (Chapter 7), how psychiatric services are organized (Chapter 8), and on the patient's characteristics, including their risk of harm to self or others (Chapter 4).

• *Communicate your understanding of the case* (Chapter 5).

Key points

• Psychiatry is a medical specialty. It mostly deals with conditions in which the symptoms and signs predominantly concern emotions, perception, thinking or memory. It also encompasses learning disability and the psychological aspects of the rest of medicine.

• Knowledge, skills and attitudes learned in psychiatry are relevant and valuable in all medical specialties.

• Be alert to the possibility of psychiatric disorder in all patients, and be able to recognize and elicit the key features.

• The major diagnostic categories are: neurosis, mood disorder, psychosis, organic disorder, substance misuse and personality disorder.

Chapter 2

The core psychiatric assessment

Approaches to psychiatric assessment

The principles and goals of psychiatric assessment were outlined in Chapter 1. A 'traditional' first assessment interview includes both an extensive search for symptoms and detailed, wide-ranging questions about the patient's life history. Though comprehensive, this approach is inefficient and can take well over an hour, which in many situations is unrealistic. Also, the content and conduct of the assessment are largely prespecified, and hard to modify or abbreviate—probably a reason why psychiatric problems are neglected in general medical practice.

We suggest a more flexible approach to assessment in which screening questions and other basic information (The Core; this Chapter) are used to identify possible diagnoses, which are then confirmed or excluded by more specific assessment (The Modules; Chapter 3). This lessens the time required for assessments and, we think, makes them more satisfying.

• To use the core and module strategy successfully you need a working knowledge of psychiatric disorders and their symptoms, in order to generate the diagnostic hypotheses that guide your assessment. This basic knowledge can be attained rapidly. A useful start is to learn Table 1.1 and to browse the key points at the end of each chapter.

The mental state examination

All psychiatric assessments include a mental state examination (MSE) as well as the history. Two aspects of the MSE can cause confusion:
• *What is the time frame?* Classically, the MSE is limited to those features present at the time of examination, with everything else being in the history. In practice, the MSE is often also used to assess the patient's report of recent (past hours or days) symptoms. Be aware that some examiners adhere to the division between history and MSE more rigidly.
• *Is the MSE the psychiatric equivalent of the physical examination in medicine?* To a degree it is, since it is where the *signs* of psychiatric disorder (i.e. observations made by the interviewer—'patient keeps looking anxiously around') are elicited. However, the MSE also includes *symptoms* (experiences reported by the patient—'I can hear an alien over there') and in this respect it overlaps with the history (Figure 2.1).

The 'core and module' psychiatric assessment

The *core* is a 'stripped down' assessment designed to:
• Obtain a clear account of the patient's main problem(s).

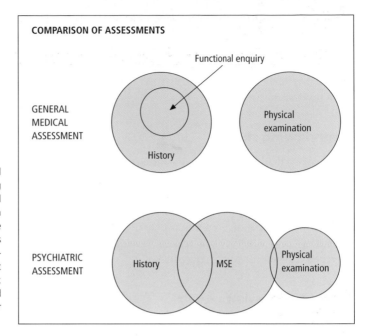

Figure 2.1 A comparison of medical and psychiatric assessments, showing the relationship of history, functional enquiry, mental state examination (MSE) and physical examination. Note the overlap between the components of the psychiatric assessment. For example, recent suicidal thoughts might be detected in the history or MSE; akathisia (Chapter 7) may be elicited as a symptom in the history or MSE or as a sign in the physical examination.

• Screen rapidly but systematically for evidence of psychiatric disorder.

• Provide the background (contextual) information needed to guide immediate management.

An assessment may then proceed to use one or more *modules* according to:

• The diagnostic suspicion(s) raised by the core assessment or other available information.

• The need to exclude a disorder that, though unlikely, would be clinically significant.

The modules cover cognitive function, psychosis, mood disorder, neurosis, eating disorder, substance misuse, somatic symptoms and the unresponsive patient. Each is designed to confirm whether a disorder in that category is present and, if so, to establish the specific diagnosis. Each module also covers contextual information needed for the overall understanding of the case.

• Assessment of childhood disorders, learning disability and sexual functioning are covered in their respective Chapters. Risk assessment is described in Chapter 4.

The way the interviewer moves from core to module, and the number of modules that are needed, will differ from case to case. It may also change as the interviewer becomes more experienced (i.e. becomes better at generating good diagnostic hypotheses). Three examples show how the assessment may develop:

• *A woman complains of tiredness. The core assessment reveals evidence of depression and a recent increase in alcohol intake, but not of suicidal intent, psychosis, or cognitive impairment. You proceed to the mood and substance misuse modules which confirm the presence of a depressive disorder, but no significant alcohol problem.*

• *A man is brought in having been found lying in the road screaming at passers by to stop persecuting him. On this basis, you proceed to the psychosis and risk assessment modules regardless of what he may report during the core assessment (since he may initially deny symptoms in case you are part of the conspiracy). Given that illicit drugs can produce this kind of behaviour, you also use the substance misuse module.*

• *A wife reports her 70-year-old husband is getting confused. Your initial suspicions are of dementia, so you administer the cognitive module. However, though concentration is poor, he does not appear demented. Returning to the core, you find evidence of depression, so you move to the mood module which shows that he is suffering from a severe depressive episode.*

If no modules have been triggered by the core assessment and review of the case, it may be concluded that there is no evidence that the person has a psychiatric disorder.

Interviewing skills

Effective psychiatric assessment comes from knowing what questions to ask when, and how to ask them. So, before proceeding to the content of the assessment we outline the skills needed to obtain the necessary diagnostic information rapidly and accurately—and which will help you develop a therapeutic relationship with the patient.

Before the interview

- Arrange the setting. Chairs are best arranged at ninety degrees to each other. If a desk is required for making notes, this should not be directly between the patient and the interviewer.
- Arrange not to be interrupted.
- Read any referral letter and previous notes. These may provide a preliminary diagnostic hypothesis, clarify the reason for the referral, and suggest lines of questioning.

Beginning the interview

- Introduce yourself, check the identity of the patient, and make him comfortable.
- Sit in a relaxed and slightly forward posture.
- Describe the reason for the interview, the time available, and the procedure to be followed.
- Emphasize confidentiality. If notes are to be taken, explain why.

Progress of the interview

- Begin by asking an open question such as: 'How have you been feeling?' or 'Could you start by telling me a bit about what you think is the problem?' Closed (but not leading) questions are used to clarify the responses (e.g. 'You say you're not sleeping well: is it that you can't get to sleep, or that you wake too early?').
- Encourage the patient to list their main problems and describe each in his own words. Ensure you understand the nature of the current problem, before asking when it started.
- Keep control of the interview, yet allow the patient sufficient time to answer questions fully and in his own way. This balance can be the hardest skill to learn.
- Get answers that are as precise as possible—for example, estimates of symptom duration.
- As well as responding to what the patient says, be sensitive to non-verbal clues—for example the patient's facial expression, posture or tone of voice.

Ending the interview

- Summarize your understanding of the case to the patient and ensure you've gained an accurate picture
- Ask if anything has been overlooked.
- Give the patient an opportunity to ask questions.
- Explain what you plan to do next.

The core psychiatric assessment

The core psychiatric assessment covers the essence of the topics in Table 2.1 and is outlined below.
- The accompanying notes provide background and rationale to the questions, plus a glossary of important terms.

The core history

Reason for referral

Who made the referral? Why?

Notes
- Clarify what questions the referrer wants addressed. This may give clues about the best way of approaching the interview and suggest initial diagnostic possibilities.
- Identify the best *informant* available—someone to supplement and corroborate the history.

Table 2.1 The core psychiatric assessment.

Core history
  Reason for referral
  Presenting complaint(s), and their history
  Psychiatric and medical history
  Alcohol and drug use

Core mental state examination
  Appearance and behaviour
  Mood
  Speech
  Thoughts
  Perceptions
  Cognition
  Insight (Attitude to illness)

Core contextual information
  Family history
  Personal history
  Current circumstances

(Risk assessment)

(Core physical examination)

Presenting complaint(s) and their history

What does the patient think is the main problem or problems?

Does the patient have any other problems? List them.

Assess the nature, duration and progression of the symptom(s).

Are there any precipitating and relieving factors? Has any treatment already been tried?

Assess the degree of functional impairment: effect on relationships, work, sleep etc.

Notes
• Getting a list of the patient's problems allows you to start generating diagnostic hypotheses. Some problems will be symptoms; others will represent the patient's predicament or provide the context of the disorder (e.g. homelessness).
• The diagnostic importance of a particular psychiatric symptom is affected by its characteristics (intensity, fluctuation, etc.) and associated features. Knowing the relevant information to elicit comes rapidly with increasing knowledge and experience.

Psychiatric and medical history

Nature of any previous psychiatric contact. Diagnosis? Treatments tried, and their effect.

Current medication and allergies.

Any serious medical illnesses or operations?

Notes
• About 50% of referrals have had prior psychiatric contact. A previous diagnosis is best seen as a strong hypothesis (i.e. it has a high pretest probability) to be tested. Past history may also provide useful information about prognosis and the patient's attitude to his disorder and its management.
• Psychiatric and medical disorders have many overlaps, hence the need to elicit any significant past or current medical history.

Alcohol and drug use

How much does the patient drink in an average week?

If patient reports that s/he drinks alcohol regularly, ask the CAGE questions:
• Have you ever felt you ought to **C**ut down on your drinking?
• Have people **A**nnoyed you by criticising your drinking?
• Have you ever felt **G**uilty about your drinking?
• Have you ever had a drink first thing in the morning (an '**E**ye-opener')?

Notes
• Alcohol and other drugs may be a cause, a component, or a consequence of many psychiatric disorders. All are common, so substance misuse should always be briefly ascertained.
• The recommended limits for alcohol intake are 21 units per week for men and 14 for women. (1 unit is half a pint of beer, a single measure of spirits, or a small glass of wine.)
• The CAGE is a useful screening tool. If three or more yes answers are given, the likelihood ratio for problem drinking is 250. If the patient answers no to all four questions, the likelihood ratio is 0.2.

Repeat questions for any illicit drugs used.

The core mental state examination (MSE)

The core MSE concentrates on aspects of the recent mental state which are commonly affected by psychiatric disorder and which have diagnostic weight.

• Much of the core MSE will have been covered in the history, from observations made in passing, or as part of a module already administered. However, the MSE is still useful to ensure that the presence or absence of all important recent phenomena are established and documented.

The headings of the core MSE are:

• *Appearance and behaviour*—much can be gleaned from careful observation of the patient's manner, movements, and dress. An underestimated source of diagnostic information.

• *Mood*—depressive symptoms are very common. This section covers them, and the associated issue of suicidal risk.

• *Speech*—abnormal speech may be present in neurological, psychotic and mood disorders.

• *Thoughts*—thought content and the way thoughts flow are affected in many psychiatric disorders. The nature of the abnormality gives important diagnostic clues.

• *Perceptions*—mainly affected in psychotic and organic disorders. Lesser alterations in sensory experiences also occur in neurosis.

• *Cognition*—cognitive impairment is characteristic of dementia and delirium. If present, it may prevent a useful history from being taken.

• *Insight*—lack of awareness of illness is classically a sign of psychosis or organic disorder, whilst the attitude to illness affects adherence to treatment and hence prognosis.

Appearance and behaviour

Note the attitude of the patient to the interview and the rapport made.

Is the patient tearful, anxious, overactive or underactive?

Are there any unusual movements or eccentric behaviour?

Note the patient's physical appearance and dress.

Notes

• Many psychiatric disorders are accompanied by characteristic changes in manner, emotional expression or physical appearance. These often provide the first diagnostic clue. So, from the moment you meet, observe closely. For example:

— An ataxic man having problems getting to his chair. Could he have a frontal lobe tumour? Is he intoxicated?

— A patient avoiding eye contact and with little facial expression—is he depressed?

— A tremor, suggesting Parkinson's disease or that the patient is on antipsychotic drugs or lithium.

Mood

• Have you been low in spirits or depressed recently?

• Can you still enjoy the things that you normally enjoy?

Ask about suicidal ideation. Use cues from the patient to broach the subject. For example:

• It sounds as if life's a bit of a struggle at the moment. Have you felt life isn't worth living?

• Have you actually thought of harming yourself in anyway?

• Have you made any plans to end your life?

Notes

• Record both how the patient reports his mood (*subjective* mood) and also how it appears to you (*objective* mood).

• Always screen for mood disorders. They are common and some patients may not be aware of, or do not complain of, mood symptoms.

• The best screening questions for depression concern the presence of persistent low mood, and the loss of pleasure (*anhedonia*).

• Always assess suicidal intent (Chapter 4). There is no evidence that asking about suicide increases the risk of it—probably the opposite.

• The mood section of the MSE can also reveal anxiety symptoms. Usually, however, these are detected more from appearance and thoughts sections.

Speech

Does the patient speak spontaneously or only in response to questioning?

Is the patient's speech hard to understand? Is it because of articulation (dysarthria) or content (dysphasia)?

Notes
- Quiet speech which tails off or is monosyllabic is typical of depression; the opposite occurs in mania.
- Dysarthria suggests a neurological disorder or side-effect of antipsychotic drugs.
- Dysphasia suggests a focal neurological disorder or thought disorder.
- Abnormalities in the content or flow of what is said are recorded in the next section.

Thoughts

Ask patient to describe current preoccupations and worries.
- Do you have particular things on your mind at the moment?

Is the patient's train of thought difficult to follow? Try and describe how?
- Have you ever felt that people were against you?
- Have there been times when you felt that something strange was going on?
- Have your thoughts been directly interfered with by some outside force or person?

Notes
Abnormalities of thoughts and thought processes occur in many psychiatric disorders, and the precise form of the abnormality can be diagnostically important. Distinguish between the *content*, *nature* and *flow* of thoughts:
- **Thought content.** Record the presence and topic of predominant thoughts. For example:
  — recurrent worries about physical health in hypochondriasis
  — a general theme of persecution in a delusional disorder
  — a preoccupation with weight in an eating disorder

- **The nature of the thoughts.** Three types of abnormal thought are recognized. Each has a very different diagnostic significance:
  — *A **delusion** is a false belief. It is firmly held despite contrary evidence and is out of keeping with the patient's cultural or religious background.* For example, a patient is absolutely convinced that he is an assassin's target and so has locked himself in his flat and adopted a disguise. There may be one delusion or many, and they may be persistent or fleeting. Delusions carry special weight in the diagnosis of psychosis, so their recognition is an important skill. During the development and treatment of psychosis, delusions may be *partial*, in that the patient realizes they might be false.
  — *An **obsession** is a recurrent thought, impulse or image that enters the subject's mind despite resistance.* The patient realizes that it originates from their own mind and may not be true, but they cannot resist thinking it and often have to act upon it (a *compulsion*). For example obsessional thoughts about having dirty hands, the compulsion being to wash repeatedly. These symptoms characterize obsessive-compulsive disorder and also occur in depression.
  — An **overvalued idea** is a belief not held quite as strongly as a delusion, and is typically more 'understandable'. It is typified by the belief of a malnourished girl with anorexia nervosa that she is fat.
- **The flow of thinking.** Even if the content and nature of thoughts are normal, the flow (form) of thinking may not be. This is called *thought disorder* or *formal thought disorder*. It is often first detected if the patient is given time to reply at length to an open question, whereupon the interviewer realizes he is having problems following the train of thought. Write down a sample of what is said. Different sorts of thought disorder characterize schizophrenia and bipolar disorder.

Perceptions

Have you ever seen or heard things that other people couldn't?

Have you ever heard voices speaking when there was nobody there?

Do things or people seem different from normal?

Notes
- *A **hallucination** is a perception experienced as real in the absence of a stimulus.* For example, hearing a voice in the corner of the room when no-one's there. Hallucinations are pathognomonic of psychosis. They can occur in any modality; auditory ones are commonest, visual hallucinations suggest an organic psychosis. Like partial delusions, there are also partial hallucinations—usually called *pseudohallucinations*—which are perceived inside the head; they have little diagnostic significance. Similarly, hallucinations are common whilst falling asleep (*hypnogogic*) or waking up (*hypnopompic*) and are not abnormal.
- *An **illusion** is a misperception*—for example seeing someone in the shadows when there's no-one there. They have an 'as if' quality and in isolation have no diagnostic significance (and so an illusion must be distinguished clearly from hallucination).
- ***Depersonalization** is a feeling of detachment from the normal sense of self*—'as if I am acting'. *Derealization* is similar, a feeling of detachment from the external world. Both are a feature of neurosis but can be mistaken for the perplexity of psychosis.

Cognition

Is the patient orientated in time, person and place?
Is there 'clouding of consciousness'?
Show the patient three items (e.g. watch, pen, shoe) and ensure they have registered them; test for recall 2 minutes later.

Notes
- If the patient can recall the three items, the likelihood ratio for cognitive impairment is 0.06.
- Cognitive impairment is the hallmark of organic disorders—especially dementia and delirium. It can also occur in depression (*pseudodementia*) and schizophrenia (previously called *dementia praecox*).
- In delirium there is *clouding of consciousness* (usually manifested as decreased responsiveness to, or awareness of, surroundings); in dementia there isn't (Chapter 13). See cognitive function and unresponsive patient modules.
- If cognitive abnormalities are detected, physical examination and the cognitive function module are essential.

Insight

Do you think anything is wrong with you? If so, what?
Do you need any treatment? If so, what sort?

Notes
- Insight is a matter of degree, and fluctuates according to the mental state. It includes the ability to recognize:
  — abnormal mental experiences as abnormal;
  — that the person is suffering from a psychiatric disorder;
  — the need for treatment.
- The patient's attitude affects management, especially the issue of compulsory admission.

Core contextual information

Recording key details of the person's background and current circumstances are part of the core assessment because they provide a *context* for the patient's problems. This helps in several ways:
- It enhances the therapeutic relationship by demonstrating an interest in the patient's problems.
- It identifies potentially modifiable contributory problems (e.g. accommodation difficulties).
- It reveals personal factors which affect management (e.g. the presence of a supportive partner).
- It is necessary for understanding why the disorder has occurred.
- It sometimes helps diagnostically. For example, asking about employment reveals that a man lost his job for being late; further questioning showed this to have resulted from an unrecognized alcohol problem.

How much contextual enquiry is needed depends on the nature of the patient's problems, and what is already known. For example, in general practice the patient's circumstances will usually be well known; for an out-patient whose marriage and business are failing, extensive questioning might be needed to clarify the relationship of these problems to her depressive disorder.

Contextual information falls into three broad categories: *family history*, *personal history* and *current circumstances*.

Family history

Family tree—at least parents, siblings, children. Their ages, occupations, health.
Nature of the family relationships.
Family psychiatric history.

Notes
• Problems in family relationships are commonly associated with psychiatric disorder.
• A positive family history is a risk factor for most psychiatric disorders—for genetic and environmental reasons.

Personal history

Childhood—health problems, maltreatment, school record.
Personality—the patient's usual attitudes, mood, beliefs, and interests.
Relationship(s)—number, duration, type.
Employment history (nature of work, problems).
Criminal offences?

Notes
• Aspects of childhood can be associated with subsequent psychiatric disorder (e.g. conduct disorder with dyssocial personality disorder; childhood abuse with later depression, and neurotic disorders).
• The premorbid personality shapes the risk, type and prognosis of psychiatric disorder. Ask simple questions about relationships, interests and prevailing mood. Offering alternatives may be helpful—for example 'Would you describe yourself as a loner or very sociable?'

• A patient's view of their personality and life may be distorted during psychiatric illness. For example, a depressed person will report themselves in an unduly negative light. Always corroborate personality details from a close informant.
• The pattern of past relationships can give diagnostic clues; for example an absence of close relationships in schizoid personality disorder.
• The nature of employment gives clues to the patient's level of functioning. A deteriorating or disrupted work record may reflect a psychiatric disorder or a personality trait respectively.
• Having a 'forensic history' (i.e. a criminal record) may be directly related to a psychiatric disorder or a coincidence. A history of violence will affect management regardless—see risk assessment (Chapter 4).
• Questions on sexual history and functioning (Chapter 11) may be necessary at this stage.

Current circumstances

Current relationships.
Current employment.
Current worries—finances, housing, relationship, etc.

Notes
• The current relationship is an important factor: it may have contributed to the disorder or have been damaged by it. Having a supportive partner improves outcome and assists management. Check the partner's gender.
• All patients with severe psychiatric disorder should have an assessment of needs (Chapter 8). Detailed information about the current circumstances is an essential component of this.
• Ongoing worries and stresses can perpetuate psychiatric disorder; their resolution is often part of management (e.g. sorting out a housing problem).

The core physical examination

The physical health of a psychiatric patient is important because:

• Medical conditions can present with psychological symptoms. For example, lethargy and low mood may signify anaemia or carcinoma.

• Patients with psychiatric disorders have increased rates of medical illness, either because of a common aetiology or because the psychiatric disorder leads them to neglect their health.

So, in every assessment take account of the patient's physical appearance, and always consider what examination is required. This may include a brief examination of all systems. However, there is no pre-specified physical examination in the psychiatric assessment since it depends upon the setting, the patient, the disorder and the treatment.

The setting. For example:

• A full examination is performed on every psychiatric admission because the psychiatrist takes medical responsibility whilst the patient is in hospital.

• In an emergency assessment, have a low threshold for examination since the possibility may not have been considered in the rush to refer the patient.

• In primary care, the GP may have examined the patient thoroughly before referral.

The patient. For example:

• Full examination if the patient has not been seen by a doctor recently.

• Full examination if homeless, since at risk of tuberculosis, malnutrition, etc.

• Examine relevant systems if there is a history of a medical disorder.

The disorder and its treatment. For example:

• If alcohol misuse is suspected, examine for the physical signs which accompany it.

• Patients on long-term antipsychotic drugs should be examined for tardive dyskinesia.

• Patients with somatic symptoms.

For patients receiving psychiatric care in the community, the responsibility for the patient's medical health should be agreed between psychiatrist and GP; usually it resides with the latter.

Core investigations

Core medical investigations do not exist in psychiatry, other than the convention that routine blood tests are performed on admission to an in-patient ward. Elsewhere, investigations should be used to test a specific diagnostic hypothesis arising from the history, MSE or physical examination. For example:

• A urine drug screen in suspected drug-induced psychosis.

• Extensive biochemical, imaging and genetic investigations in a 30-year-old with dementia.

• A brain scan in someone with delirium and a history of a fall.

• Thyroid function tests in a patient with anxiety, palpitations and weight loss.

Shrinking the core: a 'one minute screen' for psychiatric disorder

The core assessment is portable for use in all settings, not just in specialist psychiatry. However, there are occasions when only a moment can be spent on psychiatric assessment. Even this is worthwhile. The seven questions in Table 2.2 screen rapidly for psychiatric disorders common in general practice or the general hospital.

• A positive response to any question should lead to a core and module assessment.

Table 2.2 A 'one minute screen' for common psychiatric disorders.

During the past month:	Screening for:
1. Have you felt low in spirits?	*depression*
2. Do you enjoy things less than you usually do?	*depression*
3. Have you been feeling generally anxious?	*neurosis (anxiety)*
4. Are you worried about your health or other specific things?	*neurosis (health anxiety)*
5. Has your eating felt out of control?	*eating disorder*
6. Do you drink alcohol? If so, ask CAGE questions (p. 9)	*alcohol problem*
7. Present 3 items and ask patient to recall them after 2 minutes.	*dementia/delirium*

Key points

- The aim of psychiatric assessment is to gather sufficient information to make a diagnosis and set it in context.
- Most information comes from the history and mental state examination, though physical examination and investigations are sometimes important too.
- Diagnostic hypotheses should be made early in the assessment and then tested using more specific questioning.

- A flexible approach can be achieved by combining a core assessment with specific modules (next Chapter) which are only used when the likelihood of a specific diagnosis is raised.
- Psychiatric disorder can and should be rapidly screened for in all medical settings.
- Interviewing skills allow you to gather information efficiently and form an effective alliance with the patient.

Chapter 3

Psychiatric assessment modules

Using assessment modules

The purpose of the core assessment (Chapter 2) was to screen efficiently for features associated with a high probability of psychiatric disorder. The modules are used to confirm, refine or refute these diagnostic hypotheses. The modules focus on: cognitive function, psychosis, mood, neurosis and related disorders, eating disorders, substance misuse and the unresponsive patient.

- Each module contains general advice about the areas to cover, suggestions for specific questions, and explanatory notes and definitions of key terms. There is no distinction between the history and mental state examination in the modules; different headings are used as required to suit the module.
- The clinical features of psychiatric disorder are covered in Chapters 9–15. Refer to the relevant chapter in conjunction with the module.
- An adequate assessment often requires more than one module.
- Other aspects of assessment are covered elsewhere: risk (Chapter 4), sexual functioning (Chapter 11), children (Chapter 16) and learning disability (Chapter 17).

We do not suggest reading this chapter in one go. Instead, read through a module as you come across a clinical problem requiring its use.

Assessment of cognitive function

Cognitive function comprises attention, memory and language. It is the first module, since impairment in these areas interferes with the psychiatric assessment, occasionally to the point that no useful history can be obtained from the patient.

Key questions addressed by the module

- *Is clinically significant cognitive impairment present?*
- *If so, what is its cause?* The major causes are *dementia* (chronic, normal level of consciousness) or *delirium* (acute, consciousness impaired). Both have a range of specific causes, which are then investigated (Chapter 13).

Triggering the module

The suspicion of cognitive impairment may have arisen for many reasons. For example:
- The patient has scored poorly on the core cognitive screen.
- The patient is muddled, as judged by their manner or response to initial questions.
- A history of forgetfulness.
- The patient is old (e.g. >20% of 90 year olds have dementia).

Related modules

If the person can't or won't answer questions, use the *unresponsive patient* module. The *mood* module is often needed because depression can cause mild cognitive impairment. The ability to self-care may be impaired, so *risk* assessment is necessary.
- If poor cognitive functioning is longstanding, consider *learning disability* (Chapter 17).
- Deafness is a classic, but hopefully rare, cause of a misdiagnosis of dementia.

The cognitive function module

Before proceeding, revise the cognition section of the core assessment (Chapter 2). First, ask whether the patient (or their informant) has noticed a problem with memory, and characterize this. While doing so, note the patient's understanding and use of language, and their ability to attend to the questions.

• Do you find yourself forgetting things? Can you give me some examples?
• When did it begin?
• Do you have any problems finding words, or understanding what people say to you?

Sometimes it is useful to ask the patient to describe the main events and chronology of their day (especially if you can corroborate the history).

• If they give an implausible story, consider *confabulation* (the fabrication of recent events to cover gaps in memory) that occurs in *amnesic syndrome* (Chapter 13).

Then, tell the patient you want to ask some questions to assess his memory. This makes people anxious, so emphasize it's not a pass or fail kind of test. The questions comprise the *mini-mental state examination* (*MMSE*), a widely used screen for dementia (Table 3.1).

• The MMSE is distinct from the mental state examination (MSE).
• Normal MMSE score is 25–30. A score of 25–21 suggests dementia or delirium (likelihood ratio 5); 20 or less is highly suggestive (likelihood ratio 8).
• Ensure the patient has registered each question — don't be misled by sensory problems, and try to note any lack of attention or motivation.
• An alternative screen is the *seven-minute screen*, which is quicker but not so widely used. It actually takes about 12 minutes.

Assessing the cause of cognitive impairment

Assess for features of delirium.
• Is the person drowsy? Are they fully aware of their surroundings?
• Are they distractible? Irritable?

Table 3.1 The Mini-Mental State Examination (MMSE).

1. What day of the week is it? (Score 1)
2. What is the date? (1) And the month? (1) And the year? (1) What is the season? (1)
3. What country are we in? (1) The county? (1) The town [city/village]? (1) The hospital or the street? (1) The name of this ward? [Name/number of this house?] (1)
4. Name three objects (e.g. clock, table, umbrella) and ask patient to repeat them. (Score 1 for each one recalled correctly after a single presentation — maximum 3). If any failures, repeat names till all three registered.
5. Spell 'world' backwards. (Score 1 for each letter in correct order; max. 5)
6. Point to a pencil and a watch and ask patient to name them (2)
7. Now could you tell me the three objects that I named a few minutes ago? (3)
8. Repeat 'No ifs, ands or buts'. (1)
9. Tell patient to: 'Take this paper in your right hand, fold it in half, and put it on the floor.' (Score 1 for each part; max. 3)
10. Show the patient the words 'Close your eyes' and ask them to do what it says. (1)
11. Ask the patient to write a short sentence of her choice. (Score 1 if it makes grammatical sense — ignore spelling)
12. Ask patient to copy this figure:

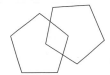

(Score 1 if both shapes are five-sided and the intersecting lines make a quadrangle)

• Do they seem to be hallucinating?
• When did the problems start?
• Any obvious cause (e.g. postictal, septic).
Administer the depression module.

Notes
• The hallmark of delirium is '*clouding of consciousness*' — drowsiness, distractibility, delusions and visual hallucinations. There is usually an acute onset and fluctuating course.
• Depression can also cause cognitive impairment and may present because of it.

- If neither delirium nor depression is present, the diagnosis is almost certainly dementia.
- Unawareness of self-identity is rare, even in severe dementia, and raises the possibility of a dissociative disorder.

Other components of the module

Do a careful physical examination. Look for evidence of vascular disease, thyroid status, alcohol abuse, infection. The neurological examination should include testing of cranial nerves and evaluation of cortical functions (e.g. apraxias, hemineglect, primitive reflexes).

Notes
- If dementia is diagnosed, proceed to assess: (a) its likely cause, (b) its effect on daily living and (c) any associated problems. These issues are covered in Chapter 13.
- Delirium is due to a variety of medical conditions, many of which need urgent treatment. It is less commonly possible to reverse dementia. Thus, a medical history and physical examination followed by appropriate investigations are essential whenever cognitive impairment is found.
- Talk to the informant first if the impairment is severe.

Assessment of psychosis

The cardinal features of psychosis (delusions, hallucinations, and lack of insight) were defined in the core assessment (Chapter 2) and relate mostly to the disorders covered in Chapter 12.

Key questions addressed by the module

- *Is the person suffering from a psychosis?* Some people with strange ideas or strange behaviour may turn out to have a neurosis, a personality disorder, or no diagnosis at all.
- *If so, which psychosis is it?* The main disorders in which psychotic symptoms occur are: schizophrenia, severe depression, mania, drug-induced psychoses, delusional disorders and organic psychoses (e.g. in dementia or delirium).

Triggering the module

Psychosis may be suspected for diverse reasons, such as:
- Possible delusions elicited in the core assessment.
- Bizarre or inexplicable behaviour.
- History of amphetamine use.
- A young adult found in a neglected state.
- Man heard talking to himself in a police cell.

Related modules

The module is usually accompanied by the *mood* and *substance misuse* modules because of the overlap of these conditions. *Risk assessment* is needed as psychoses commonly lead to a risk of harm to self and, less often, to others.

The psychosis module

The diagnosis of schizophrenia relies on detailed evaluation of symptoms and signs, especially concerning abnormalities of thought content and form, so the module is quite long.

Appearance and behaviour

Note manner and dress.

Notes
- Manner—patient may be suspicious (you may be part of his conspiracy theory), distracted (by hallucinations) or distant and uninterested (?negative symptoms of schizophrenia).
- Dress—some people with schizophrenia dress idiosyncratically. For example, a man wore a silver foil hat to prevent his thoughts being extracted.

Movements

Is there abnormality of movements or posture?
    Are there mannerisms or stereotypies?
    Is the patient restless?

Notes
- Motor abnormalities occur in psychosis and as common side-effects of antipsychotic drugs, especially the older 'typical' ones. The side-effects in-

clude *dystonia, parkinsonism, akathisia* and *tardive dyskinesia* (Chapter 7).

- A *mannerism* is a repetitive movement or gesture which is complex and seemingly purposeful. A repeated simple and purposeless one is a *stereotypy*. Both occur in schizophrenia.
- *Catatonia* describes a group of motor signs which are rare but characteristic of catatonic schizophrenia:
  — *Echopraxia/echolalia* (the patient imitates the interviewer's every action or word);
  — *Automatic obedience* (compliance with all instructions regardless of consequence);
  — *Ambitendency* (tentative movements back and forth—as if unsure what to do);
  — *Posturing* (*catalepsy*) (the maintenance of inappropriate or bizarre postures);
  — *Waxy flexibility* (limbs held in externally imposed positions—muscle tone is increased);
  — *Negativism* (seemingly motiveless resistance to all instructions or attempts to be moved).

Mood

Does the overall mood seem normal? Is it responsive?

Is the emotional expression appropriate with the topic being discussed?

Notes
- Psychosis can occur with severe depression and in mania. Here, only the abnormalities of mood occurring in schizophrenia are mentioned.
- *Flattened affect* is a decrease in emotional responsivity and expression, even when emotionally charged topics are discussed. A negative symptom of schizophrenia. Distinguish from depression and parkinsonism.
- *Incongruous affect:* emotion not in keeping with the topic being talked about.

Speech

Are made-up words (*neologisms*) used or words used idiosyncratically?

Notes
- A *neologism* is a made-up word, usually invested with a personal meaning. Be sure the patient doesn't just have a larger vocabulary than you . . .

Thoughts—content

Is there any evidence of delusions?
- Is anything bothering you at the moment?
- Do you believe or understand things differently to other people?
- Do people have a special interest in you? Are people against you? How do you know?
- Is anything on the TV referring to you particularly?
- When did you first realize this (i.e. the delusional belief) was true? How?

Notes
- Because, by definition, a delusion is believed to be true, its detection requires you to be receptive to clues and sometimes to 'go along' with implausible statements in order to elicit more details. For example, a man matter-of-factly asked one of us how we were affected by the Bulgarian mafia—the first hint of his psychosis. A non-committal reply led him to elaborate and reveal his persecutory delusional system.
- Different sorts of delusions are recognized:
  — A *delusional perception* is a delusional interpretation of a normal perception. For example, a man saw a woman sneeze and knew this meant he must leave town. It is sometimes preceded by a sense of unease or perplexity that something strange is going on (*delusional mood*).
  — In a *delusion of reference*, an event or message (often on TV) has a unique meaning for the person. An *idea of reference* is similar, but not delusional in intensity (and thus not a true psychotic symptom); it may occur in paranoid personality disorder.
  — A *secondary delusion* is one that arises understandably from another mental state abnormality (e.g. delusion of guilt in depression); a *primary* delusion doesn't.
  — Delusions may be classified by content. The commonest are *persecutory* delusions (sometimes

incorrectly called *paranoid delusions*), in which the person is the victim of perceived injustice or conspiracy. *Grandiose* delusions are seen in mania, *nihilistic* ones in depression.

Thoughts—flow and possession

Is it difficult to follow the meaning of what the patient is saying? Write down a representative sample.

Do the person's thoughts seem to flow normally?

• Do your thoughts sometimes stop suddenly? (*thought block*)

• Are your thoughts sometimes removed from your head? (*thought withdrawal*)

Does the person feel in control of their thoughts and actions?

• Do your thoughts get put into your head from outside? (*thought insertion*)

• Can other people directly influence your thoughts or actions? (*passivity; thought control*)

Are the thoughts experienced unusually?

• Are other people aware of your thoughts? (*thought broadcasting*)

• Do any of your thoughts get repeated in your mind like an echo? (*thought echo*)

Notes

• Thought disorder occurs in schizophrenia. The connections between thoughts are obscure and there is a rambling quality. Descriptive terms include *knight's move thinking* and *loosening of associations* and, in rare severe cases, *word salad*. For example, in response to a question about what the person has been up to: 'I got on the bus when I saw the man from the hostel, in the next street where I was. You know I've seen that dog again? Still, doctor, what do you think? . . .'. A different type of thought disorder occurs in mania.

• In schizophrenia, abnormalities also occur in the perceived source, ownership and fate of thoughts:

— *Thought insertion:* thoughts originate elsewhere and are put into the patient's head.

— *Thought withdrawal:* the experience of thoughts being removed from one's mind.

— *Thought broadcast:* the subject experiences his thoughts being available to and heard by others.

— *Thought block:* the flow of thoughts abruptly ends. Distinguish from thought withdrawal and from simple loss of concentration.

— *Passivity:* thoughts, feelings or actions are experienced as being under external control. For example, a schizophrenic who killed her son described being unable to resist carrying out this act because of the 'force' controlling her. Passivity phenomena are important in risk assessment (and in how resulting crimes are dealt with).

Perceptions

Does the person seem to be hearing things that are not there?

• Do you hear voices when there doesn't seem to be anyone present? (*auditory hallucinations*)

• Are the voices inside (*pseudohallucinations*) or outside (*hallucinations*) your head?

• What are they talking about?

• Do they talk directly to you or about you? (*third person hallucinations*)

• Do they comment on what you're doing? (*running commentary*)

• Do they want you to harm yourself or other people?

Repeat similar questions for hallucinations in other modalities.

Notes

• The characteristic hallucinations of schizophrenia are *third person auditory hallucinations* (i.e. hearing the voice talking *about* you). Sometimes these take the form of a *running commentary* by two or more voices.

• *Somatic hallucinations* (e.g. buzzing sensations due to a beehive implanted in the chest) and hallucinations in other modalities also occur. *Visual hallucinations* suggest an organic psychosis. *Olfactory hallucinations* and sensory distortions occur in temporal lobe epilepsy.

• Auditory hallucinations in psychotic mood disorders are *mood congruent*—i.e. critical and derogatory in severe depression; grandiose in mania.

Cognition

Is the patient disorientated?

Notes
- An acutely psychotic patient may be distracted by his experiences, or misunderstand your question in a psychotic way, and therefore perform poorly on cognitive testing. Try and distinguish from delirium.
- Patients with chronic schizophrenia may have genuine cognitive impairment as part of their illness; they characteristically underestimate their age by several years.

Other components of the module

Check insight.
- Do you think you are ill in any way? Do others? Do you need help? What sort?

Ask about complications of pregnancy or delivery, place of upbringing, academic achievements and social interests.

Ask about family history of psychosis.

Ask about past or current substance abuse.

Ask about premorbid personality and level of functioning.

Carry out a physical examination, concentrating on neurological system.

Corroborate the history from an informant.

Notes
- Insight is characteristically but variably impaired in psychosis. *Distorted awareness of reality* is a related term which conveys what is often apparent to the interviewer.
- Family history, obstetric complications, an urban upbringing, and problems at school are associated with schizophrenia.
- Alcohol and illicit drugs can induce psychosis. Consider substance abuse module.
- A decline in level of functioning (intellectually and socially) is common before and during the onset of schizophrenia.
- Organic disorders of many kinds can produce psychosis, hence the relevance of medical history and physical examination.

Table 3.2 First-rank symptoms of schizophrenia.

Delusions
Delusional perception
Hallucinations
Thought echo (audible thoughts)
Third person auditory hallucinations
Running commentary
Thought flow and possession
Thought withdrawal
Thought insertion
Thought broadcasting
Passivity
Passivity of thought, feelings or actions

First-rank symptoms of schizophrenia

A number of symptoms in this module are *first-rank symptoms*, accorded great significance in the diagnosis of schizophrenia. They are summarized in Table 3.2.

Notes
- For definitions, see pp. 19–20.
- The likelihood ratio for schizophrenia is >4 if a first-rank symptom is present. However, they are not pathognomonic—first-rank symptoms occur in other psychoses, and not all schizophrenics have had one.
- They are sometimes called *Schneiderian* symptoms after the psychiatrist who described them.
- Listing and defining first-rank symptoms is a favourite exam question.

Assessment of mood

There are separate modules for lowered mood (*depression*) and for elevated mood (*mania*).
- First, review the relevant sections of the core assessment.

Assessment of depression

Key questions addressed by the module

- *Is the person depressed?* Depression must be distinguished from normal sadness.
- *If so, is the diagnosis a depressive disorder, or are the depressive symptoms part of another disorder?* They can occur secondarily in, for example, schizophrenia and neuroses.
- *If the diagnosis is a depressive disorder, what type is it?* Depression can be a single episode, recurrent, or part of bipolar disorder. It may include psychotic symptoms. It can be caused by many organic disorders and by drugs, both prescribed and illicit.

Triggering the module

Examples of the triggers for this module include:
- Detection of a depressive symptom or suicidal thought in the core assessment.
- Unexplained fatigue.
- Any of the presentations in Table 9.2.

Related modules

Depression overlaps and coexists with so many diagnoses that any of the other modules may be necessary. The presence of mood disturbance requires risk assessment (mainly for suicide) as well.

The depression module

Appearance and behaviour

Does the patient look depressed? Is he crying? Is he agitated?

Does he exude a sense of gloom?

Is there good eye contact?

Is there a normal range of emotional expression?

Notes
- In depression there is often decreased eye contact and a lack of expression and movement—called *psychomotor retardation*. Other depressed people are *agitated*, pacing to and fro or wringing their hands.

Speech

Is the speech normal in speed, loudness and amount?

Notes
- In severe depression, speech is slow, quiet and sparse. Sentences tail off, as though the patient cannot summon the energy or concentration to continue.

Mood

Has the patient noticed a change in mood, enjoyment or in energy?
- How have you been feeling in your spirits?
- Do you still enjoy the things that you usually do? If not, can you give some examples?
- How is your energy level? Do you feel more tired or fatigued than usual?

Then:
- How long have you felt this way?
- Is your mood lower at a particular time of day? How do you feel first thing?
- Do you often feel like crying?
- Do you easily get irritable?
- In the past, have you had periods of better than usual mood, or boundless energy, or have behaved out of character?

Notes
- The duration, pervasiveness, and severity of these symptoms affect diagnosis and management.
- *Anhedonia*, the lack of pleasure from normally enjoyed activities, is a key symptom of moderate and severe depression.
- *Reactivity of mood:* in severe depression, the normal reactivity of mood to circumstances is lost.
- *Diurnal variation of mood:* mood is worst early in the morning, improving as the day goes on.
- The predominant subjective feeling in depression may be sadness, irritability, fatigue, lethargy, or lack of energy (*anergia*).
- The last question above may give a clue to mania in the past, and thus to a possible bipolar mood disorder. If any hint of a positive response, use the mania module.
- Depressive symptoms are common in the bereaved and can be hard to distinguish from normal grief (Chapter 9).

Sleep, appetite and other bodily functions

- How are you sleeping at the moment? Do you have problems getting to sleep, interrupted sleep, or of waking early?
- What is your appetite like? Do you enjoy your food? Have you lost weight?
- Are you constipated? (Are your periods regular?)
- Has your interest in sex changed recently?

Notes
- Biological rhythms and drives are frequently impaired in depression. The presence of 'biological' or 'somatic' symptoms is one way to define the boundary between mild depression and more severe cases—the latter sometimes called *melancholia*.
- Sleep is affected in several ways. *Initial insomnia* is common when there is accompanying anxiety. Sleep is shallow and unrefreshing. *Early morning waking* is the most characteristic change, often occurring with diurnal variation of mood, so the patient is awake and at his most desperate when the rest of the world is asleep.
- Appetite is reduced with resulting weight loss and contributing to constipation.
- Irregular periods or amenorrhoea occur in women.
- There is a general loss of energy and libido.

Thoughts—content

- What things are on your mind at the moment? Anything particular bothering you?
- Do you see things getting better? What would improve things?
- Do you feel guilty about anything you have done?
- Do you feel that you are of value?
- Do you have worries about your physical health?
- Do you feel that people are getting at you? If so, is it justified?

Make sure to ask in detail about suicidal thoughts and intent (Chapter 4).

Notes
- Prevailing thoughts have a negative colouring, centring upon perceived failures, worthlessness, low self-esteem, and so on.
- Hopelessness and guilt feelings are important as they lead to thoughts of suicide.
- The content of thoughts (and the person's appearance) may suggest accompanying anxiety—covered in the neurosis module.
- Worries about health and complaints of physical symptoms are common in depression, as well as in neurotic syndromes.

Thoughts—nature

Are any of the thoughts obsessional in nature?
- Do you find yourself checking things repeatedly?
- Do you like things especially clean and tidy?
Are any of the thoughts delusional?

Notes
- Obsessional thoughts and ruminations are common in depression; if prominent, consider obsessive compulsive disorder and use the neurosis module.
- Delusions are rare in depression as a whole, but characterize psychotic depression. They tend to be *mood congruent*.

Perception

Are there hallucinations? What are they like?

Notes
- Hallucinations sometimes occur in psychotic depression—usually second person voices saying derogatory things.
- Depressed people may describe that sensations are less intense than usual and they feel isolated from the normal emotions and activities of the outside world.

Cognition

Is concentration impaired?
- What is your concentration like?
- Can you read a paper or follow a TV programme?
Is there objective evidence of cognitive impairment? (Consider MMSE; see cognition module).

Notes

- Depression, especially in the elderly, can produce apparent cognitive impairment, sometimes called *pseudodementia*. This is a mixture of lack of motivation and poor concentration. Must be distinguished from dementia, as it responds to treatment of the depression.

Other components of the module

Does the patient think they are depressed?

Identify past and current stressors—marital strife, unemployment, etc.

How has the patient tried to cope with the problems?

Is there a past history of mood disorder? What has its course been? What treatment worked?

Does the person have depressive or neurotic traits in their personality?

Is there a family history of psychiatric disorder or suicide?

Notes

- Severely depressed patients may deny that their mood is abnormal and decline treatment.
- At its most severe, patients may stop eating, drinking and even moving. *Depressive stupor* is life threatening and an indication for emergency electroconvulsive therapy (ECT).
- Stressors (*life events*) can precipitate depression; identifying them helps make sense of the depression—and can be therapeutic.
- Coping strategies adopted by patients may lead to additional problems. For example, use of alcohol.
- Many patients with depression have had previous episode(s) of mood disorder. Ask about their nature, treatment and outcome.
- Depressive personality traits may affect the risk and outcome of depressive disorders. An informant should provide the personality information.
- A positive family history is a risk factor for depressive disorder and suicide.

Assessment of mania

Key questions addressed by the module

- *Is the person manic?* Mania is a pathological elevation of mood that causes substantial impairment in occupational and/or social functioning. Mania is the key syndrome in bipolar disorder. Milder manic symptoms do not necessarily cause impairment and are called *hypomania*. In hypomania, functioning may be improved but it can also precede a manic relapse.
- *Has the person been manic in the past?* Even if she is currently depressed or euthymic (normal mood), a history of mania is important because of its diagnostic and therapeutic implications (Chapter 9).

Triggering the mania module

The mania module may be triggered by:
- A hint of manic symptoms in the core assessment or depression module.
- Recent grandiose, disinhibited or disorganized behaviour.
- A past history of bipolar disorder.
- A family history of bipolar disorder.

Related modules

Most patients with an episode of mania will have, or have had, depression, so always use the *depression* module. Mania can be associated with *substance misuse*.

The mania module

Appearance and behaviour

Note manner and dress.

Is the patient distractible or irritable?

Is the patient overactive?

Notes

- Clothes and make up may be bright and garish or dishevelled.
- Look out for flamboyant or disinhibited gestures. The patient may try and hug you, snatch your notes, or challenge your qualifications.
- A manic person may be unable to concentrate enough to give useful or consistent answers. If so, focus on eliciting current symptoms and signs. Take the rest of the history later or from an informant.

- The predominant emotion can be euphoria and infectious gaiety, or sudden and extreme irritability.
- Determine if the patient's behaviour is causing them any problems in areas such as work, relationships, etc.

Speech

Is the speech fast? Excessive in amount? Hard to interrupt?

Notes
- Speech in mania is fast, loud, expansive, and hard to interrupt (*pressure of speech*). It reflects the underlying pressure of thoughts and the person's attempts to share their many wonderful ideas.

Mood

Has the patient noticed a change in mood or energy level recently? Can they describe it?
- Do you feel happier than usual? More confident?
- Are you feeling full of energy?
- Have you been very irritable or impatient

Notes
- Some people with mania deny their mood is elevated, or are too busy to think about it.
- Mood can be labile or *mixed*—simultaneous depressive and manic features.
- An increase in energy level and drive to do things almost always occurs.
- In some people, the elevated mood can be experienced as irritability.

Sleep, appetite and other bodily functions

- How are you sleeping? More or less than usual?
- How's your appetite?
- Has your interest in sex changed?

Notes
- Tiredness and sleep drive are decreased. A manic patient may stay up all night working or playing.
- Appetite may be increased, or more usually the patient is too busy to eat.

- Libido tends to be enhanced and sexual activity uninhibited.

Thoughts—content

- What's on your mind at the moment?
- Do you have special powers or abilities?

Notes
- Thoughts are expansive and grandiose. There may be a single, preoccupying scheme (e.g. to build a football stadium in the garden) but usually there is a kaleidoscope of incomplete, jumbled ideas.

Thoughts—nature

Are the thoughts delusional in nature?
  Is there any evidence of reckless or dangerous ideas?
- Have you got plans to buy anything?
- Can you do things which most people might find difficult or even impossible?
Does the train of thought jump from one topic to another?

Notes
- In mania, the grandiose ideas may become delusional. Religious themes are common—for example the patient knows he is the Messiah. Sometimes delusions are dangerous—the belief that one can drive excessively fast, fly or borrow unrealistic amounts of money. Take these risks seriously— the unpredictability of mania means they may suddenly be acted upon.
- *Flight of ideas* is a type of thought disorder characteristic of mania. Thoughts jump rapidly from one thing to another, with understandable, if unusual, connections between them. The links are often based on puns, rhymes and other associations, for example 'I'm fine, a fine wine, whining and moaning like Jonah . . . Jonah the whale . . . in Wales . . .'. Write down a snippet.

Perceptions

Is there any evidence of hallucinations?

Notes

• Mood-congruent auditory and occasionally visual hallucinations occur. For example, voices telling the person what special powers they have and how they can save humanity.

Other components of the module

Does patient think they are unwell or need treatment?

Corroborate recent history, especially with regard to unusual and inappropriate beliefs and actions.

Check recent use of illicit drugs or alcohol

Ask about past history of mania or depression

Has patient ever been prescribed lithium or other mood stabilizing drug? Is he supposed to be taking it now?

Ask about family history of mood disorders.

Do a physical examination.

Notes

• Insight fluctuates in mania. A person may seem aware of their condition and agree the need for treatment one moment but not the next.

• An informant usually paints a more dramatic picture of recent behaviour than does the patient. Gather evidence of specific dangerous or out-of-keeping behaviours, since they affect management—for example whether patient should be detained, or needs a pregnancy test.

• Manic episodes can be caused by drugs, such as amphetamines and steroids, and sometimes by alcohol.

• Bipolar disorder is often treated long term with lithium to prevent relapse, and sudden discontinuation can precipitate mania. Ask the patient if they take lithium, and check the plasma level.

• Bipolar disorder is strongly familial.

• Physical examination is indicated since mania can be due to an organic disorder (e.g. frontal lobe tumour), especially if the first episode occurs in middle age or beyond.

Assessment of neurosis (including stress-related and somatoform disorders)

Neuroses are emotional disorders, usually involving anxiety, and manifesting as psychological, cognitive and physical (somatic) complaints. As discussed in Chapter 10, for various reasons the neuroses are classified together with *stress-related disorders* (where neurotic symptoms are attributed to a particular stressor) and *somatoform disorders* (where medically unexplained physical symptoms predominate). The next module concerns neurotic and stress-related disorders; the following one covers somatoform disorders.

• This is a notoriously confusing area, and we suggest you read Chapter 10 in conjunction with this module.

Assessment of neurosis and stress-related disorders

Key questions addressed by the module

• *Does the person have a neurosis?* A distinction must be made from (a) worries and emotional distress which are within normal limits or part of the person's personality, and (b) from neurotic symptoms occurring in depression or other diagnostic categories.

• *If a neurosis is present, which one?* There are many types of neurosis, including panic disorder, phobias, obsessive–compulsive disorder, and hypochondriasis (Table 10.1). Occasionally, but importantly, anxiety disorders can be organic in origin (e.g. phaeochromocytoma).

Triggering the module

Neurotic symptoms are extremely common. The module might be triggered, for example, by:

• A woman who is preoccupied or clearly worried about something.

• A person distressed by a recent trauma.

Related modules

Neurotic symptoms often coexist with depression, so the *depression module* will nearly always be necessary. Use the *substance misuse* module if there is evidence of alcohol or drug use as a cause of, or response to, the symptoms. Worries about food or body image will trigger the *eating disorders* module. If the presentation is predominantly with somatic concerns (e.g. pain, fatigue) use the *somatoform disorders* module.

The neurosis module

Appearance

Does the patient look tense, anxious or worried?

Notes
• Anxiety is a state of arousal and may be apparent from the person's appearance and behaviour. With practice, it is usually possible to distinguish this from the agitation of depression.

Anxiety

Start with open questions:
• Have you been worrying a lot about things recently? What about?
• Do you feel wound up or tense?
• Do you suffer from aches and pains?
Characterizing the anxiety:
• Are the feelings there most of the time, or in specific situations?
• What thing or situation makes you most anxious?
• Do you get sudden 'attacks' of anxiety? How does your body feel then?
• Can you put your worries out of your mind?
• Do you avoid doing things because of your worries?

Notes
• Anxiety consists of *psychological* symptoms (e.g. tension, fear) and *bodily* symptoms (e.g. palpitations, sweating), described in detail in Chapter 10. Either can predominate.
• Anxiety is usually *situational* (*phobic*), occurring in response to a specific stimulus. Less commonly it is *generalized* or *free floating*.
• Anxiety can also be paroxysmal—a *panic attack*: a discrete episode of severe anxiety which builds rapidly then gradually subsides over about an hour.
• People rapidly learn to *avoid* situations in which they feel anxious or uncomfortable. They may first present for help because of the practical problems which avoidance produces.

Obsessions and compulsions

• Do you get repeated unpleasant images or thoughts?
• Do you have to keep checking things, or keep things very clean and tidy? What do you do? How often?
• Do you try to resist the thoughts or the urge to respond to them? If so, what happens?

Notes
• *Obsessions* and *compulsions* are characteristic of obsessive-compulsive disorder and also occur in depression and anankastic personality disorder.
• Severe obsessions can, in practice, be difficult to distinguish from delusions. Stick to their strict definitions (Chapter 2).

Other symptoms of neurosis

Enquire about somatic symptoms:
• How is your health generally?
• Do you suffer from severe tiredness or exhaustion?
• Have you ever lost your memory, sight, or the use of part of your body?
• Have you felt detached or distant from yourself or your surroundings?

Notes
• Unexplained physical symptoms (e.g. palpitations) are common in anxiety disorders, and in depression. If they are prominent, and not explained by depression, then consider a *somatoform disorder* (see below).
• Medically unexplained fatigue is the main feature of *neurasthenia* (*chronic fatigue syndrome*). Fatigue and lethargy also occur in depression.
• *Dissociative disorders* are rare neuroses in which there is loss of function (e.g. amnesia, paralysis). They are usually encountered in medical settings (e.g. after admission for neurological investigation).
• Feelings of detachment from self or surroundings (*depersonalization-derealization*) are a common symptom of neurosis, may occur in healthy people when tired, and are occasionally a diagnosis in its own

right. Such feelings are hard to describe (e.g. 'It's as if there is glass between me and the world') and must be distinguished from psychotic symptoms.

Other components of the module

When did the symptoms start? Did they seem related to recent events?

How has the person coped? Have they had any treatment?

How do the symptoms interfere with daily life?

Is there a family history of neurosis?

● Are you under particular recent stress?

● Have there been major events or difficulties in your life recently?

● Have you ever been in a major accident or trauma? If so, how has it affected you?

Notes

● Many people have had neurotic symptoms for years before seeking help. If similar symptoms have been present since adolescence, consider personality disorder.

● Whilst all neuroses are made worse by stress, sometimes the symptoms are best understood as a response to a major stress or life change—a *stress-related disorder*. If the stress was within the past few days, then consider an *acute stress reaction*. If the stressor was weeks or months ago, the category is *adjustment reaction*. *Post-traumatic stress disorder (PTSD)* is a form of stress-related disorder in which a *significant* event (e.g. rape, serious accident) is followed by reliving of the trauma in flashbacks or nightmares, and avoidance of similar situations.

● People turn to alcohol and other maladaptive strategies (e.g. avoidance) to cope with anxiety and other neurotic symptoms—these responses may exacerbate the situation and should be dealt with as part of treatment.

● The presence of dysfunction is one criterion used in diagnosing neurosis, so assess the symptoms' effects—for example on relationships and work performance.

● There is a modest genetic contribution to neurosis, and there may also be relevant learned behaviours from neurotic relatives.

Assessment of somatic symptoms and somatoform disorders

Somatic symptoms and concerns about health can of course be a presentation of a medical condition and should be assessed accordingly. They may also occur in any psychiatric disorder, particularly neuroses. *Somatoform disorders* really apply to patients where the somatic symptoms are most prominent, and none of these other categories seems applicable (Chapter 10 and 18).

Key questions addressed by the module

● *Are the patient's somatic symptoms medically unexplained?*

● *If so, is the diagnosis somatoform disorder of a depression or other neurosis?*

● *If the diagnosis is somatoform disorder, what type is it?* Somatoform disorders can manifest predominantly with somatic symptoms, or predominantly with concerns about health or appearance.

Triggering the module

Examples of triggers include:

● Detection of somatic symptoms that appear unexplained by a medical condition in the core assessment.

● Preoccupation with health or disease.

● Repeated and excessive seeking of medical assessment or treatment.

Related modules

Because somatic symptoms can occur in many disorders, any other module may be needed, especially those covering *neurosis*, *depression*, and *eating disorders*.

The somatoform disorders module

Appearance and behaviour

Does the patient emphasize somatic complaints?

Are they unduly preoccupied with their health?

Do they have evidence of many previous operations?

Do they hide aspects of their body or appearance?

Are they repeatedly seeking reassurance from you that they do not have disease?

Is there evidence that they have deliberately made themselves ill (e.g. by picking open a wound or omitting their insulin?)

Notes

• In somatoform disorders the patient emphasizes somatic over other symptoms and often seeks tests and treatments that are not medically indicated.

• Patients with chronic *somatization disorder* may have had many unnecessary operations.

• Patients with *body dysmorphic disorder* (*dysmorphophobia*) may seek to hide aspects of their appearance because they perceive themselves as ugly.

• Repeated reassurance seeking about disease suggests *hypochondriasis*.

• Rarely, patients deliberately make themselves ill (or apparently so) to justify medical care—called *factitious disorder*, or in order to gain some advantage (e.g. money)—*malingering*.

Mood

Is there evidence of depressed or anxious mood?

Notes

• Depressed or anxious mood are often apparent or suspected but may be denied by the patient. If you conclude either is present and significant, then the somatic symptoms will usually be viewed as symptoms of a depressive or anxiety disorder.

Sleep, appetite and other bodily function

• How is your health?

• Do you have many aches and pains, or other bodily symptoms?

• Do you have medical problems your doctor can't explain?

Notes

• Patients with somatoform disorder typically perceive their health as poor even when it is objectively good.

• Many bodily concerns and symptoms may be reported. The more somatic symptoms they have the less likely they are to have a medical condition. Many chronic symptoms suggest somatization disorder.

Thoughts—content

• What do you think causes your symptoms?

• Are your fearful that you have a particular medical condition?

• What do you think about your appearance?

• What do you think should be done about your symptoms?

Notes

• Patients may have unlikely or bizarre theories about what causes their symptoms, but these should not be delusional—if so, the patient has a psychosis of some kind.

• A strong fear of a medical condition is typical of hypochondriasis.

• Preoccupation with appearance suggests body dysmorphic disorder.

• The patient with a somatoform disorder will often want extensive investigation, and may not be reassured by negative results.

Other components of the module

What is the nature and quantity of the medical history?

Will the patient co-operate with a psychiatric assessment?

What does the patient want done?

Notes

• A frequent medical attender and 'thick notes' suggest a chronic somatization disorder.

• Many patients want medical not psychiatric treatment. They may minimize distress to lessen the probability of a psychiatric diagnosis. The assessment usually proceeds more smoothly if you pay due attention to and make it clear that you accept their somatic symptoms before asking about psychological ones.

• Patients do not necessarily want treatment. Some want validation that they are ill, others want you to complete insurance claims. Conflict can be avoided if you ask what they want.

Assessment of eating disorders

Key questions addressed by the module

• *Does the patient have an eating disorder?* The core feature is an over-evaluation of shape and weight. The disorders must be distinguished from problems of weight, shape or diet occurring in other psychiatric disorders or secondary to a medical disorder.

• *If so, is the diagnosis anorexia nervosa or bulimia nervosa?* The former is characterized by low body weight, the latter by repeated binges which punctuate the dietary restriction. However, many patients with an eating disorder do not fit into either of these classic categories, but have an eating disorder not otherwise specified.

When using the module, note that:

• People with eating disorders can be difficult to engage and tend to minimize their problems, so take the opportunity to form a good relationship, and plan to corroborate the history.

• Physical complications of anorexia nervosa are frequent and can be life-threatening.

• The disorders do occur in men.

Triggering the module

The eating disorder may be triggered by:

• A patient saying she has problems controlling her eating.

• Medically unexplained weight loss.

• A teenage girl with fatigue or amenorrhoea.

• A patient who looks thin or is wearing a baggy sweater on a hot day.

Related modules

The *depression* and *neurosis* modules will invariably be necessary given the overlap between these conditions. Risk assessment is important since deliberate and accidental self-harm can occur.

The eating disorder module

Eating, bingeing and weight

Ask about diet:

• Describe a typical day's food intake.

• Are you on a diet? If so, what sort? How strict?

Ask about binges:

• Do you ever feel out of control and eat a large amount of food rapidly ('binge')?

• If so, what do you eat in a binge? Afterwards, how do you feel? What do you do?

Ask about weight:

• What is your current weight? How often do you weigh yourself?

• Have you ever been very overweight or underweight?

Notes

• A description of a typical day's intake is an informative way of discovering the patient's eating patterns and the quantity and type of food being consumed. But, as with alcohol histories, interpret with caution.

• Dieting in someone who is not overweight raises suspicion of an eating disorder.

• A person's response to being asked about their diet or current weight can itself give clues.

• A past history of obesity and dieting is common.

• Bingeing followed by induced vomiting is the main feature of bulimia nervosa.

Attitude to weight and shape

• Do you think you are fat? How much would you like to weigh?

• How do you feel about your body? How would you like it to be?

• Do other people say you're too thin? Do you believe them?

Notes

• *Preoccupation with weight and diet* and *distortion of body image* are key diagnostic features, so explore fully her views on the subject. The woman may be convinced that she is overweight despite being demonstrably underweight. These beliefs are overvalued ideas (p. 11).

• A low body weight is seen as an accomplishment not a problem to a person with anorexia nervosa. Asking how the person would feel if she weighed a normal amount (a body mass index [BMI] of 18; see below) can be useful.

Physical symptoms of weight loss

Ask about menstrual history: (check if taking oral contraceptive pill)

• Are your periods regular?

- When was your last period?
- When did your periods begin?
- Have you been more tired or weaker than usual?

Notes
- Amenorrhoea (or scanty, irregular periods) is a feature of anorexia nervosa. If the disorder began in early teens, menarche may never have occurred.
- Fatigue, lethargy and weakness are consequences of starvation and should alert the doctor to the need for physical examination and investigation.

Additional methods of weight control

Has the patient tried other ways of losing (or maintaining) weight?
- What exercise do you do? How often?
- Do you use laxatives, diuretics or slimming pills?

Notes
- Misuse of diuretics increases the risk of hypokalaemia.

Physical examination

Weigh the patient and measure them. Calculate the body mass index.
  Examine the mouth and hands. Are there calluses? Poor state of teeth?
  Check the cardiovascular system.
  Note secondary sexual characteristics.
  Is there lanugo hair?
  Are there scars suggestive of self-cutting?

Notes
- Patients may wear very baggy clothes, or ensure they have a full bladder, to give a misleading impression of their weight. Weigh them in their underwear.
- The *body mass index* (BMI) is weight (kg)/[height (m)]^2. BMI should be 18–25. In anorexia nervosa, the BMI is below 17.5—sometimes well below.
- Always examine the *cardiovascular* system. Arrythmias occur due to hypokalaemia. *Bradycardia* and *peripheral oedema* are common in anorexia.
- There are various signs in the skin, mouth and

teeth of people with eating disorder (Table 11.1). Lanugo is fine downy hair on the arms, back and face in anorexia nervosa.
- Self-cutting occurs in a small subgroup of people with bulimia nervosa.

Other components of the module

Obtain a history of the development of the eating disorder.
  Ask about past medical and psychiatric history.
  Ask about premorbid personality.
  Corroborate history from an informant.
  Perform relevant investigations.

Notes
- People with eating disorder often minimize their problems. Always try and confirm the history about dieting, bingeing, etc.
- The medical differential diagnosis of eating disorder includes inflammatory bowel disease, hypopituitarism, and neoplasms. Each is rare, but important.
- The psychiatric differential diagnosis includes depression and body dysmorphic disorder.
- Eating disorder is commoner than expected in people with diabetes mellitus.
- Investigations may be needed to rule out other causes of anorexia and weight loss and to check for *complications* of weight loss (Table 11.1).
- Perfectionism is a common personality trait in eating disorder, especially anorexia nervosa.

Assessment of substance misuse

Key questions addressed by the module

- *Which substance(s) are misused and in what way?* This includes establishing the duration, quantity and pattern of use.
- *Is the person dependent on the drug?* Physical dependence on alcohol, opioids and some other drugs, is the most serious form of misuse.
- *What are the complications of the misuse?* Substance misuse produces diverse medical, psychiatric and social harms.

Continued

Triggering the module

Examples of triggers for this module include:
- Identification of significant alcohol intake in the core assessment.
- Insomnia in a stressed and depressed executive.
- Acute psychotic symptoms in a young person.
- Unexplained recurrent episodes of irritability or low mood.

Related modules

The module will be used particularly in association with the *psychosis, mood* and *cognitive function* modules, given the diagnoses that arise from or coexist with substance misuse. *Risk assessment* is also necessary as substance misusers have high rates of deliberate and accidental self-harm.

Note: You cannot psychiatrically assess someone who is intoxicated. Though you may be pressured to do so (e.g. by nursing staff in the emergency department), it must be deferred till the person is sober.

The substance misuse module

The questions below refer to alcohol; modify for other substances as required.

The quantity and the pattern of consumption

- How much do you drink in the average week? What do you drink?
- Do you sometimes drink much more than that?
- Do you drink every day?

Ask the patient to describe a typical day.

Ask about how long the current pattern has been present.

Notes
- Self reports of consumption are underestimates (by half, as an unproven rule of thumb). The description of a typical day can be more revealing and accurate. Also ask about the associated behaviours and feelings.
- Check the type of beer drunk—the alcohol content varies considerably.

- Some people misuse alcohol in a steady fashion, others do so intermittently.
- Regular drinking that began in early adolescence is common amongst alcohol misusers.
- Ask CAGE questions (p. 9) if not asked already.

Dependence and withdrawal

- Do you have to drink more than you used to in order to get the same effect?
- Have you ever got into trouble due to your drinking?
- Have you tried to cut down the amount you drink? What happened?
- Do feel that you have lost control over your drinking?
- Do you drink more than you intend to?
- Do you ever have a drink in the morning to get you going?

Ask the patient to rate the importance of drinking compared to other activities.

Identify if the patient continues to drink despite awareness that it is harmful.

Notes
- *Dependence* is a cluster of physiological, behavioural and cognitive features arising from sustained use of alcohol, opioids, amphetamines and some other drugs (Chapter 14). Its features include: a *compulsion* to take the substance, *tolerance* (the need for increasing doses of the substance to achieve the same subjective effect), and *withdrawal*. Dependence is associated with serious medical and psychiatric complications.
- Withdrawal symptoms are a physiological reaction to lack of the dependent substance. Benzodiazepines and some antidepressants can produce them.
- The symptoms of alcohol withdrawal includes tremor, retching, sweating and muscle cramps. If severe, it is called *delirium tremens*.

Associated psychosocial problems

Ask whether drinking has caused any psychological or social problems.

• Have you got into financial problems due to your drinking?

• Have you ever missed work or lost a job due to your drinking?

• Has drinking interfered with your relationships?

• Have you ever been in trouble with the police (e.g. drink driving) due to your drinking?

Notes

• This section is an example of an extended *contextual history*. It is necessary because substance misuse leads to many psychosocial problems.

Psychiatric and medical complications

• Has drinking affected your physical health? For example, jaundice, shakes, hepatitis?

• Have you ever had blackouts while drinking?

Ask about the patient's medical and psychiatric history.

Notes

• Misuse of alcohol and other substances leads to a range of psychiatric and medical disorders, the characteristics of which depend on the substance being misused.

• Psychiatric disorders associated with alcohol misuse include depression, psychosis, delirium, and dementia, as well as suicide and sexual dysfunction. Use screening questions from core assessment and then other relevant modules to investigate these areas.

Physical examination

Examine the patient for the stigmata of alcohol dependence (Table 14.4).

If the patient has symptoms or history of a physical illness, examine the appropriate systems.

Notes

• A physical examination is essential with alcohol misuse because of its many effects on the body.

• Many medical disorders result from unsuspected alcohol misuse.

• Opioid use produces its own physical signs.

Investigations

Many may be indicated, for example breath or blood alcohol, full blood count, liver function tests, urine or hair analyses.

Notes

• Medical problems of alcohol misuse, suspected from the history or physical examination, may need investigation and liaison with the GP or a physician.

• The mean corpuscular volume (MCV) and hepatic gamma-glutamyl transpeptidase (GGT) are raised in 60–70% patients with alcohol misuse. If other causes of their elevation are excluded, they are useful markers of alcohol misuse and for monitoring progress.

• Hepatitis B or HIV testing may be indicated in intravenous users.

• Urine screens pick up some drugs of abuse. Hair analyses are more sensitive but not widely available.

Use of other substances

The same kinds of question should be repeated for each class of misused drug.

Notes

• Many people who misuse one drug misuse at least one other.

• Use similar questions as those used for alcohol to establish the drugs used, the pattern of use and the associated problems.

• Ask about the route of administration.

• Patients may need reassurance about confidentiality when discussing drug use.

• Not all misused drugs are illegal—for example analgesics.

Assessment of the unresponsive patient

Key questions addressed by the module

- *Why is the person unresponsive?* Nonco-operation with the assessment, due to inability or unwillingness, is uncommon but causes obvious problems. The main diagnostic questions are:
- *Is there clouding of consciousness?* If so, consider delirium, stupor and their various causes.
- *If not, is there evidence of psychosis, severe mood disorder or dissociative disorder?* These disorders can all present with unresponsiveness.
- *Is the person intentionally uncooperative?* This may be a sign of malingering or simply a belief that they are better off keeping quiet.

Note that:
- By unresponsive, we mean a person who does not participate in the assessment, not one who is unconscious.
- Because the module is for use when communication is limited, it focuses on appearance, behaviour, and on a physical examination.
- Unresponsive patients can be aggressive, and any physical examination will be without their consent. So, ensure the environment is safe and be accompanied — you may need a witness to confirm what took place.

Triggering the module

By definition, the module will be triggered when a patient does not co-operate (fully) with the assessment. For example:
- A patient found standing rigidly in the street staring at the sky.
- A patient who sits there but does not speak.
- An aggressive patient who does not reply to any questions and demands to leave.

Related modules

Complete the assessment when the patient becomes responsive. The *cognitive function* and *psychosis* modules will almost certainly be needed.

The unresponsive patient module

Background information

Is there an informant? Get as many details as possible, covering:
- Onset, course and duration of current episode.
- Past medical and psychiatric history.
- Medication, drug and alcohol history.

Check person's pockets and possessions for other clues.

Check hospital and GP records in case there is a past history.

Notes
- Your problems are largely solved by a good informant or past records. For example, the patient may be known to have catatonic schizophrenia, a recent head injury, or be wanted by the police.

Level of consciousness

Is the patient responsive to her surroundings?

Ask her to nod or open her eyes.

Does she move? Do her eyes follow a moving object? Is she paying attention to what's going on?

Notes
- Establishing if there is clouding of consciousness is crucial since it indicates delirium and the need for urgent medical treatment.
- *Stupor* describes a condition in which the patient does not speak, move or respond, but appears fully conscious. Amongst psychiatric in-patients, stupor is caused mainly by catatonic schizophrenia, severe depression, organic disorders such as drug-induced states, akinetic mutism, and by dissociative disorder. In other populations (e.g. neurology wards) the proportions — and even the definition of stupor — are different.

Facial expression and communication

Does her expression change?

Does she seem fearful, depressed, preoccupied or hostile?

Does she speak spontaneously or in response to questions?

Can she communicate in other ways, for example by writing or hand signals?

Notes
- Facial expression and behavioural responses give diagnostic clues. For example: the characteristic appearance of a severely depressed patient; per-

plexity and fear in someone with psychosis or delirium; the focussed hostility of someone with a personality disorder who does not want to be interviewed.

• In *elective mutism*, usually seen in children, the unresponsiveness is limited to speaking—other forms of communication are intact.

Motor system

Is posture abnormal? Is it awkward or bizarre?

Is muscle tone normal? Is there resistance when you try and make a movement?

Is there spontaneous movement?

Are there stereotyped movements or mannerisms?

Notes

• These questions are aimed mainly at detecting *catatonia* (see psychosis module), which usually occurs in catatonic schizophrenia but is also caused by some rare neurological syndromes.

• Increased muscle tone, decreased consciousness and hyperthermia suggest neuroleptic malignant syndrome (Table 7.7).

• Surreptitious observation may reveal that the patient behaves differently when unaware she is being observed—indicating feigned unresponsiveness.

Other components of the module

What is the patient's attitude to being examined?

Do a neurological examination in addition to aspects mention above—include cranial nerves, reflexes.

Do a general physical examination—for signs of recent hygiene, trauma, intoxication, etc.

Notes

• Examine the neurological system in as much detail as possible. Consider asking for an urgent neurological or general medical consultation if no clear psychiatric cause for unresponsiveness is found.

Chapter 4

Risk: harm, self-harm and suicide

Risk in psychiatry

In psychiatry, *risk* refers to the probability that an adverse event such as self-harm, suicide, or harm to others will occur. Public and professional concern about such events makes *risk assessment* and *risk management* an important part of psychiatric practice. A brief evaluation of risk, especially of suicide, is always part of the core assessment, but often a more detailed risk assessment is required. For example, in someone with:

- Current suicidal intent.
- A history of mood disorder, psychosis or substance abuse.
- A history of self-harm or violence to others.

This chapter covers the assessment and management of risk in general, and self-harm and danger to others in particular.

- Harmful outcomes can never be eliminated. However, competent risk assessment and management can decrease their likelihood.

Risk assessment

When assessing the risk of harm to self or others, look for features associated with an increased risk. Try and gather the information from different sources—patient, informants, medical records, social services, police, etc.

In the *history*:

- Previous harm to self or others—the past is the best predictor of the future.

- Recent actions suggestive of impending harm (e.g. buying a hosepipe, making a will).
- Recent major stresses or losses.
- Depressive disorder, psychosis, substance abuse or personality disorder.

In the *mental state*:

- Suicidal or violent thoughts.
- Significant mood disturbance.
- Psychotic symptoms, especially passivity.

In the *context*:

- Demographic factors (Table 4.1).
- Abuse of drugs or alcohol.
- Social restlessness—for example few relationships, frequent changes of address.
- Easy access to potential weapons or victims.

Formulation of risk

After completing the risk assessment, document the findings:

- What potential harmful outcome, if any, has been identified?
- What is your estimate of its probability?
- How immediate and long lasting is the risk?
- What factors may increase or decrease the risk?
- What can be done to reduce the risk?

Mr J is referred for a psychiatric opinion because he has threatened to kill his wife and himself. He has convictions for bodily harm and theft. You find no evidence of depressive disorder, psychosis or violent thoughts. However, he admits to drinking heavily at weekends, whereupon he becomes threatening and

Table 4.1 Risk factors for suicide.

Factor	Comment
Demographic factors	
Male	
Increasing age	Though the rate in young males has increased in recent years
Living alone	
Unemployed	
Recent life crisis	
Previous DSH	Increases suicide rates 100-fold
Occupation	Vets, doctors, nurses, pharmacists and farmers have increased rates
Illness-related factors	
Chronic medical problems	
Psychiatric disorder	Present in 70% of suicide victims, usually depression
Depressive disorder	15% suicide rate in severe depression
Schizophrenia	>10% commit suicide
Substance misuse	Especially alcohol and opioid dependence
Personality disorder	Higher suicide rate, especially borderline type
Being in psychiatric care	75% of suicides have been in psychiatric treatment
In-patient	5% of suicides
Recent discharge	See p. 38
Mental state factors	
Depressed mood	
Expressed wish to be dead	
Detailed suicide plans	
Hopelessness	
Absence of reasons to go on living	e.g. bereavement

low in mood. His wife and the police (with his permission) corroborate the history. Your preliminary conclusion is of an alcohol-related problem and possibly personality disorder. His risk of harm or self-harm is low when sober but quite high when intoxicated or stressed. This fluctuating pattern of risk will continue as long as his drinking problem does. Marital strife is the other factor increasing risk.

Risk management

Risk management aims to:
- Reduce the level of immediate risk.
- Maintain it at an acceptable level.
- Set up a process for reviewing the risk.

Risk management strategies can be divided into immediate and longer term interventions. *Immediate interventions* include:

- Psychiatric admission, if necessary under the Mental Health Act.
- Acute sedation.
- Ensuring there is adequate community support.
- Lowering of tension and provision of reassurance as a result of the assessment itself.
- Making the family and significant others aware of risk.
- Removing access to weapons.
- Notifying the police.

Longer term interventions include:
- Effectively treating associated psychiatric disorder.
- Implementing the care programme approach (Chapter 8).
- Alleviating psychosocial stresses.
- Enhancing positive coping strategies.

In all cases, ensure that:
- The management plan is documented and

communicated to others involved in the case (Chapter 5).

● A date is set for reviewing the case and the plan — this may be within hours for an acutely suicidal in-patient, or every year in a stable patient in the community.

You discuss Mr J with your colleagues and draw up a risk management plan. A copy is given to Mr J, his wife and GP. Mr J is given advice to help him cut down his drinking. The couple refer themselves to Relate to try and reduce conflicts between them. It is made clear to Mr J that he will be held responsible should he harm his wife. He agrees to record his alcohol intake and to return in 6 weeks.

Suicide and deliberate self-harm

Definitions

● *Deliberate self-harm (DSH)* is the umbrella term for self-inflicted non-fatal harm. Self-cutting is the commonest form, though self-poisoning accounts for 90% of medical presentations of DSH.

● *Attempted suicide* may be used where there was a definite attempt to take one's life, and *parasuicide* when the degree of suicidal intent associated with the act is not clear.

● *Suicide* is the taking of one's own life. Although suicide is clearly defined by death, establishing intent retrospectively is often difficult — some suicides are expressions of distress that went tragically wrong.

Deliberate self-harm (DSH)

DSH is important because:

● *It is common.* There are approximately 150 000 presentations to general hospitals with DSH each year, and DSH accounts for 10% of all acute medical admissions. It is the commonest reason for acute admission of women and the second commonest for men. A GP may expect five of his/her patients to commit DSH each year.

● *It is a risk factor for repeated DSH and suicide.* About 20% present with DSH in the following year, and 1–2% will commit suicide.

● *It can be the presenting feature of serious psychiatric*

disorder. However, most patients seen after DSH have a mild depressive disorder, adjustment reaction, personality disorder, or no psychiatric diagnosis. Substance misuse is commonly associated.

Motivations for DSH are various and mixed. Only a minority have clear and sustained suicidal intent. Many acts are an impulsive response to what is perceived as an intolerable situation, or an attempt to affect the behaviour of others. DSH is often carried out under the influence of alcohol.

● DSH can also represent a failed outcome of a determined attempt at suicide. Though rare, recognition of this small group is important.

Suicide

Though not a common cause of death, suicide is the third biggest cause of lost years of life because, relatively, it often affects young adults. People who successfully commit suicide are often depressed, and perceive the future as both intolerable and hopeless. Occasionally, this perception may be shared by others (e.g. in terminal cancer), but usually it is strongly biased by depressed mood. Suicides are usually planned. The risk factors for suicide are shown in Table 4.1.

● An increased risk of suicide in the weeks after discharge from a psychiatric hospital should be taken into account when planning management.

● Suicide rates in young men increased in the UK in the 1980s and 1990s, before plateauing. The reason is unknown.

● In depression, suicide may occur during the initial recovery phase — some people are so depressed that, until then, they lack the motivation to kill themselves despite a wish to be dead. Suicide risk assessments and interventions should therefore not stop just because improvement has begun.

Assessment of suicide risk

Assessing suicide risk is part of the core psychiatric assessment. If present, a full assessment is then essential. This follows the general principles of risk assessment, taking into account the risk factors for suicide (Table 4.1). Particular attention is paid to:

- The person's expressed intent.
- Their mental state.
- Recent DSH.

Never omit to assess suicide risk because you think (a) it might precipitate suicide, or (b) someone really planning to kill himself will deny it. Neither is true—the evidence is that recognition and active management may prevent suicide. Many people who kill themselves have been in contact with a doctor in the days before the fatal act.

Assessment following DSH

All patients who have self-harmed should be psychiatrically assessed, even if only briefly, to determine their risk of a repeat attempt and to identify the presence of a significant psychiatric disorder. Certain characteristics of DSH predict a high suicidal intent, and a high risk of subsequent suicide:

- The attempt was planned.
- Affairs put in order beforehand.
- The person took precaution to avoid discovery.
- They did not seek help afterwards.
- The used a method that the patient believed to be dangerous.
- They left a suicide note.

Management after DSH

General management

The number of patients seen after DSH is large and their management presents a challenge to medical and psychiatric services, especially if these are not well integrated (Chapter 18).

- For most cases, no specialist care is indicated, and the patient is discharged to the GP. Ensure the GP receives clear and prompt communication about the assessment (Chapter 5).

Ms S was seen in casualty having taken 20 paracetamol tablets earlier that night. She had been drinking and had taken them after a row with her boyfriend. She had not planned to kill herself and now felt foolish about her behaviour. She was unaware that paracetamol could be lethal. She was offered an appointment for out-patient counselling but declined, preferring to see her GP.

- A minority of patients are found to be at acute risk of suicide and require immediate and intensive management. The priority is to keep the person safe, often by psychiatric admission, and sometimes under the Mental Health Act. Serious suicidal intent is sufficient grounds for admission under the Act, even if the presence of a psychiatric disorder has yet to be established. If admission is not used, ensure relatives are aware of the severity of the situation and know how to contact services urgently if necessary.

Mr P was found in his fume-filled car in an isolated field and resuscitated. He was angry at being saved and still wished to die. He was suffering from psychotic depression and had previously taken a serious overdose. He was admitted under the Mental Health Act and treated with ECT.

- Another important principle for all those at acute risk of suicide is to form a positive therapeutic relationship and begin to instil hope for the future.
- Recognizing and treating depression effectively is also a sensible priority, given the importance of depression as a factor in suicide—though there is little evidence that doing so does decrease suicide rates.
- Many DSH patients have personal, relationship or social problems for which they may be offered help, e.g. by counselling or problem solving therapy, or by referral to community mental health psychology services.

Management of patients who repeatedly self-harm

A small number of people, mostly young women, present repeatedly with DSH from overdoses or wrist cutting. A diagnosis of personality disorder (dramatic cluster; Table 15.1) is often made, and a history of childhood sexual abuse or other trauma may emerge. Management includes:

- Psychological support which is not contingent on acts of DSH.
- Checking for emergent depressive disorder.

Table 4.2 Prevention of suicide.

Individual interventions
Better detection and management of:
   suicidal intent in patients attending medical services
   depressive disorder
   substance misuse

Population interventions
Public education and discussion
Education of doctors and others (e.g. teachers)
Easy, rapid access to psychiatric care or support groups
   (e.g. Samaritans)
Make it harder to commit suicide by:
   limiting access to paracetamol—smaller bottles,
      blister packs
   make exhaust pipes harder to fix a hose over
   safety nets around high buildings and bridges
Decreasing societal stressors—unemployment,
   domestic violence, etc.
Decreasing substance misuse

Suicide as a public health problem

Prevention of suicide in the population has been a priority for health policy, but it is difficult to achieve, in part because social and political factors, and not just medical ones, are important (Table 4.2).

Risks to others

Despite the public perception, psychiatric patients are more likely to be recipients than perpetrators of violence, and most aggressive acts are committed by persons with no psychiatric disorder. Nevertheless, knowing when and how to assess and manage potential harm to others is an important aspect of psychiatric practice.

- In response to public concerns, the UK government has proposed the category of *dangerous and severe personality disorder* (p. 166).

Assessment of risk to others

The disorders most associated with increased risk of violence are substance abuse, schizophrenia and mania, as well as some personality disorders. These disorders act cumulatively—so the risk is greater in a person with more than one of these diagnoses.

- Harmful acts are occasionally *directly* due to the disorder. For example, passivity experiences in schizophrenia, or nihilistic delusions in psychotic depression, may lead to harm to others without any wilful intent. More commonly, violence results *indirectly* from the same combination of frustrations and personality that determine such acts in anybody. The disorder merely decreases the threshold (and perhaps increases the chances that the aggressor is caught.)
- As with most behaviour, the strongest predictor of future violence is previous violence.

Management of risk to others

After identifying a risk to others, the clinician should do all they reasonably can to prevent the harmful outcome.

- Check access to weapons and whether there are specific plans or identified victims.
- Warn a potential target—the risk to others can over-ride patient confidentiality, for example in morbid jealousy (p. 134).
- If there is known or suspected psychiatric disorder, consider admission, if necessary to a secure unit and discuss with a forensic psychiatrist.
- Conversely, if psychiatric assessment reveals no evidence of psychiatric disorder, this conclusion should be clearly recorded.

Key points

- Risk in psychiatry particularly refers to the risk of self-harm and the risk of harm by the patient to others.
- Assessment of suicide risk should be included in every psychiatric assessment.
- Detection of risk should lead to active management of the risk.
- DSH is very common. All patients who have self-harmed should be screened for suicidal risk and for psychiatric disorder.
- The majority of people committing suicide have depressive disorder or other chronic psychiatric disorder. However they also occur, especially in young men, in people with no known psychiatric history.
- Most psychiatric patients are not violent. Most violence is not committed by psychiatric patients.
- Substance misuse, personality disorder, schizophrenia and mania are all associated with increased risk of harm to others, especially if they coexist.

Chapter 5

Completing and communicating the assessment

Completing the assessment

The process of psychiatric assessment described in Chapters 2 to 4 provides diagnostic information and an understanding of the patient in context. These facts are now combined to allow you to:

- Make a (differential) diagnosis.
- Identify the factors which have contributed to the disorder.
- Plan your initial management, and think about the longer term.
- Think about the prognosis.
- Summarize and present the case.

This chapter covers these areas in turn. An overview of the process is given in Figure 5.1.

- Remember that making a psychiatric diagnosis is not a neutral act—it has drawbacks (e.g. for job prospects, stigmatization) as well as benefits (e.g. effective treatment).

The diagnostic process

Assuming the core and module approach has worked, you will have eliminated most possible diagnoses for your patient. Sometimes, one overwhelmingly likely diagnosis will remain, but usually there is a differential diagnosis that requires further investigation. Either way, draw up a list of the key features in favour of each plausible diagnostic possibility.

- Weighing the diagnostic evidence helps clarify your own thoughts about the case. It is also useful to others who may refer back to your assessment— for example, if there is a subsequent review of the diagnosis.
- Throughout the chapter, a single vignette will be used, to show how different aspects of a case are highlighted depending on the stage in the diagnostic process and the clinical situation.

Mr K, 60, was referred after a suicide attempt. You have elicited many depressive symptoms, some anxiety symptoms, and an alcohol intake of 40 units/week. There are no features suggestive of psychosis or personality disorder, nor of imminent suicide risk. Your provisional diagnosis is depressive disorder, plus alcohol misuse.

It is now time to add in the contextual information collected during the core and modules, particularly those factors that appear to help explain the origins and evolution of the disorder.

The context and cause of the case

When considering causative factors in psychiatry, the two key variables are:

- The *type* of factor—usually divided into biological, psychological and social.
- The *time* at which the factor operates. A useful mnemonic for this is 'the three Ps': predisposing, precipitating and perpetuating.

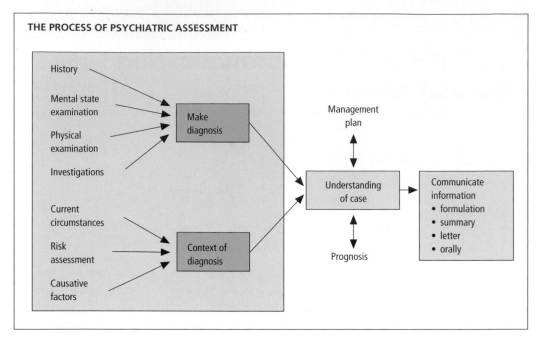

Figure 5.1 The process of psychiatric assessment.

Types of causes: biological, psychological and social

The development of psychiatric disorders is influenced by biological (genetic and environmental), psychological and social factors (Chapter 6). Sometimes one predominates, sometimes another, but all three always contribute something to each disorder. Hence the *biopsychosocial model* of psychiatry, which requires that due attention is paid to all three areas and which encourages an equally eclectic approach to treatment.

- The biopsychosocial model should seem obvious and essential. However, psychiatry has at times been guilty of focusing too closely on one or other of its components. This has led to mindless psychiatrists (who see only the molecules) and brainless psychiatrists (who see only minds and the social issues). We hope we are neither, but we could be both.

Mr K was made redundant 6 months ago. He is gay and his partner left him around the same time, after which he had several casual homosexual encounters.

He has no close friends or relatives. Mr K had a stroke 2 years ago which left him with a mild hemiparesis. He has had two past depressive episodes. His father committed suicide when Mr K was 5.

Applying the biopsychosocial approach to Mr K, several causative factors can be proposed, based on evidence from what is known about the origins of mood disorder (Chapters 6 and 9). Not all factors may be relevant, and some may be not be 'provable' facts, but all merit consideration (Table 5.1).

Timing of causes: predisposing, precipitating and perpetuating

In terms of timing, causal factors can be:
- Predisposing: factors which exert a long-term or distant causal effect, such as family history and early childhood experiences.
- Precipitating: factors which explain why the disorder has occurred now. They include recent life events, injuries and new medical conditions, and discontinuation of medication.

Table 5.1 Biological, psychological and social factors.

Biological
Genetic predisposition (his father had a depressive
    disorder)
Cerebrovascular disease (associated with depressive
    disorder)
Alcohol misuse (associated with depressive disorder)

Psychological
Stress of being gay (a secret?)
Recent breakdown in a serious relationship
Guilt about recent sexual liaisons

Social
Social isolation (has his stroke stopped him driving?)
Unemployment affecting his self esteem or causing
    financial worries

Table 5.2 Predisposing, precipitating and perpetuating causes.

Predisposing
    Genetic predisposition
    Psychological effects of father's suicide
    Guilt about his sexuality
    Alcohol misuse
    Stroke
    Past history of depression

Precipitating
    Ending of long-term relationship
    Increased alcohol intake
    Being made redundant

Perpetuating
    Social isolation
    Stressors continue
    Excess alcohol intake

• Perpetuating: factors affecting the course of a disorder. Ongoing marital and social problems and non-adherence with treatment are two common ones. The nature of the disorder itself is also relevant; for example, Alzheimer's disease requires no external perpetuating factors.

Table 5.2 summarizes the causative factors for Mr K according to the three Ps.
• Note that the same factor (in this case alcohol) can be involved in all three aspects of aetiology.
In practice, a useful tip is to combine the 'type' and 'timing' approaches to causative factors in a 3×3 box. This provides a template that can be filled in as details of the case emerge.

Having hypothesized the causal factors, try and substantiate them. For example, in this case:
• Examine for neurological deficits.
• Find out more about his alcohol misuse.
• Discover his views on his sexuality.
• Consider an HIV test.
• Investigate how he feels about the redundancy, and its financial consequences.
• Get hold of his case notes and review his past history.

You find that Mr K has only minimal physical impairment, but does have mild hypertension and a carotid bruit. He has misused alcohol intermittently for many years; the recent increase in consumption seems to have been a response to his low mood. His sexuality conflicts with his religious beliefs. He feels he was made redundant unfairly because he had taken sick leave, and has been left with serious financial problems. He is HIV negative. His notes reveal a similar picture during previous episodes, with a good response to ECT and antidepressants. You conclude that he has a recurrent depressive disorder.

Another way to clarify the role of causal factors and the interplay between them is to create a *life chart*. This is most useful when the history is long and complex, to show whether illness episodes, or recovery from them, are related to specific factors, and whether there is any pattern of treatment response.
• A life chart may be time consuming, but is usually worthwhile—and always impressive.
Table 5.3 shows a life chart for Mr K.

The future context

Having: (a) made a diagnosis and (b) investigated the causative factors; it is time to consider the management and the prognosis—the *future context*. These will follow directly from your current understanding of the case, and both will need to be mentioned in the summary, letter or phone call which will follow the assessment.

Table 5.3 A life chart.

Age	Events	Psychiatric disorder	Treatments
0	Complicated delivery		
5	Father commits suicide		
10	Mother remarries		
15	Turbulent home life	First depressive episode, severe	ECT × 6; amitryptiline 150 mg/d for 6 months
20	Joined navy; binge drinking		
25	'Came out', left navy		
30	Met long-term partner		
35	Became storeman	Depressive episode, moderate	Amitryptiline 150 mg/d for 9 months
40	Mother dies		
45		Intermittent heavy drinking	Counselling
50	Hypertension		β-blocker, continuing
53	Mild stroke		Physiotherapy
54	Made redundant		
55	Relationship ends	Current depressive episode, severe	

Management

Management in psychiatry involves making a number of decisions, several of which need to be made soon after the initial assessment. For example:

- *Does the person need treatment?* Some assessments produce no evidence of psychiatric disorder and no indication for treatment—other than reassurance and a clear statement of your conclusions.
- *How urgent is the problem?* Acute psychosis and severe mood disorders generally need immediate treatment. Serious risk of self-harm or harm to others is a major determinant of urgency. Is the patient sufficiently ill or at risk to need compulsory treatment?
- *Where should treatment take place, and from whom?* Most psychiatric disorders are treated by GPs; some will be referred to psychiatrists; a few need admission.
- *What management is indicated?* Treatment decisions depend primarily on the diagnosis. However, they are also affected by the context—another reason why contextual information was collected in the assessment. For example, is the patient motivated enough for a psychological treatment? Does his job mean I should avoid sedative antidepressants? What did she respond to last time?

Prognosis

Once you have a diagnosis and a reasonable understanding of the context, a provisional judgement about prognosis should be possible. Together with the diagnosis, it's the prognosis that is of most concern to the patient, their relatives and the referrer.

Short-term prognosis depends mainly on the natural history of the disorder and, particularly, the treatment response. It is usually possible to give a rough estimate of the likelihood of improvement and its timing.

Long-term prognosis is much more difficult to predict, and opinion on this issue may be deferred. It may be easier to estimate after an initial response to treatment has been observed. There are several non-specific factors which identify people at higher risk of a poor outcome:

- Insidious onset.
- Longer duration of disorder prior to treatment.
- Comorbid personality disorder.
- Comorbid substance misuse.
- Lack of close relationships.
- History of poor adherence to treatment.

Summarizing and communicating cases

In the assessment process, you have generated and tested diagnostic hypotheses, collected contextual information and have considered the management and prognosis. If it is to be useful, the understanding of the case that you have obtained must be communicated effectively to others. These are the GP and other agencies, those who may use the information in the future and, last but not least, the patient. When planning this communication, ask yourself:

• *What does the recipient want to know?* This can vary from a detailed discharge summary for the psychiatric case notes, to a brief letter informing a GP that the dose of a drug has been changed. Avoid unnecessary information—it obscures the important bits. On the other hand, always include important negatives (e.g. 'He is not suicidal', 'She is not currently psychotic'). Similar rules apply to oral presentations.

• *What does the recipient know already?* If you are summarizing a person's tenth admission, information about the previous nine is likely to be available to and known by everyone, and may not need to be repeated. Conversely, a psychiatric court report should be written assuming that the recipient knows nothing about the person and nothing about psychiatry (or psychiatric terminology).

• *What does the patient need to know?* Informing the

Box 5.1 A psychiatric formulation

Opening statement
Mr K is a 60 year old unemployed storeman. He was seen in clinic last week following an overdose and was admitted voluntarily because of suicidal intent and many depressive symptoms. Relevant factors included recent redundancy, break up of a long-term relationship, and alcohol abuse.

Differential diagnosis:
1. *Depressive disorder.* In favour: subjectively and objectively low mood, suicidal ideation, recent self-harm, poor sleep, loss of appetite, feelings of guilt and worthlessness; two prior depressive episodes. Against: his depressive symptoms are secondary to diagnoses 2–4.
2. *Anxiety disorder.* In favour: worrying about his health, feeling tense, socially phobic, and lies awake worrying. Against: the depressive symptoms began first, and are clearly more prominent.
3. *Alcohol misuse.* In favour: drinking 40 plus units/week; long history of harmful intake; describes withdrawal symptoms when in the navy (30 years ago). Against: intake over past few years has averaged 25 units/week; recent increase post-dated onset of symptoms; normal LFTs and MCV.
4. *Organic mood disorder.* In favour: stroke last year. Against: this seems insufficient to explain his symptoms; no focal neurological signs; preceding history of depressive disorder.

Diagnosis: Major depressive disorder—severe.

Context and cause:
Predisposing factors. Father had depression and committed suicide when Mr K aged 5. Alcohol misuse. Guilt about his sexuality. Stroke 2 years ago. Two other depressive episodes (age 16, 34), one requiring ECT.
   Precipitating factors. His partner left him 3 months ago after 20 years. Increased alcohol intake. Made redundant 6 months ago.
   Perpetuating factors. Social isolation—no close friends or family. Feeling guilty about recent casual homosexual affairs—and risk of HIV. Continuing high alcohol intake. Financial worries.

Management plan:
1. Further investigations: repeat LFTs; HIV test; get old notes; phone GP for background. Needs a medical opinion regarding hypertension and treatment.
2. Monitor mental state daily. Continue nursing observations whilst actively suicidal.
3. Observe for signs of alcohol withdrawal.
4. Start antidepressant (specify drug and dose). Benzodiazepine if required for sedation.
5. As mental state settles, assess further the current stressors—employment, finance, sexuality.
6. Longer-term will need continuing support—begin care programme approach assessment.

Prognosis:
His history predicts a good response to antidepressants. However, if stressors continue, recovery will be compromised and he will be vulnerable to relapse.

patient (and family) of the outcome of the assessment is the beginning of effective management. Patients are now entitled to know what is written about them; indeed it is expected that the patient will receive copies of all correspondence between doctors. This has many potential benefits, but may be particularly challenging in psychiatry because of the nature of the patients illness or the content of the letter (e.g. in an acute psychosis, or if there is a potential risk to others). In these (rare) circumstances, you may prefer to convey the information to others by phone.

Here we outline different types of communication—a formulation, a case summary, a problem list and a GP letter.

Formulations

A formulation is a concise, informative way of summarizing a psychiatric assessment. It is also educational for the reader since it involves weighing up the evidence and showing how you came to your conclusions. The formulation consists of:

• *An opening statement*—patient's name, age, occupation, presenting complaint and *brief* summary of main findings.
• *The differential diagnosis*. Put the most likely diagnosis first. Include the factors for and against each diagnosis. Remember that more than one diagnosis may be needed (comorbidity).
• *The context and cause of the problem*. Summarize the causative factors and relevant context. This can be done in different ways, as outlined above.
• *The management plan*. This should be clear and indicate the role of each party in implementing it. Include investigations and immediate interventions.
• *Prognosis*. Short and longer term.
An example of a formulation, for Mr K after his admission, is shown in Box 5.1.

Case summaries

A psychiatric case summary is equivalent in most respects to a medical one. It is useful:

• At the end of a psychiatric admission.
• On discharge from psychiatric care.

Table 5.4 Headings for a psychiatric case summary.

Demographic details
  Name, age, sex, occupation
  Dates: of referral, assessment, admission, discharge,
    Mental Health Act status.
Presenting complaint(s)
  Nature, onset, progression, treatments to date
Mental state at presentation
Past psychiatric history
  Diagnoses, admissions, treatments
Personal history
  Childhood, academic and job record, relationships,
    children
  Premorbid personality
  Use of alcohol and drugs
Mental state examination
Risk assessment
Physical examination
Investigations
Differential diagnosis
Management and progress
  Current symptoms and problems
Prognosis

• When the patient is being transferred to other psychiatric services.
Suggested headings are shown in Table 5.4—they overlap with those of the core assessment.

Problem lists

Once the background to a case is familiar, the emphasis usually switches to current problems and their solution. *Problem lists* ensure that the key issues are identified and dealt with. A problem list for Mr K is shown in Table 5.5.

Letters between psychiatrists and GPs

Letters from psychiatrists to GPs should be as concise as possible. Remember you are offering the GP advice, not giving instructions. Also bear in mind that the GP will often know at least as much as you about the person's history and circumstances. Take into account the purpose of the referral: was it for an opinion or for continuing care? Has the GP asked a specific question or requested a particular

Table 5.5 A problem list.

Problem	Action	Agent	Review
Suicide risk	Close observation	Nursing staff	Daily
Depression	Start amitriptyline 50 mg	Psychiatrist	One week—plan to increase dose
Insomnia	Sleep hygeine; hypnotics	Psychiatrist	One week
Social isolation	Investigate supports	Social worker	One week
Guilt about sexuality	Get contact number of local gay groups	Social worker	One week
HIV status	Consider HIV test	GUM clinic for advice	Two weeks
Alcohol misuse	Counselling (when mental state improved)	Specialist nurse	Unspecified

intervention? Generally the GP is most interested in:

• Your formulation of the case, including a clear diagnosis.

• A specific management plan, including the date of review and what he or she is expected to do.

• What the patient/relative has been told. If the patient has been copied into the correspondence, as mentioned above, this should be made clear.

• What the patient and GP should do if matters unexpectedly deteriorate (or improve).

As a final visit to Mr K's case, Box 5.2 is a letter to his GP, a year later. Letters from GPs to psychiatrists should follow the same principles. The psychiatrist wants to know:

• The presenting complaint(s), the chronology and the GPs provisional diagnosis.

• What is the reason for the referral—for a diagnostic opinion, treatment advice, ongoing care, etc?

• Is there an acute crisis? If not, why refer now?

• Past psychiatric and medical history.

• Key personal and social details (e.g. recent stressors, drug misuse).

• Any specific issues to be aware of (e.g. language difficulties, history of violence).

Box 5.2 Psychiatric discharge letter to GP

Dear Dr,
Re: Mr J.K., d.o.b 1.1.44, 24 Easy Street, Anytown

Diagnosis: severe depressive disorder, now in remission.

Course and current situation
Mr K has made a good recovery from his illness which was detailed in the summary sent to you on his discharge from the ward 6 months ago. Since then, he has continued to make a good recovery though, as you know, he required augmentation with lithium for full recovery. At review in clinic today he was again entirely free of symptoms.

Management and prognosis
Thank you for prescribing his medication (amitriptyline 150 mg nocte; lithium carbonate 800 mg nocte), which he has taken as prescribed. His lithium level will need to be checked in 6 weeks and maintained at 0.5–0.8 mmol/l—it was stable at 0.72 mmol/l last week. He should continue

the medication for at least another 6 months. At that time he intends to stop it, but he is aware that his risk of relapse will be lower if he remains on amitryptiline. When he does decide to stop, it should be tailed off over a few weeks.

Mr K is fully aware of the diagnosis and our formulation of its causes (especially the relationship break-up, guilt about his sexuality, and the increased alcohol intake). We have addressed these issues, and they appear largely resolved. His drinking is now within normal limits, and his LFTs have remained normal. Also on the positive side, he is in a new and seemingly stable relationship, and his financial worries have evaporated having been left money in his aunt's will.

We have not arranged to see him again. Please get in touch if you wish to discuss his case further, or if problems recur.

Yours etc
cc Mr J.K.

Key points

- Completing the psychiatric assessment involves using the information you have collected to make a diagnosis, understand its likely causes, plan management and estimate prognosis.
- When thinking about causation, divide the factors according to timing (predisposing, precipitating and perpetuating) and type (biological, psychological and social).
- A formulation is a useful way of summarizing a psychiatric case. It comprises: an introductory statement, the diagnoses and evidence for and against each differential diagnosis, the causative factors, the management plan, and the prognosis.
- Tailor the content and format of any communication to the needs of the recipient. Be concise, structured and emphasize the points relevant to diagnostic and management decisions.

Chapter 6

Aetiology

Aetiological factors in psychiatry

In this chapter we examine general principles for understanding the aetiology of psychiatric disorders. The key point is that psychiatric disorders (like all illnesses) are caused by multiple and diverse influences—some known, some unknown. Some factors will be more important than others for a particular disorder or individual.

For example, we might hypothesize that a teenager's eating disorder arises from:

- Inheritance of a genetic predisposition.
- Childhood obesity.
- Wanting to be a ballerina.
- Peer pressure to be thin.
- Disturbed 5-HT neurotransmission.
- A hypothalamic tumour.

The study of aetiology in psychiatry has to be equally diverse (Table 6.1).

- The only exceptions to the 'multifactorial' rule are a few, very rare, familial dementias which are caused by single gene mutations.
- A given causal factor often contributes to several different disorders.
- Longitudinal, prospective studies, starting with healthy but 'at risk' individuals and following them up until illness develops in some, are a powerful design. They help distinguish 'state' from 'trait' changes, and other problems of retrospective or cross-sectional studies of illness. Obviously they are more feasible in some situations than others.

- Aetiological conclusions should be just as evidence-based as therapeutic and diagnostic ones.

Epidemiology

Epidemiological methods are a tool that can be applied to social, psychological or biological studies. They have contributed in two main ways to psychiatry:

- Population surveys have provided good information about the *prevalence* and *incidence* of the major psychiatric disorders, their sex and age distribution, and so on. This basic demographic information underpins most other kinds of aetiological research.
- Cohort and case control studies have identified *risk factors* for psychiatric disorders—ranging from urban birth to autoimmune diseases to viral infection and drug side-effects. An example is the finding that head injury increases the risk of dementia. Sometimes, as in this example, the causality of an epidemiological finding is clear, but often it is not (e.g. the association of unemployment with depression), and further studies must be carried out to see which way the causal arrows point.

Social factors

Social factors are important both in the cause and shaping of psychiatric disorder. They can operate at different levels:

49

Table 6.1 Approaches to studying the aetiology of psychiatric disorders.

Field	Approaches
Epidemiology	Prevalence and incidence studies
	Risk factor studies
Sociology	Life events
	Family influences
	Cultural factors
	Illness behaviour
Psychology	Behavioural theories
	Cognitive theories
	Psychodynamic theories
	Personality theories
	Neuropsychology
Biology	Genetics
	Biochemistry and pharmacology
	Brain imaging
	Neuropathology
	Animal models

• *The immediate environment*. One's surroundings act as non-specific risk factors for illness. For example, psychiatric disorders are twice as common in those living in deprived conditions. Many mechanisms are involved, including social conflict, substance misuse, noise and overcrowding; there may also be factors that contribute independently to poverty and psychiatric disorder. In addition, having a psychiatric disorder may make it harder for the person to improve their circumstances and make continuing poverty more likely.

• *The social and family group*. Parents, siblings and others close to us are important influences on our development and functioning—for better and worse. For example, childhood emotional deprivation predisposes to later depression, whereas being in a close relationship protects against the effect of stressors.

• *The wider environment*. Environment in a broader sense is also relevant. For example, societal attitudes contribute to the prevalence of eating disorders, whilst political decisions affect the types and quantities of substances misused. Sociologists have also investigated trans-cultural differences in the occurrence of psychiatric disorders—many are uni-

versal, but some are much commoner in particular populations.

• Some of these apparently 'social' influences actually involve genes too—because genes and environment interact. In other words its 'nature plus nurture', not 'nature versus nurture'.

Life events

Life events are specific external stressors. They include marriage, bereavement, unemployment and moving house. Life events, especially negative ones, lead to an increased risk of psychiatric disorder, notably depression, in succeeding months.

• The impact of the life event on hypothalamo–pituitary–adrenal (HPA) axis is often implicated to explain this relationship.

• If a recent life event is the predominant, understandable trigger for a psychiatric disorder, the diagnostic category of *stress reaction* or *adjustment reaction* may be appropriate (Chapter 10).

The social origins of depression

A classic example of the role of social factors in psychiatry is depressive disorder. Researchers wondered why depression was particularly common in women of low socio-economic status, and why some women did not get depressed despite similar circumstances. They identified several factors (examples of the 'three Ps' approach to causation introduced in Chapter 5):

• Women who as children had suffered emotional deprivation or death of a parent were at greater risk of depression. Other *vulnerability (predisposing) factors* included not having a supportive partner or close friend, and being stuck at home with several young children.

• In the women who had one or more of the vulnerability factors, depressive disorder was *precipitated* by a single major life event or by an accumulation of minor stressors.

• Continuing stress and lack of support acted as *perpetuating* factors.

A similar combination of social factors is now known to be associated with depression in other environments and groups.

Family theories

Family theories view psychiatric disorder in one member as reflecting an abnormality in the whole family. They are applied particularly to childhood psychiatric disorders, where the theories have inspired a treatment approach—*family therapy*. However, it has been hard to confirm the aetiological role of the family, for two main reasons:

• Recent research shows that resemblances between family members are influenced by genes at least as much as by the family environment. An example where family factors (in a sociological sense) were wrongly invoked is autism, which was attributed to parents being aloof or obsessional but in fact it is highly genetic.

• How do you show that family abnormalities are causal? In the 1950s, schizophrenia was explained in terms of parenting styles (the 'schizophrenogenic mother') and patterns of family communication ('double bind', 'schism and skew'). Such abnormalities, if they occur, seem more likely to be the result, not the cause, of having a schizophrenic relative in the house.

The sick role and illness behaviour

The *sick role* describes four processes that occur when someone is ill:

• Exemption from normal obligations (such as earning a living).

• A right to receive care.

• An obligation to co-operate with care.

• A desire to recover.

Illness behaviour refers to the behaviour of the person in the sick role.

Both the sick role and illness behaviour are sociological concepts that describe normal processes. They can also be excessive or maladaptive, and then are relevant to understanding the presentation and persistence of psychiatric (and medical) disorders.

• People differ markedly in their response to symptoms—that is, they vary in their illness behaviour and readiness to adopt the sick role. Some are stoical and are reluctant to see a doctor, others dramatize symptoms and have a low threshold for medical consultation. These individual differences are compounded by society's views about psychiatric disorder—including stigma and ignorance about their nature and treatability. As a result, psychiatric patients may have more difficulty than medical patients in negotiating a sick role.

• Patients with medical complaints who appear to adopt the sick role unnecessarily or excessively (i.e. have *abnormal illness behaviour*) may have depression or a somatoform disorder.

• The benefits of the sick role (sometimes called *secondary gain*) play an especially important role in dissociative and somatoform disorders (Chapter 10).

Antipsychiatry

Some sociologists, and a few psychiatrists, have argued that psychiatric disorders are not medical illnesses, but merely social constructs to deal with deviant behaviour. This thesis—*antipsychiatry*—was influential in the 1960s. Whilst antipsychiatry was important in drawing attention to the limitations of psychiatric knowledge and the dangers of stigmatization and institutionalization, there is little evidence to support its tenets, and it is not helpful to ill patients.

• A watered down version ('critical psychiatry') is currently advocated in some quarters. It sees psychiatric disorders as predominantly social in origin and requiring psychosocial interventions. It is influenced by philosophical and political beliefs. The importance of medical and neuroscientific aspects of causation and management are minimized.

Psychological factors

There are various psychological models of psychiatric disorder, differing in their theoretical background and experimental support, but sharing two features:

• They are extensions of theories of normal psychological processes.

• There is a psychological treatment based upon the theory.

Behavioural theories

Many of our actions are explicable in terms of learned behaviours or *conditioning*. There are two types of conditioning, *classical* and *operant*. These underlie contemporary *behavioural theories* of normal and abnormal behaviours.

- Behavioural theories have given rise to *behavioural therapy* (p. 73), an effective intervention for several childhood disorders and anxiety disorders.

Classical conditioning

In classical conditioning, we unconsciously associate two stimuli that regularly occur together. In Pavlov's classic experiments, dogs were given food when a bell was rung. After a while the dogs began to salivate when the bell rang, even if no food was there. This conditioning gradually wears off (*extinction*). People are classically conditioned in many ways: for example, men may become aroused at the sight of lingerie if they have come to associate it with impending sexual gratification.

- Conditioning is important in the development of some psychiatric disorders. For example, agoraphobia developing in a woman who was twice assaulted in the street; she associates leaving the house with the fear of attack, which she avoids by staying at home.

Operant conditioning

A behaviour will occur more frequently if it is rewarded (*positive reinforcement*), and decreases if it is not (*negative reinforcement*) or if it has unpleasant consequences (*punishment*). This is called *operant conditioning*. Rats learn to press a lever if it gives them food but not to press it if they don't, or if they receive a painful shock. Children will shout and scream if they learn that this behaviour gets them an ice cream; on the other hand they learn to be polite if that is effective in obtaining one. Adults are equally conditionable, though might not like to think so.

- *Learned helplessness* is an example of operant conditioning. Animals subjected to inescapable stresses (electric shocks) eventually give up trying to avoid them. A similar mechanism is proposed to explain why childhood adversity predisposes to depression in adulthood.

Cognitive theories

The core assumption of cognitive theories is that cognitions (thoughts, patterns of thinking, and ways of processing information) influence our mood, behaviour and physiology, and that inaccurate or distorted cognitions can lead to inappropriate or abnormal mood and behaviour.

- Cognitive theories of depression and anxiety disorders are especially well developed. The cognitive model explaining how panic disorder develops is summarized in Figure 6.1.

A woman gets a twinge of chest pain whilst reaching for a tin of beans in the supermarket. She has the thought that it might be a heart attack. She becomes more anxious and develops the physiological changes associated with anxiety. She interprets these sensations as confirming that she is having a heart attack, the anxiety increases, and she has a panic attack. The next time she is in the supermarket she recalls the episode, becomes hypervigilant for bodily sensations, and a second panic attack occurs more readily than before. As the cycle continues, her cognitions and the associated symptoms are repeated until she has established panic disorder.

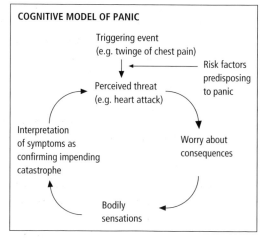

Figure 6.1 Cognitive model of a panic attack.

- In the equivalent cognitive model of depression, the central abnormality is the presence of dysfunctional assumptions and negative thoughts that lead to a vicious cycle of lowered mood and more negative thoughts.
- Cognitive distortions can arise for different reasons. For example, the lady above may be concerned about a heart attack because of childhood illness, the experience of a relative's death or health education programmes.
- Cognitive theories are well validated and are clinically important because they have led to an effective and widely used form of psychotherapy— *cognitive therapy* (p. 73).

Psychodynamic theories

Psychoanalysis, associated with Sigmund Freud, is a complex theory of psychological processes and the origins of psychiatric disorders, especially neurosis. It also refers to the therapy inextricably linked to the theory. Psychoanalysis has changed a lot since the time of Freud and the generic term *psychodynamic* is usually used to describe theories that combine Freudian elements with later ideas. Key features include:

- Feelings and memories of which we are unaware, especially those arising from early in life, shape our current thoughts and feelings.
- The mind is partitioned; some is conscious but much is unconscious. In Freud's final model, the components of the mind were the ego, superego, and id: the ego is the part of us in contact with reality; the superego is our conscience; and the id is our instinctive drives and desires. Its energy is called *libido*, which is primarily sexual in nature.
- Neuroses result from a failure to progress through normal stages of mental development.
- We use unconscious *defence mechanisms* to reduce tensions which exist between our conflicting desires (Table 6.2). These mechanisms may be healthy or dysfunctional.

Psychodynamic theories have been influential but have declined in importance for several reasons:

- They are not true scientific theories.
- When elements of the theories have been tested they have not been supported by evidence.

Table 6.2 Defence mechanisms.

Defence mechanism	Definition
Repression	Suppressing desires and memories from consciousness
Denial	To behave as though genuinely unaware of external reality
Projection	Attributing your own feelings to someone else
Displacement	Shifting emotions from the appropriate object or person to a more acceptable target, e.g. kicking the dog rather than your father
Reaction formation	Behaving in a way opposite to your (unacceptable) instincts
Regression	To regress to an earlier pattern of behaviour, e.g. to become more dependent on others to cope with an insoluble problem
Sublimation	Finding a socially acceptable alternative outlet for emotions
Intellectualization	Thinking about your emotions rather than feeling them

- Psychodynamic psychotherapies are of unproven efficacy.

Nevertheless, psychodynamic insights are still clinically useful in:

- Emphasizing that early experiences and unconscious processes affect our feelings and actions.
- Outlining psychological defence mechanisms— strategies we automatically use to cope with real or perceived stresses (Table 6.2).
- Identifying *transference* and *counter-transference*, relevant to all doctor–patient relationships (p. 72).

The role of personality

Personality describes our persistent pattern of thoughts, attitudes and behaviours. As such, it is critical to psychiatric disorder (as introduced in

Chapter 5), but the very fact that the two are so intertwined makes it hard to identify the specific aetiological relationships between them. It is clear, though, that:

• Different personality types predispose to different psychiatric disorders.

• Personality affects the clinical picture of psychiatric disorder (i.e. acts as a *pathoplastic* factor).

• Personality affects the prognosis of psychiatric disorders.

These issues are discussed in Chapter 15.

Biological models

Genetics

A genetic contribution to a psychiatric disorder may be suspected for one of four reasons:

• If the disorder clusters in families. Familial aggregation can be shown to reflect shared genes not shared environment if twin studies show a higher concordance rate in monozygotic than dizygotic twin pairs, because MZ twins have identical genomes but DZ twins share 50% of genes.

• If the incidence of the disorder remains increased in adopted-away children (though this doesn't control for prenatal environment—which may be relevant for some disorders, such as schizophrenia).

• If there is a known chromosomal (*cytogenetic*) aberration, e.g. Down's syndrome, fragile X syndrome.

• If there is a known pathological or biochemical abnormality, then the underlying gene is a *candidate gene* for the disorder. For example in Alzheimer's disease, the β-amyloid protein in senile plaques led to the discovery of amyloid gene mutations. The lack of definitive lesions in most psychiatric disorders means there are few convincing candidate genes.

Apart from a few dementias (e.g. Huntington's disease) and developmental disorders (e.g. tuberous sclerosis), psychiatric disorders are not caused (determined) by gene mutations. Instead, there are genetic variants (*polymorphisms*) that act as risk factors, influencing susceptibility to the disorder (usually with odds ratios of less than 3). *Heritability* refers to the size of the genetic predisposition; it de-scribes the proportion of the disorder in the population that is attributable to genes. It is best measured in epidemiological twin studies. Heritability estimates for psychiatric disorders (for which good data are available) are shown in Table 6.3.

• Heritability is a population average figure. Any given individual's disorder may be much more or less 'genetic'.

• The rest of the 100% not explained by heritability denotes the environmental contribution, usually divided into individual-specific and shared environmental factors.

Although there is a substantial heritability for many psychiatric disorders, it is proving difficult to complete the next step (Figure 6.2)—to locate the chromosomal loci and susceptibility genes—despite using the molecular techniques being applied successfully elsewhere in medicine. There are several possible reasons for this slow progress:

Table 6.3 Heritability of psychiatric disorders.

Disorder	Heritability (%)
Addiction	40
Alzheimer's disease	50
Anxiety disorders	30
Bipolar disorder	80
Depressive disorder	40
Schizophrenia	80

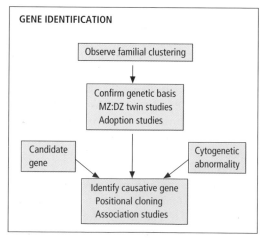

Figure 6.2 Finding genes for psychiatric disorders.

• There are probably many genes, each conferring a small amount of the risk for a psychiatric disorder. If so, the genes will be hard to find, and population genetic association studies (looking for genetic variants associated with a differential risk) are most likely to reveal them.

• Whilst there may be a major gene, a second gene or an environmental factor is also needed—a *two-hit* model.

• The disorder may be caused by different genes in different people (*genetic heterogeneity*).

• The causative genes may not map onto the currently defined clinical syndromes. That is, the wrong patients, genetically speaking, are being grouped together.

Biochemistry and pharmacology

Biochemical theories propose that psychiatric disorders are caused by a disturbance in the level or activity of an enzyme, neurotransmitter or receptor.

• Many of these theories are based on the mechanisms by which psychotropic drugs work. For example, antipsychotics treat schizophrenia and were found to block dopamine receptors; this observation led to the dopamine hypothesis of schizophrenia (p. 131). This has proved to be true, to some degree, but the line of reasoning is flawed: diuretics treat heart failure, but heart failure is not usually due to renal disease.

Measurements in the brain

Biochemical studies of the brain were crucial in the understanding of Alzheimer's disease. In particular, the discovery of cholinergic deficits and the β-amyloid protein. Similar approaches have revealed abnormalities in schizophrenia and mood disorders, though no comparably clear picture has emerged. Part of the problem is that studies of post mortem brains have many limitations, such as the effects of dying, death, and a bias towards old, medicated, chronically ill cases. This makes it difficult to establish whether alterations occurred early or late in the disease, and to exclude ageing or treatment effects.

Functional imaging overcomes these problems. It allows first-episode and unmedicated subjects to be studied. Various imaging modalities are being applied:

• Positron emission tomography (PET) and single photon emission tomography (SPET) use radioactive ligands to measure brain receptors. They have shown, for example, that people with schizophrenia do not have elevated dopamine D2 receptors (as one version of the dopamine hypothesis had proposed).

• PET, SPET and functional magnetic resonance imaging (fMRI) can be used to measure regional brain metabolism and cerebral activity. Such information points to the specific brain regions that may be involved in the pathophysiology of a disorder.

Peripheral markers

The brain is relatively inaccessible, so many biochemical measurements have been made in cerebrospinal fluid, blood or urine. A robust finding is that people who are impulsive and aggressive have low CSF levels of the metabolite of 5-HT, suggesting impaired functioning of the central 5-HT system. However, it is often unclear whether peripheral markers reflect the situation in the brain.

• In a *neuroendocrine challenge test*, a substance known to produce a change in the plasma level of a hormone is administered. The size of the change is used as a marker of the sensitivity of the system which mediates the response in the brain. For example, in the *dexamethasone suppression test* (DST), plasma cortisol is measured after a dose of dexamethasone, to assess HPA axis function. Many people with severe depression fail to suppress cortisol—leading to a 'steroid hypothesis' of depression

Brain structure

Structural brain imaging

Computerized tomography (CT) and MRI allow brain structure to be investigated *in vivo*. For example, they show that patients with schizophrenia have enlarged lateral ventricles, and that mood disorder in the elderly is associated with focal abnormalities in the white matter.

• Longitudinal MRI studies are increasingly used. For example, they show that some differences in brain structure long precede the onset of symptoms in schizophrenia.

Neuropathology

Many dementias have a known neuropathological basis—indeed, neuropathology provides the diagnostic criteria. Most other psychiatric disorders do not. Nevertheless, recent studies using sensitive and molecular techniques suggest that there may be histological changes in schizophrenia, mood disorder and autism.

Animal models

No one would suggest that a rat can get schizophrenia—and how would we know if it did? However, animal studies have contributed to psychiatric research in various ways—Pavlov and learned helplessness have already been mentioned—and they continue to be of use:

• To assess the effects of an experimental intervention (e.g. maternal separation, neonatal hippocampal damage) upon relevant behaviours (e.g. cognitive performance, social interactions) and biology (e.g. receptor sensitivity).

• *Transgenic* animals allow the role of specific genes in brain function and dysfunction to be investigated. For example, mice containing a mutated human amyloid precursor protein gene develop cognitive impairment and histological features of Alzheimer's disease; mice without a prion protein gene are resistant to prion disease (p. 143).

Key points

• The cause of most psychiatric disorders is multifactorial. It involves biological, psychological and social factors.

• There is a genetic predisposition to most disorders. The number and identity of the genes involved remain unknown.

• Other biological aetiological factors include head injury, drugs and viral infections.

• Important psychological factors are early experience, cognitive style and conditioning.

• Social influences include childhood deprivation, relationship problems, family structure and unemployment.

Chapter 7

Treatment

Psychiatric treatments may be categorized as *biological*—drugs and electroconvulsive therapy (ECT), *psychological*—the psychotherapies, and *social*. A combination of approaches is usually used. Sometimes *compulsory* treatment is given.

- This is the longest and most 'fact packed' chapter. We suggest you read about a particular treatment as you encounter it in your clinical work.
- Table 7.1 gives a chronology of the major treatments currently in use.
- Chapter 8 considers how treatments are delivered and services organized.

Evidence-based treatment

As in the rest of medicine, there is excellent evidence for some psychiatric treatments and rather less for others. We have endeavoured to use an evidence-based approach to our recommendations, and point out areas where the evidence is lacking and there is clinical uncertainty.

- Appendix 2 summarizes useful sources of evidence regarding psychiatric treatments.

Drug treatments (psychopharmacology)

Principles and practice of prescribing

Drugs used in psychiatry can be grouped into eight main categories (Table 7.2).

- Consult a more detailed text for complete information about individual drugs, doses, side-effects, drug interactions and contraindications.
- Always check the British National Formulary or similar before prescribing any drug with which you are not wholly familiar.
- Box 7.1 summarizes the important principles that govern the prescription of all psychiatric drugs. Bear these in mind as you read on, and try to put them into practice.
- Many patients—maybe even the majority—do not take their drugs regularly. This is variously called *compliance*, *adherence* or *concordance*, and the lack of it is a major reason for apparent non-response to medication. Box 7.2 lists the main reasons for the problem and how to minimize it.

Antidepressants

Antidepressants are effective, readily available and a first-line treatment for depressive disorders. Some are also used to treat other disorders. The major classes are shown in Table 7.2. The efficacy of antidepressants is well established. Selective serotonin reuptake inhibitors (SSRIs) and tricyclic antidepressants (TCAs) have similar efficacy, with about 60% of patients responding after 6 weeks. Over the same period, 30–40% respond to placebo.

- Patients often want to stop antidepressants too soon. Antidepressants usually produce some reduction in symptoms by 4–6 weeks, but it may take

	Physical therapies	**Psychotherapies**
1800s		Medical psychotherapy
1900s		Psychoanalysis
1930s	Psychosurgery	Group therapy
	Electroconvulsive therapy	
1950s	Antipsychotics	Brief psychodynamic therapy
	Monoamine oxidase inhibitors	
	Tricylic antidepressants	
1960s	Benzodiazepines	Family therapy
		Behaviour therapy
1970s	Lithium	Cognitive therapy
1980s	Selective serotonin	Cognitive behaviour therapy
	reuptake inhibitors	Interpersonal therapy
		Cognitive analytic therapy
1990s	Atypical antipsychotics	

Table 7.1 When current psychiatric treatments entered regular use.

Table 7.2 Drug treatments in psychiatry.

Type	Example	Main indications
Antidepressants		Depression, neuroses
TCAs	Amitriptyline	
SSRIs	Fluoxetine	
MAOIs	Phenelzine	
Other	Venlafaxine	
Mood stabilizers	Lithium	Bipolar disorder
	Valproate	
Hypnotics and anxiolytics		Anxiety, insomnia
Benzodiazepines	Diazepam	
Antipsychotics		Schizophrenia, mania, psychotic depression
Typical antipsychotics	Haloperidol	
Atypical antipsychotics	Clozapine	
Anticholinergics	Procyclidine	Extrapyramidal side-effects of antipsychotics
Drugs for dementia		Alzheimer's disease
Cholinesterase inhibitors	Donepezil	
Glutamate antagonist	Memantine	
Drugs used in substance dependence		Detoxification, abstinence
Alcohol	Disulfiram	
Opiates	Methadone	
Stimulants	Methylphenidate	ADHD

TCAs: tricyclic antidepressants; SSRIs: selective serotonin reuptake inhibitors; MAOIs: monoamine oxidase inhibitors; ADHD: attention deficit hyperactivity disorder.

Box 7.1 Principles of psychiatric prescribing

- *Choose the right drug.* This requires an adequate assessment, diagnosis and consideration of other factors such as comorbid medical conditions.
- *Give the right dose.* Antidepressant doses are often inadequate, antipsychotic doses excessive. Each poses risks: lack of efficacy and unnecessary side-effects respectively.
- *Give the drug for the right duration.* Antidepressants tend to be given for too short a period and anxiolytics for too long. Again, the trade off is between incomplete response and adverse effects, including the potential for dependence.
- *The efficacy of each drug in a class is similar.* Consequently the choice of drug is determined largely by side-effects (e.g. sedative profile), strength of evidence and your own experience. We tend to use well-tried drugs rather than the most recent and heavily advertised, unless there is good reason to do so.
- *Avoid combinations of drugs from the same class.* There is no evidence for greater efficacy, and often more side-effects.
- *Psychiatric drugs are better than placebo . . . but not always by much.* Due humility is essential, along with a clear grasp of how and when to prescribe appropriately—and an awareness of, and willingness to use, alternative strategies.

Box 7.2 Non-compliance in psychiatry

Major causes are:
- Reluctance to accept the need for treatment.
- Lack of belief in drug efficacy.
- Concern about drug side-effects, including worry about becoming 'addicted'.
- Stigma.
- Forgetfulness.
- Expense.
- As an effect of the disorder being treated. For example, a psychotic patient may be convinced you want to poison him; a severely depressed person may feel they do not deserve to recover.

Improve concordance with medication in several ways:
- Establish a good therapeutic relationship.
- Discover the patient's own views about their illness and its treatment. Correct any misapprehensions, but respect their views if they disagree with yours.
- Share information about the evidence for (and against) the drug. Give simple, clear advice and figures. For example, 'You have a 60% chance of being a lot better after a month'; 'There is a small chance you'll feel nauseous at first'. Give the patient a chance to ask questions or dispute the evidence. And make sure that you include discussion about the risks and benefits of *not* taking the treatment.

---

many months for the patient to recover fully. Continued treatment maintains the improvement in the medium term (6 months after getting better). Prolonged use halves the chances of relapse in those at risk.

- All antidepressants are thought to work by enhancing activity of the monoamine neurotransmitters noradrenaline (NA) and/or serotonin (5-HT; Figure 7.1). The various classes achieve this in different ways.
- The focus here is on the drugs; see other chapters for discussion about their use in management. Chapter 9 discusses the treatment of depression, including combination therapies and treatment resistance.

Selective serotonin reuptake inhibitors (SSRIs)

SSRIs are the usual first line antidepressant. Compared to TCAs, previously the main class used, they have several advantages, though there are some disadvantages too (Table 7.3).

- *Mode of action.* Selectively inhibit synaptic 5-HT reuptake transporters, thereby increasing synaptic 5-HT concentration (Figure 7.1).
- *Practical usage.* Usual to start at full dosage, once daily with breakfast. Like all antidepressants, take 7–14 days for onset of antidepressant efficacy. However, side-effects (see below) occur in first few days—remember to warn the patient of this. Consider giving a hypnotic (e.g. trazodone) for the first few weeks to aid sleep. Always withdraw an SSRI slowly at the end of treatment.
- *Individual SSRIs.* There are few major differences in properties between the various SSRIs. *Fluoxetine* (20–40 mg/day) has a long half-life, so useful if compliance is poor, and withdrawal reactions are rare (but drug interactions also persist longer). *Citalopra*m (20–40 mg/day) and *sertraline* (50–

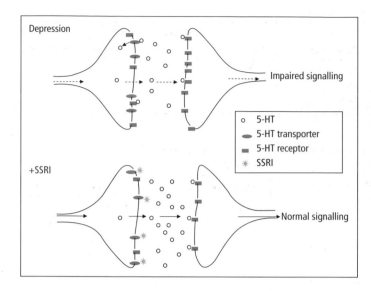

Figure 7.1 How SSRIs work. In depression, there is thought to be a relative 5-HT deficiency, and up-regulation of 5-HT receptors. The net effect is abnormal signalling and functioning of the postsynaptic neuron. SSRIs block the 5-HT transporter, and increase 5-HT in the synapse. The antidepressant effect takes several days to occur, because other adaptive changes have to occur too (to restore normal firing of the neuron, down-regulate receptors, and other secondary effects). TCAs work similarly, but act upon the presynaptic receptors and noradrenergic synapses too.

Table 7.3 SSRIs versus TCAs.

	SSRIs	**TCAs**
Dose regimen	Simple	Variable
Side-effect burden	Moderate, often light	Often marked
Main side-effects	Gastrointestinal, headache, sexual dysfunction, insomnia	See Table 7.5
Overdose	Safe	Dangerous— cardiotoxic
Other indications	Anxiety disorders Bulimia nervosa	Chronic pain Anxiety disorders

100 mg/day) have a 'clean' profile, and few interactions with other drugs.

- *Side-effects.* Usually well tolerated, though 15% have nausea, abdominal discomfort, diarrhoea, insomnia and agitation, mainly in early stages. Sexual dysfunction (lack of libido, anorgasmia) is common in women and also occurs in men. SSRIs may increase the risk of upper gastrointestinal bleeding. Some people experience discontinuation symptoms (insomnia, nausea, dizziness, agitation) when stopping the drug, hence withdraw over a few weeks.

- *SSRIs and suicide.* Some evidence suggests a small increase in suicide risk with SSRIs in the early stages of treating depression. Patients should always be monitored for suicide risk carefully at this time. However, any such risk must be set against the benefits of effective treatment in reducing the unequivocal suicide risk associated with depression.

- *Overdose.* Few effects; rarely if ever fatal.

- *Cautions and contraindications.* Few. May increase seizures in epilepsy. Avoid combining with monoamine oxidase inhibitors (MAOIs); and use with lithium only with caution.

Tricyclic antidepressants (TCAs)

Despite the overall advantages of SSRIs, TCAs retain an important role, especially for people intolerant of, or unresponsive to, SSRIs. They may also have slightly greater efficacy in severe depression and in chronic pain.

- Not all drugs in this class are actually tricyclic in structure. Semantically strict people call them *heterocyclic antidepressants*.

- *Mode of action.* Inhibit presynaptic NA and 5-HT transporters. Some TCAs are more selective for

Table 7.4 Comparison of three usefully different TCAs.

Drug	Dose (mg/day)	Main action	Sedation	Anticholinergic side-effects	Toxicity in overdose
Amitriptyline	75–250	NA, 5-HT	+++	+++	+++
Lofepramine	140–280	NA	+	++	+
Clomipramine	75–250	5-HT	++	+++	+++

one monoamine than another—e.g. clomipramine mainly acts on 5-HT; desipramine on NA (Table 7.4). Unlike SSRIs, TCAs also block various receptors, contributing to their side-effect profile (Table 7.5).

• *Practical usage.* Usually given at night (due to their sedative action) or in divided doses. Delayed onset of action as for SSRIs, though reduction in anxiety (anxiolysis) and sedation occur rapidly. To minimize initial side-effects, start at low dose and increase over 10 days.

• *Side-effects.* See Tables 7.4 and 7.5. The ability to drive and use machinery may be impaired due to drowsiness.

• *Individual TCAs.* Lofepramine is an effective TCA and generally well tolerated. *Amitriptyline* is very sedating and anxiolytic.

• *Overdose.* Dangerous in overdose causing tachyarrhythmias, seizures, coma, death.

• *Cautions and contraindications.* Avoid in glaucoma, prostatism, recent myocardial infarction, cardiac failure, and porphyria. Increase seizure frequency, so caution in epilepsy. Avoid combining with MAOIs.

Monoamine oxidase inhibitors (MAOIs)

MAOIs (e.g. *phenelzine*) are third-line antidepressants; their use is limited by toxicity and by their lesser efficacy than TCAs or SSRIs.

• *Mode of action.* Prevent breakdown of monoamines in presynaptic terminals by the enzyme MAO, thereby increasing transmitter availability.

• *Uses of MAOIs.* The main indication is atypical depression (Table 9.4). Also used in depression unresponsive to other treatments, either alone or in combination.

• *Practical usage.* Ensure patient is aware of the necessary dietary restrictions and drug interactions

Table 7.5 Receptor blockade by TCAs and their side-effects.

Receptor blocked	Side-effects produced
Muscarinic cholinergic	Dry mouth, urinary retention, constipation, blurred vision, glaucoma, tachycardia, delirium, sexual dysfunction
Alpha-1 adrenergic	Postural hypotension, drowsiness, sexual dysfunction
Histamine H1	Drowsiness, weight gain
Other or unknown	Arrythmias, seizures

(see below). Wait 2 weeks after stopping a TCA and 5 weeks after an SSRI. Prescribe in divided doses.

• *Side-effects.* Postural hypotension, insomnia, ankle oedema, dry mouth, dizziness, agitation, and headache.

• *Overdose.* Hypertension, delirium, coma, death.

• *Cautions and contraindications.* Prescribe with caution. MAO also metabolizes tyramine, so eating tyramine whilst on MAOIs can cause a hypertensive crisis ('*the cheese reaction*')—headache, palpitations, fever, convulsions and coma. Certain food and drinks must consequently be avoided, e.g. cheese, red wine, broad beans, pickled herrings, game, Marmite. There are also dangerous interactions with many drugs including opiates, insulin, cold remedies, antiepileptics, SSRIs and some TCAs. Avoid MAOIs in cardiac or hepatic failure or porphyria.

• *Reversible MAOIs.* Unlike classical MAOIs, *moclobemide* (300–900 mg/day) is virtually free from the cheese reaction and associated risks (because it only inhibits one form of MAO, and does so reversibly) although its effectiveness may be less.

Selective serotonin and noradrenaline reuptake inhibitors (SNRIs)

Venlafaxine (75–375 mg/day) is the only member of this group.

- *Mode of action*. Like TCAs, venlafaxine potently blocks 5-HT and NA reuptake. Unlike TCAs, it doesn't block cholinergic receptors.
- *Practical usage*. Slightly more effective than SSRIs. Its main indication is for SSRI non-response. Give twice daily, though a long-acting (once daily) form is available. Also has pain relieving properties.
- *Side-effects*. Resemble those of SSRIs, but may be worse. At high doses, hypertension may occur and should be monitored. Not sedative. Avoid MAOIs.

Other antidepressants

Various other antidepressants are available which do not fall readily into a specific class. None are more effective than SSRIs or TCAs, and they are not widely used.

- *Reboxetine* is a selective NA reuptake inhibitor. It is non-sedating and may improve social functioning.
- *Mirtazapine* and *trazodone* have complex pharmacologies. Both are very sedating. Low-dose trazodone (50–100 mg at night) is a useful (non-addictive) hypnotic, often used in conjunction with SSRIs in the early stages of treatment.
- *St. John's Wort* is an extract of the plant *Hypericum perforatum*, available without prescription and tried by many patients. It is an effective but weak antidepressant. Though a 'natural' remedy, it has side-effects, drug interactions, and there are reports of toxicity.

Mood stabilizers

A *mood stabilizer* is a drug used to prevent mood swings in bipolar disorder. Lithium was the first. The others are all antiepileptic drugs; it is not known why they have mood stabilizing properties.

Lithium

- *Mode of action*. Unknown. May act on second messenger systems to enhance neuronal plasticity.
- *Uses*. Usually given as lithium carbonate. The main indication is to prevent relapse in bipolar disorder; it is most effective in preventing mania. Needs to be given for at least 18 months for the benefit to be clear. Also effective in acute mania (though antipsychotics work faster) and as an adjunctive treatment for depression (Chapter 9). It is sometimes used to treat behavioural disturbance in learning disability.
- *Side-effects*. At therapeutic levels (0.5–1.0 mmol/l): fine tremor, metallic taste, dry mouth, thirst, mild polyuria, nausea, weight gain. Hypothyrodism in 20% of women; rarer in men. Renal impairment may occur after prolonged use, but rare if toxicity has been avoided.
- *Overdose*. Toxic symptoms occur above 2.5 mmol/l: coarse tremor, agitation, twitching, thirst and polyuria. Above 4 mmol/l: polyuric renal failure, seizures, coma and death. Toxic levels can result from even mild dehydration, or with low salt diets. Fatalities after overdose are not uncommon; survivors may be left with renal failure or brain damage.
- *Practical usage*. Before prescribing, a detailed discussion about the commitment and potential dangers is necessary. Do a physical examination and measure electrolytes, creatinine clearance, thyroid function, and also ECG if indicated. During treatment measure lithium levels regularly (weekly at first, then 3 monthly once stable). Titrate dose (usually 400–1200 mg/day) to keep the plasma level at 0.5–1.0 mmol/l. Test thyroid and renal function every 6 months. Withdraw gradually, in order to avoid rebound mania.
- *Cautions and contraindications*. Many. Avoid if adherence likely to be variable or short lived. Avoid in renal failure and pregnancy. Do not combine with diuretics, angiotensin converting enzyme inhibitors, or high dose antipsychotics. Use cautiously with anti-inflammatories and anaesthetics.

Valproic acid

Valproic acid (prescribed as sodium valproate or valproate semisodium) is the other leading mood stabilizer. It is of comparable efficacy to lithium (though this is still being studied), and possibly more effective against depressive relapses and in rapid cycling bipolar disorder.

- *Mode of action*. In epilepsy, works by blocking sodium channels and increasing GABA turnover.
- *Practical usage*. Dose depends on the drug formulation. Valproate semisodium is started at 250–500 mg/day and titrated upwards every few days, depending on adverse effects. The usual maintenance dose is 750–1250 mg/day. Plasma levels can be measured, but no therapeutic range for mood stabilization has been established.
- *Side-effects*. Sedation, tiredness, tremor, and gastrointestinal disturbance may occur. Reversible hair loss in 10% of patients. May cause thrombocytopenia.
- *Cautions and contraindications*. May increase plasma levels of other protein-bound drugs (e.g. other antiepileptics). Avoid in pregnancy, and use with caution in women of childbearing potential.

Carbamazepine

Carbamazepine is less effective than lithium or valproic acid, but may be used when these are contraindicated, ineffective or not tolerated.

- *Mode of action*. In epilepsy, works by blocking sodium channels.
- *Practical usage*. Start at low dose (200 mg bd) and build up to 600 mg bd. Measure plasma levels if signs of toxicity (ataxia, confusion, blurred vision) emerge. Check white cell count after a week.
- *Side-effects*. If erythematous rash or leucopenia occur, stop the drug. Other side-effects are nausea, dizziness, drowsiness and hyponatraemia.
- *Cautions and contraindications*. Carbamazepine is a potent enzyme inducer, so other drugs will be metabolized faster—e.g. the Pill. Avoid MAOIs or if there is evidence of hepatic failure, arrhythmias or pregnancy.

Lamotrigine

Lamotrigine is a newer antiepileptic drug. It is more effective than lithium against depressive relapses, but probably ineffective against manic relapses. Its position in the therapeutic hierarchy is not yet clear.

- *Mode of action*. In epilepsy, blocks sodium and calcium channels.
- *Practical usage*. Start very gradually, initially 25 mg daily for 2 weeks then 50 mg daily for 2 weeks. The usual dose in bipolar disorder is 100–300 mg daily.
- *Side-effects*. A rash occurs in 3–5% of patients, requiring that the drug be stopped. The risk is reduced by a gradual increase in dose. Other side-effects include nausea, headache, tremor and dizziness.
- *Cautions and contraindications*. Plasma levels are increased by valproate, and a combination of lamotrigine and carbamazepine may cause neurotoxicity.

Anxiolytics

These drugs are also known as *hypnotics* and *sedatives* if being used to help sleep. Benzodiazepines are the main class and in the 1960s and 1970s were very widely prescribed. With the awareness of their potential for dependency and withdrawal problems (Chapter 14), SSRIs or TCAs have replaced benzodiazepines as the usual drugs for anxiety. However, anxiolytics still have a role for short-term use.

Benzodiazepines

The former popularity of benzodiazepines is understandable: they are highly effective and relatively free of unpleasant side-effects.

- *Mode of action*. Potentiate inhibitory transmission via the benzodiazepine binding site of the $GABA_A$ receptor.
- *Uses in psychiatry*. Relief of acute anxiety and treatment of panic disorder, phobic anxiety and insomnia. Also used for delirium tremens, and to augment antipsychotics for sedation in acute psychosis.

● *Practical usage. Diazepam* (2–5 mg bd) is the standard anxiolytic. For intramuscular or intravenous administration use lorazepam (1–4 mg 4 hourly). *Temazepam* (20 mg) is shorter acting and used for insomnia. In the USA, *alprazolam* (250 μg tds) is widely used for panic disorder.

● *Side-effects.* Drowsiness, 'hangover effects', headache, nausea, ataxia, dysarthria and delirium. Occasionally, disinhibition or aggression. Should not normally be prescribed for longer than 4 weeks, to prevent dependency. Withdrawal symptoms include rebound anxiety, insomnia, visual and auditory hallucinations and seizures. This is managed by switching from short-acting benzodiazepines to diazepam, and by tapering dose over several weeks or longer.

● *Overdose.* Very rarely fatal in healthy people. *Flumazenil* can be used to acutely reverse the effects.

● *Cautions and contraindications.* The sedative effect may interfere with driving ability, especially if combined with alcohol.

Other anxiolytics

● *Propranolol* reduces the somatic symptoms of anxiety (tachycardia, tremor) but has a limited role. Avoid in asthmatics as it can cause bronchospasm.

● *Buspirone* is a non-sedating anxiolytic, used in generalized anxiety disorder. It is said not to be addictive, and takes several days to work.

● Chloral hydrate is a hypnotic frequently used in the elderly.

● The 'z-drugs' (*zolpidem, zopiclone* and *zaleplon*) are newer hypnotics, claimed to produce fewer hangover effects and less tolerance than the benzodiazepines, although the evidence for this is limited.

● Low-dose TCAs also have anxiolytic and hypnotic effects—e.g. *amitriptyline* (25 mg) or *trazodone* (50 mg) and are not addictive.

Antipsychotics

Antipsychotics (also called *neuroleptics* or *major tranquilizers*) are the mainstay of treatment for schizophrenia and all other psychoses.

● Antipsychotics have a range of chemical structures—a common if tedious exam question (Table 7.6).

A more important classification is into two main groups: the older, *conventional* (typical) antipsychotics, and the newer *atypical* ones (Box 7.3). There are differences between them (see below) but the fundamental properties are the same for all antipsychotics:

● All antipsychotics work primarily by blocking D2 dopamine receptors. This reverses the excessive dopamine activity in the mesolimbic system that is

Table 7.6 Chemical structures of antipsychotics.

Chemical class	Example
Phenothiazines	
Aliphatic side chain	Chlorpromazine
Piperazine side chain	Fluphenazine
Thioxanthines	Flupenthixol
Butyrophenones	Haloperidol
Dibenzodiazepines	Clozapine, olanzapine
Benzisoxazoles	Risperidone
Substituted benzamides	Amisulpride

Box 7.3 Conventional and atypical antipsychotics

The term 'atypical' was applied to *clozapine* (see below), the first antipsychotic that did not produce extrapyramidal side-effects (EPS). This is the correct usage of the term: an antipsychotic that does not produce EPS at clinical doses. Since clozapine, many other antipsychotics have been marketed as atypical. However, the terminology is confusing because:

● Atypical is sometimes wrongly thought to imply greater efficacy, because clozapine also proved to be more effective than other antipsychotics. This property is not shared by other atypical antipsychotics.

● Atypicality is a spectrum, with clozapine at one end and haloperidol at the other; many antipsychotics are in the middle (e.g. sulpiride). This means that the distinction is blurred—bear this in mind when reading this section.

● Several mechanisms have been proposed to explain 'atypicality'. One is that the drugs block D2 receptors only intermittently; another is that they also block 5-HT2 receptors.

thought to cause the symptoms of psychosis. D2 receptor blockade also contributes, along with antagonism at other receptors, to their side-effects.

• Antipsychotics are effective against positive psychotic symptoms, i.e. delusions, hallucinations and thought disorder, regardless of diagnosis, in about 70% of patients within 6 weeks. *Clozapine* is the only antipsychotic with a greater efficacy (see below). Their onset of action is gradual, over 1–2 weeks. Antipsychotics are also used in prevention of relapse of psychosis, in delirium, and in severe depression.

• There are several serious side-effects (see below). Knowing how and when to explain the potential side-effects is difficult if a patient is acutely psychotic. It should be done properly as soon as the mental state permits.

• Avoid the use of high doses (above recommended limits), either for non-response or to produce sedation. There is no evidence of greater efficacy and good evidence of harm.

Side-effects of conventional antipsychotics

These are many and serious (Table 7.7). Their prevalence and severity vary from one drug to another, depending on their pharmacological profile. The main features of two widely used conventional antipsychotics, *haloperidol* and *chlorpromazine*, are summarized in Table 7.8.

Extrapyramidal side-effects (EPS) are a major problem. EPS are motor abnormalities related to the dopaminergic receptor blockade in the basal ganglia. There are four types:

• *Acute dystonia*—painful contractions of muscles in the neck, jaw or eyes. Young men given high doses are particularly vulnerable. Onset is within hours or days. They are treated with intramuscular or intravenous anticholinergic agents.

• *Parkinsonism*—decreased facial movements, shuffling gait, stiffness and sometimes tremor. Common in early weeks of treatment. Managed by

Table 7.7 Side-effects of conventional antipsychotics.

Side-effects	Comments
Common	
Extrapyramidal (EPS)	See text; due to D2 receptor blockade in basal ganglia
Acute dystonia	
Parkinsonism	
Akathisia	
Tardive dyskinesia	
Hyperprolactinaemia	Due to D2 receptor block in the pituitary; may lead to osteoporosis in women
Galactorrhoea	
Amenorrhoea	
Sexual dysfunction	
Anticholinergic	As for TCAs; see Table 7.5
Antiadrenergic	As for TCAs; see Table 7.5
Weight gain	Due to histamine H1 or 5-HT2C receptor blockade
Rare or idiosyncratic	
Neuroleptic malignant syndrome	Dangerous; see text
Photosensitivity	Especially chlorpromazine
Cholestatic jaundice	Especially chlorpromazine
Retinal pigmentation	
Blood dyscrasias	
Seizures	
Tachyarrythmias	
Hypothermia	

Table 7.8 Side-effect profiles of selected antipsychotics.

	Typical dose (mg/day)	EPS	Prolactin elevation	Anticholinergic side-effects	Sedation	Weight gain
Conventional						
Haloperidol	2–12	+++	+++	+	+	–
Chlorpromazine	50–400	++	++	++	++	++
Atypical						
Risperidone	2–8	+	++	–	–	++
Olanzapine	5–20	–	–	–	+++	+++
Clozapine	300–900	–	–	+	+++	+++

reducing the dose or temporarily adding an anti-cholinergic. Easily mistaken for depression or negative symptoms in schizophrenia.

- *Akathisia*—a feeling of restlessness and a need to walk around. It is very unpleasant and occurs in the first months of treatment. May be mistaken for psychotic behaviour. Treat by lowering the dose or temporarily giving propranolol.
- *Tardive dyskinesia (TD)*—uncontrollable grimacing movements of face, tongue or upper body. This is both distressing and disabling. TD occurs in 20% of patients taking antipsychotics for 2 years. There is no way of predicting who will develop it. Neither is there any reliable treatment, and it can be irreversible. Vitamin E is ineffective.

Two other rare but life-threatening adverse effects to note are:

- *Neuroleptic malignant syndrome* (NMS). The features are pyrexia, stiffness, autonomic instability and seizures leading to coma. The incidence is about 1 in 500. It is fatal in about 10% of cases and requires urgent medical care. Stop antipsychotics temporarily if a fever develops without a clear cause. NMS can occur with any antipsychotic, especially the high-potency ones (e.g. haloperidol). After an episode of NMS, restart treatment gradually, using an atypical antipsychotic, and with careful monitoring.
- Prolongation of the QTc interval on the ECG, which predisposes to a serious arrhythmia called *torsade de pointes*, has been associated with some antipsychotics. It may explain the low but increased incidence of sudden death reportedly associated with antipsychotics.

Table 7.9 Atypical compared to conventional antipsychotics.

Advantages of atypical antipsychotics
  Fewer EPS (definite)
  Greater overall tolerability (probable)
  Lower risk of tardive dyskinesia (probable)
  More efficacy against cognitive symptoms (possible)
  More efficacy against depressive symptoms (possible)

Disadvantages of atypical antipsychotics
  Weight gain more likely (probable)
  Type II diabetes mellitus more likely (possible)
  Stroke more likely in the elderly (possible)
  No long-acting (depot) preparations, except risperidone

Specific advantages of clozapine
  Efficacy in treatment-resistant schizophrenia (definite)
  Reduced risk of suicide in schizophrenia (probable)

Specific disadvantages of clozapine
  Risk of agranulocytosis (definite)
  Need for regular blood tests (definite)

Atypical antipsychotics

Atypical antipsychotics are increasingly used as first-line agents instead of the conventional drugs because of several probable advantages (Table 7.9). A range of atypical antipsychotics is now available. Side-effect profiles that differentiate three of them are shown in Table 7.8.

- *Risperidone* has the best long-term evidence for efficacy and, unlike other atypical antipsychotics, is available as a depot injection.

- *Olanzapine* has the next largest body of evidence for its effectiveness; its sedative effects can be useful.
- *Amisulpride* may have some efficacy against negative symptoms.
- *Aripiprazole* is the latest atypical antipsychotic. It is claimed to have a different mode of action, as a dopamine partial agonist. This means it 'stabilizes' dopamine—antagonizing it when levels are high and mimicking it when dopamine is low. It is not yet clear whether this translates into tangible clinical benefits.

However, atypical antipsychotics also have potential disadvantages (Table 7.9):

- *Weight gain.* This varies between drugs, and also occurs with typical antipsychotics. Clozapine and olanzapine are the worst culprits, with mean weight gains of about 5 kg over 6 months. A genetic polymorphism in the 5-HT2C receptor may contribute to individual vulnerability to weight gain.
- *Type II diabetes.* There is an increased incidence of type II diabetes in patients with schizophrenia, and their relatives, and in people taking antipsychotics. It is unclear how much of the excess is caused by medication, and if so, whether one drug is worse than another. Practice guidelines on this issue are awaited; we suggest a random blood glucose and questioning about diabetic symptoms should be done before starting antipsychotic treatment, and 6 monthly thereafter.
- *Stroke.* Atypical antipsychotics should not be used in dementia because of some evidence that they increase the risk of stroke (Chapter 13). Caution should also be applied in all elderly patients.

Clozapine

Clozapine is a unique antipsychotic, being effective in 30% of patients with schizophrenia resistant to, or intolerant of, all other antipsychotics. It may also reduce suicide risk in schizophrenia.

- It is not clear how clozapine achieves its greater efficacy. It may block dopamine receptors in a different way, or it may be the particular combination of additional receptors that it blocks.
- Clozapine does not have clearly greater efficacy against negative or cognitive symptoms.

Unfortunately, clozapine causes agranulocytosis. Although rare (1–2%), it means that:

- Clozapine is reserved for patients with schizophrenia who have not responded to, or are intolerant of, at least two other antipsychotics.
- Regular (weekly) blood tests are mandatory to monitor the white cell count, and patients must be registered with a monitoring service. This means the drug often needs to be (temporarily) stopped if white cell count falls; it also makes the drug expensive.

Other important side-effects of clozapine are weight gain, hypersalivation and sedation. Seizures can occur at high dose. Plasma levels can be monitored.

Anticholinergics

These drugs are used to counteract EPS resulting from the use of antipsychotics.

- *Mode of action.* Block muscarinic receptors. Their use may seem paradoxical given that other side-effects of antipsychotics are attributed to the same action (Table 7.5). The rationale is that they restore a dopaminergic–cholinergic balance in the basal ganglia.
- *Practical usage. Procyclidine.* Can also be given parenterally to reverse acute dystonias.
- *Side-effects.* Can exacerbate psychosis and cause delirium, memory impairment and euphoria. The anticholinergic side-effects of the antipsychotic may be worsened.
- *Cautions and contraindications.* Prophylactic and long-term use, though widespread, should be avoided for three reasons: (1) the efficacy of antipsychotics is maximal at a dose below that at which EPS occur, so reducing the dose is the logical response to these side-effects; (2) the long-term use of anticholinergics may increase the risk of tardive dyskinesia; and (3) anticholinergics may be misused because of the euphoric effect.

Drugs for dementia

Several drugs are now licensed to treat Alzheimer's disease (Chapter 13). They have a small beneficial effect on cognition in the short to medium term, but do not modify the course of the disease.

Cholinesterase inhibitors

Acetylcholinesterase inhibitors (e.g. donepezil, rivastigmine, galantamine) are used in the treatment of mild to moderate Alzheimer's disease.

- *Mode of action.* Inhibit the synaptic breakdown of acetylcholine, which is decreased in Alzheimer's disease and necessary for memory and cognitive functioning. Galantamine also stimulates nicotinic cholinergic receptors.
- *Practical usage.* Limited to specialist clinics and requires formal assessments before and during treatment, including tests of cognitive, global and behavioural functioning, and activities of daily living.
- *Side-effects.* Anorexia, nausea, vomiting and diarrhoea can occur.

N-methyl-D-aspartate (NMDA) receptor antagonists

Memantine is licensed for moderate and severe Alzheimer's disease.

- *Mode of action.* Memantine blocks the effects of glutamate at the NMDA receptor, decreasing the potential neurotoxic effects of increased glutamate that may occur in Alzheimer's disease.
- *Practical usage.* As for cholinesterase inhibitors.
- *Side-effects.* Usually well-tolerated but may cause dizziness, headache and hallucinations.

Drugs for substance dependence

Drugs are available to help withdrawal, maintain abstinence or control intake of various substances. The beneficial effect of these drugs is relatively modest.

Alcohol dependence

Disulfiram (Antabuse):

- *Mode of action.* Interferes with alcohol metabo-

lism by blocking one of the enzymes involved. If alcohol is consumed, acetaldehyde accumulates leading to flushing, headache, choking sensations, rapid pulse and anxiety.

- *Uses.* As a deterrent to drinking alcohol in people motivated to use the drug.
- *Practical usage.* Usually employed in specialist practice in combination with non-drug treatments.
- *Side-effects.* Sedation and nausea.
- *Cautions and contraindications.* Avoid in heart disease, suicide risk, psychosis or severe liver disease.

Acamprosate:

- *Mode of action.* Unknown, probably acts via GABA and glutamate receptors.
- *Uses.* Used to reduce craving in abstinent patients.
- *Practical usage.* Used in specialist practice, in combination with other non-drug treatments.
- *Side-effects.* Diarrhoea, nausea.

Opiate dependence

Opiate agonists:

- *Mode of action. Methadone* is an opiate agonist and an effective substitute for other opiates such as heroin. *Buprenorphine* is a partial agonist, effective in patients with moderate dependence, but which may precipitate withdrawal in patients with severe dependence.
- *Uses.* To reduce craving and withdrawal symptoms.
- *Practical usage.* Used by specialists in combination with other medical and psychological treatments.
- *Side-effects.* Drowsiness, nausea and vomiting, constipation, respiratory depression.
- *Cautions and contraindications.* Acute respiratory depression or raised intracranial pressure.

Opiate antagonists:

- *Mode of action. Naltrexone* blocks the effects of opiates and precipitates withdrawal symptoms.
- *Uses.* To block the effect of opiates in patients after withdrawal.
- *Practical usage.* Used only in specialist clinics at a usual dose of 50 mg daily.
- *Side-effects.* Nausea and vomiting.

• *Cautions and contraindications.* Do not use in patients currently dependent on opiates or with acute hepatitis or liver failure.

Prescribing in specific groups

Special care is needed when prescribing for patients who are pregnant, breastfeeding, children or elderly. Many drugs are not approved for use in these groups, but nevertheless are widely used. As a rule:

• Choose a well-established drug.
• Consult the British National Formulary first.
• Review the need for, and contraindications to, every drug.
• Ensure patient (or carer) is aware of possible side-effects.
• Monitor closely. If in doubt, stop drug and review.

Pregnancy

Strike a balance between the wish to avoid all drugs for the sake of the foetus, and the potential adverse effects on mother (and foetus) of leaving the psychiatric disorder untreated. Few drugs are established as completely safe in pregnancy or when breast feeding, so use all drugs cautiously and ensure that the mother is fully aware of the known risks and benefits, and also the uncertainties.

• *Antidepressants.* TCAs and SSRIs (and ECT) are not contraindicated. There is no good evidence of increased obstetric complications, or impaired development, but the use of TCA near term may result in a 'twitchy' baby. The dose requirement increases in the third trimester. There is most evidence for the safety of amitriptyline and fluoxetine.
• *Mood stabilizers.* As a rule, avoid lithium and valproic acid, especially around conception and first trimester, due to a small but clear teratogenicity risk. Use of lithium near term may result in neonatal hypothyroidism.
• *Anxiolytics and hypnotics.* These are best avoided.
• *Antipsychotics.* EPS may occur in the baby if these are taken near term.

Breast feeding

Most drugs are excreted into the breast milk. Therefore weigh up the need for medication against the mothers wishes to breast feed and the risks of doing so. As in pregnancy, always proceed with caution and seek expert advice.

• *Antidepressants.* TCAs (especially amitriptyline, imipramine) and SSRIs are probably safe. MAOIs are not recommended.
• *Mood stabilizers.* If lithium is used the baby should be monitored. Carbamazepine, valproate and lamotrigine are probably safe.
• *Anxiolytics and hypnotics.* Avoid benzodiazepines as they can make the baby lethargic and cause failure to thrive.
• *Antipsychotics.* These can sedate the baby and are not recommended.

Children

The prescribing of psychotropic drugs for children is best left to child psychiatrists. See Chapter 16.

The elderly

In general, prescribe at lower doses or increased intervals to compensate for the slower metabolism and excretion in the elderly. Always consider medication as a cause of delirium.

• *Antidepressants.* TCAs may cause delirium (due to their anticholinergic effects) and falls (due to postural hypotension). SSRIs are therefore preferable if sedation is not needed.
• *Mood stabilizers.* These are not contraindicated.
• *Antipsychotics.* Avoid atypical antipsychotics in dementia, and caution with other antipsychotics.
• *Anxiolytics and hypnotics.* Notorious for causing delirium and falls. Avoid.

Other biological treatments

Electroconvulsive therapy (ECT)

ECT is an effective and safe treatment for severe depression. Its bad press reflects understandable fears, misinformation and its past misuse. Current guidelines are intended to ensure its use is limited, and made as safe, effective and acceptable as possible.

- *Mode of action.* Unknown. ECT has many effects in the brain. It may act on monoamines, producing the same result as antidepressants.
- *Clinical indications.* ECT is mainly used for, and has the best evidence of effectiveness in, severe depression including depressive stupor and depressive psychosis. The response is often better than drug therapy and may be dramatic. It is also used for puerperal psychosis and treatment-resistant depression and mania.
- *Practical usage.* Obtain informed consent, or use the Mental Health Act. Always do a physical examination, and obtain an ECG and routine blood tests first. During a brief general anaesthetic with muscle relaxant, an electric charge (~300 mC) is passed across the head to produce a generalized seizure of 30–60 seconds. Treatment can be bilateral, with one electrode on each temple, or unilateral into the non-dominant hemisphere. Bilateral ECT is slightly more effective but causes more short-term memory impairment. ECT is usually given twice a week for 6–12 treatments. A good response is predicted by a greater severity of depression and a past response to ECT.
- *Side-effects.* Anaesthetic effects—nausea, dry mouth, headache. Memory loss for the hours surrounding the seizure. Significant long-term memory loss is sometimes reported by patients; objectively, subtle deficits in recall of personal memories may occur (but it is unclear if this is due to ECT or to the depressive disorder). Nonetheless, it should be discussed when obtaining consent. No neuropathological effects of ECT have been found, even following multiple treatments.
- *Cautions and contraindications.* Few, and mainly related to anaesthetic risk. Avoid if the patient has a suspected intracranial lesion (as intracranial pressure rises during seizure). ECT can be given in conjunction with antidepressants and antipsychotics. ECT is extremely safe, with a mortality rate of 5 per 100 000 treatments.

Psychosurgery

In the 1940s and 1950s—prior to the introduction of antidepressants and antipsychotics—thousands of patients each year were operated on to sever pathways between frontal lobes and limbic structures. Psychosurgery is still used very occasionally for intractable obsessive–compulsive disorder and depressive disorder, but only after wide consultations under the Mental Health Act and never without informed consent. Modern stereotactic procedures avoid most of the earlier complications (haemorrhage, seizures and death).

- Recent case series suggest worthwhile improvement in a third of patients—at the expense of some frontal lobe impairment and with continuing ethical concerns about the principle.

Psychological treatments (the psychotherapies)

All medical treatments take place in the context of a therapeutic relationship between doctor and patient. This interaction is a major determinant both of the patient's satisfaction with the consultation, and of their subsequent adherence to treatment recommendations. 'Psychotherapy' in a generic sense is consequently a part of all medical practice, whether the doctor realizes it or not. However, the term is normally used to apply to a range of *specific* psychological treatments, the main ones being *psychodynamic psychotherapy*, *behaviour therapy* and *cognitive therapy*. Here, we first consider the factors common to all psychotherapies, and then describe the characteristics of each one.

- Box 7.4 is a historical note on the position of psychotherapy in medicine.

Factors common to all psychotherapies

All psychotherapy is based on a number of general or *non-specific* factors:

- The therapist is empathic and interested, and both listens and talks.
- The structure and boundaries of therapy are established (e.g. time, place, content).
- A therapeutic relationship is formed.

Box 7.4 Psychotherapy in medicine

Before there were effective treatments for most diseases, physicians paid great attention to the psychological aspects of the medical consultation. Accounts of medical practice in the late 1800s clearly describe psychological methods as an integral part of medicine, including listening carefully to the patient's account of their suffering, instilling hope and encouraging patients toward a graded return to activity. At this time, psychotherapy as a specialist treatment also began, attributed to Freud with *psychoanalysis* (*psychodynamic psychotherapy*), and later with *behaviour therapy* and *cognitive therapy* (Table 7.1). Each was based upon a psychological theory and each is in use in psychiatry today. However, despite the good evidence for efficacy of several psychotherapies in various disorders, in general, there has been a neglect of psychological aspects of medicine as compared to our Victorian predecessors. Now, as patients become interested in holistic care and more concerned about the limitations of physical treatments, there is a renewed focus on psychological aspects of all illnesses, and attempts to introduce effective psychotherapies into all medical settings (Chapter 18)

- The therapeutic effect takes time, and requires effort by the patient.
- An explanation for the specific form of treatment is given.
- There is an expectation that the person's problems can improve.

Successful psychotherapy

Successful psychotherapy, of any type, requires attention to several practical issues.
- *Select the right psychotherapy for the right patient.* Take account of the features predictive of good outcome to psychological treatment in general: being motivated, articulate, able to tolerate emotional arousal, and successful in some areas of life, as well as the indications, and contraindications for each specific therapy.
- *Prepare the patient for therapy.* Many people have either no idea, or the wrong idea, of what psychotherapy involves. Ensuring a patient knows what to expect and what will be required helps avoid inappropriate referrals and weeds out those unlikely to stay the distance.

- *Ensure the therapy is available.* Many psychotherapies are not widely available, or have a long waiting list. During this time, the referring doctor should offer continuing support or use the time for a trial of medication.

Evidence-based psychotherapy

Psychotherapies have been less well evaluated than drugs, due to the practical difficulties of doing so, and the absence of pharmaceutical funding. However, there is good quality evidence for several specific psychotherapies, especially cognitive and behaviour therapies, in several disorders, as outlined below.

Adverse effects of psychotherapy

Like all medical treatment, psychotherapy can have adverse effects. These are more likely with poorly trained therapists, or therapists in a position to deliberately exploit the patient.
- Even well delivered therapy can be ineffective or harmful. An example is early debriefing for people who have suffered a trauma (p. 106).

The main psychotherapies

The major psychotherapies can, just about, be divided into two classes: either they are descendants of psychoanalysis (i.e. psychodynamic psychotherapy), or they are based upon behavioural and cognitive theories. The key differences are highlighted in Table 7.10.

Psychodynamic psychotherapy

With the arrival of the more evidence-based (and more widely available) psychotherapies outlined below, psychodynamic psychotherapy now has a lesser role, and its provision on the NHS is very limited. Nevertheless it remains important to know about its principles and its contemporary indications. Several psychodynamic concepts also remain useful throughout medicine (Box 7.5).

The principles of psychodynamic psychotherapy are:

Table 7.10 Comparison of the two major classes of psychotherapy.

	Psychodynamic psychotherapy	Other psychotherapies
Examples	Psychoanalysis	Behavioural therapy
	Psychodynamic therapy	Cognitive therapy
Focus	Unconscious phenomena	Observable phenomena and behaviour
Time focus	The past (as evidenced in the present)	The present
Aim	Insight and self-understanding, thence altered interpersonal behaviour	Direct, practice-driven change in behaviour and/or cognitions
Practical issues	Therapist listens and interprets	Therapist explains
	Sessions unstructured	Sessions highly structured
Therapist	Extensive training (years)	Briefer training (months)
	Usually psychiatrists	Psychologists, psychiatrists, nurses
	Key is therapist's skills and attributes	Key is adherence to treatment manual
Duration	Unspecified, can be prolonged (years)	Agreed number of sessions (e.g. 8)
Efficacy	Unknown	Proven
Main indications	Difficulties with relationships	Depressive disorder
	Some personality disorders	Neuroses
		Eating disorders

Box 7.5 Psychodynamic concepts of continuing value

- *Transference.* The feelings and attitudes a patient develops for their therapist. They represent emotions transferred to the therapist from the person to whom they were originally attached (usually a parent). Consider transference during any doctor–patient relationship if a patient starts to behave in an unexpected or unusual way (e.g. inappropriate signs of affection, or threatening self-harm if an extra appointment is not given).
- *Counter-transference.* The feelings a patient produces in the therapist (e.g. excessive involvement, attraction or dislike). Counter-transference is influenced by the therapist's own past experiences and relationships, but also gives clues to unconscious processes in the patient. More generally, it is valuable for all doctors to be aware of the emotions evoked by patients, to try and understand their origins, and ensure they do not affect their ability to treat the patient effectively.
- *Psychological defence mechanisms* (Table 6.2).

- Emotional and interpersonal problems result from *unconscious* processes, driven by psychological mechanisms and internal representations (of people and things) developed earlier in life.
- These processes can be revealed and resolved by gaining access to the unconscious mind. The therapist can do this in various ways (e.g. free association, hypnosis, dream analysis).
- The therapist is particularly interested in the patient's pattern of relationships, evidenced most directly by the way the patient interacts with the therapist (*transference*; Box 7.5).
- The therapist makes *interpretations* about what the patient says, and draws connections between events and feelings that he conveys to the patient.
- During therapy, the patient is expected to *gain insight* into their emotions and behaviour as a result of the interpretations.
- The therapeutic effect may emerge directly from the self-understanding, and be promoted (reinforced) by new patterns of behaviour and relating which arise from it.

Psychodynamic therapy is now used mainly for 'personality difficulties', especially recurrent problems with relationships. It also has a role in chronic neuroses and depressive disorders resistant to other drug and psychological treatments. It should be avoided in paranoid or dyssocial personality disorder, and psychosis.

- *Brief psychodynamic psychotherapy* compresses a psychodynamically-oriented therapy to a more feasible 10–20 sessions. The therapist takes a more active role than in traditional psychoanalysis and focuses on particular issues. There is evidence for efficacy in depression.

Behaviour therapy

Behaviour therapy arose from the behavioural theories of experimental psychology (p. 52). It is effective in anxiety disorders (especially phobias and obsessive–compulsive disorder) and in learning disability. The central idea is that adaptive behaviours can be learned and maladaptive behaviours unlearned. In turn, good behaviour leads to good feelings.

Exposure is a key component of treatment. Either the patient is reintroduced (re-exposed) to a situation or behaviour he has come to avoid (e.g. an agoraphobic leaving the house), or he learns to stop an inappropriate, excessive response (e.g. recurrent hand washing in OCD). Exposure is usually graded (*graded exposure*).
- Sudden and prolonged exposure (*flooding*) — such as shutting a claustrophobic in a lift until the panic subsides — also works, but is too unpleasant for routine use.

The elements of graded exposure are:
- The therapist assesses the problem behaviour, its antecedents and consequences. He explains the nature of the treatment and its rationale to the patient.
- A step-by-step programme is developed jointly with the patient. Homework tasks are set which re-expose the patient to the situation to a degree that produces a tolerable level of anxiety. The patient finds that each extra exposure increases anxiety, but that it then subsides. In this way the patient is *desensitized* to the stimulus.
- Subsequent sessions review progress and problems, and set the next series of tasks.

*Mr Q had not been out of his house for 2 years, fearful he might faint in the street. His therapist elicited a detailed account of the problem, how it started, and its effect on Mr Q. She explained what behavioural treatment was and expressed optimism. They agreed a plan for Mr Q to do a task he felt he could just manage: to walk to his front gate and stand there briefly. He felt anxious doing so, but achieved this goal sev-*eral times in homework sessions. He moved to the next steps: remaining there longer, then walking increasing distances. He was able to do the shopping, which reinforced his feeling of success. During the agreed 12 sessions he made steady progress, maintained thereafter.*

Many other treatments and techniques are also based on the premise that changing behaviour and other bodily functions such as muscular tone and posture, helps mental well-being. They include *relaxation training, assertiveness training, biofeedback* and *social skills training*. They are available in occupational therapy and physiotherapy departments, by private therapists, and from self-help manuals.

Cognitive therapy

The aim of cognitive therapy is to correct inaccurate or unhelpful ways of thinking, usually in order to improve mood or reduce anxiety. The main components are:
- The therapist obtains a detailed description of the problem, paying particular attention to the thoughts (cognitions) and interpretations that have generated or are exacerbating the problem.
- The therapist formulates the problem in a way that makes sense to the patient.
- The patient is taught how to challenge negative and inaccurate ways of thinking which are maintaining the problem, and to practise thinking in more accurate and helpful ways.
- Therapeutic techniques include education about the role of cognitions and their consequences; confirming the occurrence of particular thoughts and inferences using diaries; and simulation of events during the session. Patients are encouraged to do 'experiments' to test their beliefs and behaviour against alternatives.
- The patients applies these techniques when the problem symptoms occur or recur (*self-monitoring*).

Ms R had a depressive disorder. Her therapist helped her identify a number of negative thoughts such as 'Nobody likes me', 'I won't do things as I keep making mistakes' and 'There's no point trying to change anything, it won't help'. The therapist formulated the depression as being maintained by the effect of this thinking on her mood and behaviour. He helped Ms R become aware of the distorted and negative slant of her thoughts and explained their possible origins and self-defeating consequences. They role-played alternatives and she practised challenging the thoughts and replacing them with positive ones. She became skilled at doing this. Her depressive thoughts and symptoms improved. At follow up a year later she remained well, and was using the techniques whenever she felt negative cognitions or low mood creeping back.

Cognitive behavioural therapy (CBT)

In practice, cognitive and behavioural treatments are usually combined as *cognitive behavioural therapy (CBT)*. In phobic anxiety, for example, this would involve both graded exposure and intervention at the underlying thoughts and beliefs.

There is good evidence for the efficacy of CBT (with varying proportions of C and B) in several disorders:
• In mild to moderate depressive disorder, CBT is at least as effective as antidepressants.
• In panic disorder and phobic anxiety, CBT is probably the most effective treatment; benefits are more persistent than with anxiolytics, and avoid the problems of the latter.
• There is good evidence of efficacy in other neuroses, including somatoform disorders and obsessive–compulsive disorder.
• CBT is the most effective treatment in bulimia nervosa.
• CBT has some effect against psychotic symptoms in schizophrenia.

Other psychotherapies

Hybrid therapies

The distinction between the two types of therapy in Table 7.10 is, in reality, over-simplified and blurred. There are several hybrid therapies (Figure 7.2), and other therapies that have additional components. None is widely available in the UK.
• *Cognitive analytical therapy* (CAT) uses a cognitive approach to analyse earlier events and their influence on current feelings and behaviours. It is used in depression and other conditions.
• *Interpersonal therapy* (IPT) uses cognitive, behavioural and psychodynamic concepts and techniques to focus on the patient's relationships and the problems arising from them. Limited evidence suggests similar efficacy to CBT in depression and bulimia nervosa.
• *Dialectical behaviour therapy* (DBT), developed specifically for borderline personality disorder. It combines psychoeducation with behavioural skills training.
• *Eye movement desensitization and reprocessing* (EMDR), used in post-traumatic stress disorder.

Group therapy

Many of the psychotherapies have been adapted to treat several people at once. *Group therapy* originated from the view that it is therapeutic to share experiences and feelings, and to examine the relationships that form in a group.
• CBT can be given effectively in a group format for the same indications as individual CBT.

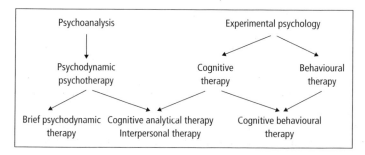

Figure 7.2 Links between the psychotherapies.

- A *therapeutic community* is a form of psychodynamic group therapy where the participants are resident for 6–12 months. It is mainly used in attempts to treat personality disorder.

Family therapy

Family therapy is based upon the theory that the problem is located in the family rather than in the (child) patient. The family 'system' is therefore the therapeutic target. Psychodynamic, behavioural and other concepts are used. There is some evidence for its efficacy in conduct disorder, substance misuse and eating disorders.

Simple psychotherapies

In addition to the 'formal' psychotherapies described above, informal or *simple psychotherapies* are important too. They merge imperceptibly into the therapeutic component of all doctor–patient relationships, as mentioned in Chapter 1 and at the start of this section.
- *Counselling* is a loosely defined activity whereby people are helped to overcome or cope with life's problems. The counsellor serves as a support, a facilitator of emotional expression, a source of information, and as someone off whom ideas can be bounced. Counselling is provided in many settings, mostly non-psychiatric. There is modest evidence for it effectiveness in mild neuroses and stress-related disorders.
- *Problem solving therapy* is a structured mix of counselling and CBT. It helps the patient learn to deal with life's problems—by specifying them, selecting an option for tackling each one, trying out solutions, and reviewing the effect. It is effective in mild neurotic and depressive disorders and can be given effectively by GPs and nurse practitioners in primary care.
- *Supportive psychotherapy* describes the supportive element of a therapist–patient relationship. All health professionals—as well as relatives and friends—provide supportive psychotherapy whether they realize it or not. It does not aim to produce change, but to help people cope with adversity or insoluble problems over a sustained period—in part by maintaining of a sense of hope and a focus on achievable goals, however modest.

Social treatments

Social factors have major roles in the aetiology and maintenance of psychiatric disorders (p. 49). Social factors also determine the environment in which therapy is given and affect its outcome. Equally, social treatments—intervening to change some aspect of the person's circumstances—are themselves important therapeutic interventions.

Acute social interventions

Psychiatric admission is a major social intervention. It may relieve a crisis at home which is exacerbating the psychiatric disorder, or represent the best means of ensuring a homeless person gets a decent assessment.

Crisis intervention also involves practical things like finding temporary accommodation, helping get emergency benefits, or daily home visits. Crisis intervention services are currently being introduced, in part to reduce acute admissions.

Social interventions during psychiatric care

Practical social interventions are needed at some stage in most patients' care.
- Accommodation and financial problems are common. Help with housing, rescheduling debts, etc., etc., are therapeutic by reducing stressors maintaining the disorder. Involvement of the patient in these processes can itself be therapeutic by giving them a sense of mastery over circumstances and improving practical social skills.
- Family support and education is an important part of the overall social package of care, even if specific family therapy is not being carried out.
- Isolation is often a problem. This can be addressed by home visits, attendance at day centres, putting the person in touch with self-help groups, etc.
- In chronic psychiatric disorder, social and occupational skills and self-confidence are often

damaged. *Rehabilitation* involves continuing support of the kinds outline above, as well as more extensive interventions such as sheltered accommodation and supported employment.

The wider social environment

Preventing domestic violence, child abuse and unemployment would no doubt improve the psychological well-being of the population. Whilst such utopian ('primary prevention') goals are not relevant for the management of individual patients, there are measures that can affect their prevalence or impact:

• *Public education.* To increase awareness of psychiatric disorders, and decrease the stigma attached to them and to their treatment.

• *Social policy.* Political decisions alter the social fabric and influence behaviours associated with psychiatric disorder. For example, taxation affects alcohol consumption and legislation determines the extent of compulsory treatment. Some events are, however, beyond control — e.g. the effect of national soccer results on deliberate self-harm rates.

Compulsory treatment

The nature of psychiatric disorders means that some people refuse help, even though to do so puts their health or that of others at risk. Psychiatrists in most countries thus sometimes treat people against their will.

• There is continuing debate about balancing the benefits of treatment against infringement of civil liberties.

Common law

Treatment without informed consent is technically an assault. However, in an emergency, a doctor may treat a patient without consent if rapid action is called for to save life – e.g. to maintain an airway in a comatose patient or to sedate an uncontrollably delirious patient. Such actions are carried out under the 'common law'.

• The limits of what can and should be done under common law are governed by the principle of doing what the public would consider reasonable (or where failing to act would be considered unreasonable). When in doubt, take advice from a senior colleague or your defence organization.

Mental Health Act (1983)

Apart from these specific emergencies, compulsory psychiatric treatment in England and Wales is carried out under sections of the 1983 Mental Health Act (Box 7.6 and Table 7.11).

• All doctors need to know about Section 5(2).
• General practitioners are involved in most Sections.

Box 7.6 Key aspects of the Mental Health Act (1983)

• The person must have refused voluntary treatment.
• The person must be at acute, significant risk of self-harm, self-neglect, or harming others.
• The behaviour must be the result of a known or suspected psychiatric disorder. Disruptive behaviour, intoxication, drug abuse, etc. are not of themselves grounds for detention.
• For Sections lasting a month or less, a loose definition of psychiatric disorder is adopted. For the longer lasting Sections, one of the following categories must apply: *mental illness* (not actually defined in the Act), *psychopathic disorder*, or *mental impairment (learning disability)*.
• Implementing most Sections involves an *application* from an Approved Social Worker (ASW) or the nearest relative, and a *medical recommendation* from a psychiatrist (Consultant or Specialist Registrar, approved under *Section 12* of the Act). (Relatives are rarely called upon in practice).
• Detained patients can appeal to hospital managers or to a Mental Health Review tribunal for the Section to be discharged. A Section is discharged by the responsible psychiatrist once the patient's mental state no longer justifies it, and/or when he adheres consistently to treatment.
• The Act only covers treatments for psychiatric disorder. It cannot be used if a patient refuses treatment for a medical problem — such as a stomach washout after an overdose or to set a fracture.

Table 7.11 Key Mental Health Act Sections and their uses.

Situation	Section
Psychiatric admission, for assessment	2
Psychiatric admission, for treatment	3
Psychiatric admission, psychiatrist not available	4
Stopping an in-patient leaving a hospital	5(2)
To allow police to find and take person to a safe place	135
To allow police to take person from public place to safe place	136
Psychiatric assessment or treatment of person on remand	35 and 36
Psychiatric treatment of convicted person	37 and 41

- *A new Mental Health Act for England and Wales is imminent. When it becomes law, most of this section will no longer apply.*

Section 2: Admission for assessment

- *Uses.* Assessment of suspected psychiatric disorder. It would apply, for example, to a man who set fire to his car because he believed it was demonically possessed or to a depressed woman who has tried to kill herself. Drug treatment can be given without consent, but use Section 3 once treatment becomes the main reason for in-patient care.
- *Applied for by*: Approved Social Worker (ASW) in consultation with nearest relative. Medical recommendation from a psychiatrist and another doctor (usually the GP). The ASW must have seen the person within the past 14 days, the doctors within 5 days.
- *Duration*: 28 days.
- *Right of appeal*: In first 14 days.

Section 3: Admission for treatment

- *Uses.* For an established psychiatric disorder (usually schizophrenia) where admission is intended to improve the condition or prevent deterioration.

- *Applied for by*: as for Section 2. Cannot normally proceed if the nearest relative objects.
- *Duration:* 6 months, renewable. Section 3 patients can go on leave for up to a month on a *Section 17*. Before discharge, a *Section 117* meeting is held to discuss future management; there are statutory responsibilities for subsequent care (p. 83).
- *Right of appeal:* One per 6 months. Reviews are instituted anyway if no appeal is made.

Section 4: Admission in an emergency

- *Uses.* For compulsory admission when a psychiatrist is not available and delay would be dangerous. Cannot be used just because it is easier to organize than a Section 2.
- *Applied for by*: ASW or nearest relative. Medical recommendation by any doctor, usually GP.
- *Duration:* 72 hours, during which a full assessment for a Section 2 or 3 is made. No right of appeal.

Section 5(2): Emergency detention of an in-patient

- *Uses.* A '5-2' prevents a patient leaving *any* hospital where to do so would put their health in jeopardy. For example, a patient who is confused postoperatively and tries to run off, drip stand in tow, can be stopped at first under common law but if the attempt to leave persists, a Section 5(2) should be used. A Section 5(2) does not allow treatment to be enforced. (A Section 5(4) is used by psychiatric nurses to detain a psychiatric in-patient for 6 hours if no psychiatrist is to hand).
- *Applied for by*: the responsible consultant or named deputy (not preregistration house officer). In a general hospital, this means the physicians managing the patient, ideally in consultation with a liaison psychiatrist.
- *Duration*: 72 hours, during which a full Mental Health Act assessment is carried out. Once completed, the Section 5 is converted to a Section 2 or 3, or it lapses. No right of appeal.

Table 7.12 Key Scottish Mental Health Care and Treatment Act (2003) Sections.

Situation	Section	Duration	Applicants
Emergency detention	36(1)	72 hours	Registered doctor, plus MHO if available
Nurses holding power	299	2 hours	Registered specialist nurse
Short-term detention	44(1)	28 days	Approved doctor and MHO
Compulsory treatment order	64(4)	6 months	Two doctors, one approved, plus MHO plus approval of mental health review tribunal

Registered doctor = any doctor registered with the General Medical Council.
MHO = Mental Health Officer, a specially trained social worker.
Approved doctor = psychiatrist approved under the Act.

Other sections

- *Section 135* allows the police to enter private property and take a person to a place of safety (usually a hospital) for 72 hours. It is requested by an ASW and granted by a magistrate.
- *Section 136* empowers the police to take someone in a public place who they suspect has a psychiatric disorder (e.g. because of bizarre behaviour) to a safe place (police station, hospital). Lasts for 72 hours.
- *Sections 35–38* are used by a Court to send offenders to hospital for psychiatric assessment or treatment. *Section 47* allows for transfer of a prisoner to hospital.
- ECT may not be given without consent to detained patients, except the first treatment in an emergency. A second opinion must be obtained and *Section 58* completed before the course of ECT proceeds.

Mental Health Act in Scotland

Compulsory treatment is covered by the 1984 Mental Health Act (Scotland), but new legislation, the 'Mental Health Care and Treatment Act (Scotland) 2003' is being phased in (Table 7.12).

Other aspects of the law and psychiatry

Forensic psychiatrists specialize in the law (p. 85), but all psychiatrists find themselves involved with the law from time to time. Not all issues are strictly related to treatment, but they are summarized here for convenience.

- *The law and child psychiatry.* Children under 16 are subject to different laws and conventions. The main legislation is the Children's Act (1989). Consult a child psychiatric team or social services for advice.
- *Writing legal reports.* Psychiatrists may be asked to write a report on a patient who has been charged with an offence, usually to give an opinion as to whether psychiatric factors contributed to the offence or influence how it should be dealt with. They may also be asked to write a report concerning the psychiatric consequences of an accident as part of a compensation claim.
- *Fitness to enter into contracts.* Psychiatric opinion may be sought regarding the person's competence to make a will, get married, etc.
- *Fitness to drive.* Psychiatric disorders and medications can impair driving by affecting judgement or concentration. Psychiatrists should warn patients of this and of their duty to inform the relevant authority. A person may not drive for 6 months after a psychotic episode. People with dementia (even mild cases) have an excess of accidents and should be discouraged from driving.
- *Confidentiality.* There are exceptional circumstances that override the principle of medical confidentiality in psychiatry. For example, if a patient tells you he is going to murder his wife (perhaps because of morbid jealousy; p. 134), or if you suspect a colleague is unfit to practise, you have a duty to act. If unsure, always seek advice and keep notes.

Key points

- Psychiatric disorders are treated with drugs (psychopharmacology) and/or psychological methods (psychotherapy). Social interventions are also important; remember hospital admission is a major social intervention.
- The main classes of drugs are antidepressants, antipsychotics, mood stabilizers, and anxiolytics. The commonest form of psychological treatment in primary care is simple counselling, and in psychiatric services is CBT.

- The choice of treatment depends upon the diagnosis and on other contextual factors, including the patient's preference and treatment availability.
- There is good evidence for the efficacy of most commonly used drugs, but all also have limitations and side-effects. CBT is of proven benefit for several disorders but has limited availability.
- Involve patients fully in treatment decisions.
- A small minority of patients require compulsory treatment under the Mental Health Act.

Chapter 8

Psychiatric services

This chapter covers the main features of how specialist psychiatric services are organized, and how the treatments discussed in Chapter 7 are delivered. However, as introduced in Chapter 1, remember that psychiatrists see only a small and unrepresentative fraction of all psychiatric disorders, and its services are 'biased' accordingly. In particular, the perspective from general practice— where most patients with psychiatric needs are managed—is very different. This important issue is covered in Chapter 18.

Psychiatric specialties

Psychiatric subspecialties are delineated by the patients' age and/or type of disorder:
- General adult psychiatry.
- Psychogeriatrics (psychiatry of old age).
- Child and adolescent psychiatry.
- Liaison psychiatry (psychological medicine).
- Substance abuse.
- Forensic psychiatry.
- Learning disability (Chapter 17).

General adult psychiatry

Adults with psychiatric disorders are looked after by general adult psychiatrists unless their problems come into the domain of another subspecialty, and their care transferred to it. The boundaries are blurred, and depend on local factors. Psychosis re-

mains the focus of most general psychiatry services although they increasingly work in relation to primary care and assist general practitioners in the management of patients with the more common psychiatric disorders.

Trends in service delivery and organization

Over the past 30 years, psychiatric services have progressively moved to the other settings shown in Figure 8.1. The shift of psychiatry to the community has occurred for several reasons:
- The community is where psychiatric disorders present, and provides their context.
- Public preference and social attitudes.
- Long-term in-patient care is rarely necessary and sometimes harmful.
- Economic and political pressures.

Despite these trends, in-patient care remains an important component of psychiatry for several groups:
- Assessment of suspected severe psychiatric disorder.
- Those at significant risk of suicide.
- 'Asylum' for those in crisis.
- Those dangerous to others as a result of psychiatric disorder.
- Treatment of acute schizophrenia, mania and severe depression.
- Longer-term care of some patients with

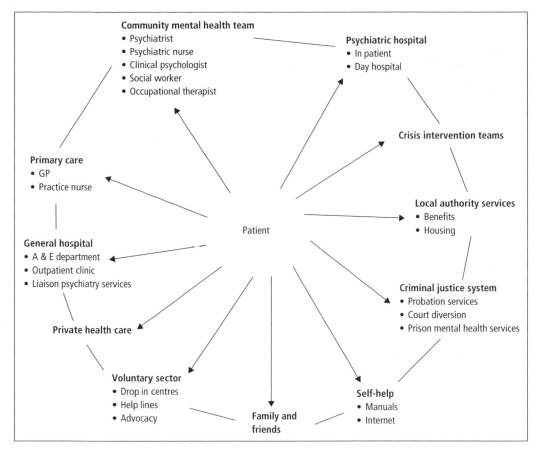

Figure 8.1 Psychiatric services.

dementia, chronic schizophrenia and mental retardation.

As the number of psychiatric hospital beds has fallen, the threshold for admission has risen and an increasing percentage of in-patients are psychotic, disturbed and detained compulsorily. This is especially true in inner cities, and has stimulated efforts to ease the pressure on in-patient facilities. Research suggests that admission can be avoided in approximately 40% of cases by using day hospitals or 'crisis teams'.

• Crisis intervention services are currently being set up in many areas.

Making the move from hospital to community-based care has posed problems and has led to a gap between the intention and reality of community care:

• Hospitals have closed before community services are fully in place.

• Community care is not a cheap option, and has been under-resourced.

• A considerable burden is placed upon relatives.

• It is difficult to provide care for people often most at need—the homeless, those with complex psychiatric and social problems, and those whose illness interferes with treatment adherence.

Community care

Logically, this term should refer to the management of all psychiatric problems outside hospital; numerically this would mainly comprise emotional disorders looked after by GPs. Usually, however, community care means care *within psychiatric services*—patients who tend to be more severely and chronically ill, especially with schizophrenia, severe mood disorder and comorbid conditions.

The main features of contemporary community care in psychiatry are:

• Psychiatric problems are managed at the patient's home, in GP surgeries or in local mental health centres. To facilitate this, the psychiatrists usually divide workload into geographical sectors.

• Care is provided by a community mental health team (CMHT; see below).

• Management includes social interventions as well as drug and psychological treatments.

• Admission is reserved for severe episodes and crises. Transitions between in-patient and community care should be as smooth as possible.

• Most patients are treated with their consent. A few need some form of legal coercion, which will be increased in scope in the UK by forthcoming mental health legislation.

Multidisciplinary teams

As psychiatry has moved to the community, it has also become less medically dominated. Most psychiatrists (except in some subspecialities described below) now work in *multidisciplinary teams*, called *community mental health teams* (CMHTs), as one amongst many mental health professionals. The psychiatrist may or may not be the team 'leader'. The psychiatrist's particular roles in the team generally centre on:

• Making diagnoses.

• Prescribing medication.

• Use of Mental Health Act.

• Taking medicolegal responsibility.

The other members of multidisciplinary teams usually comprise:

• *Community psychiatric nurses* (CPNs). CPNs perform much of the day-to-day psychiatric work of the CMHT. CPNs are often the designated *key worker* (see below), they do many of the initial and follow-up assessments, and they give medication. Some have additional therapeutic skills (e.g. in cognitive therapy) and are called *nurse practitioners*.

• Social services departments have statutory responsibilities affecting psychiatric patients which *social workers* attached to the team fulfil. For example, the social worker takes the lead role in assessing social circumstances and arranging accommodation, helping with benefits, etc. *ASWs* (*Approved Social Workers*) are specialized in psychiatric issues and have a key role in Mental Health Act applications.

• *Secretary/administrator*. Teams generate a lot of paperwork and its members are often out and about. A central person who handles the administration, takes messages and arranges meetings is therefore a key figure.

• *Clinical psychologist*. Many teams have a clinical psychologist, who helps in assessments and in providing psychological treatments.

• *Other team members* may include occupational therapists, accommodation officers, befrienders, etc.

• *Voluntary organizations* and *self-help groups*, though not formally part of the CMHT, provide important additional sources of support and help for many people—including those with needs but who are not receiving formal psychiatric care.

The key worker

Every patient under the care of more than one member of a multidisciplinary team has a *key worker* (the actual term used may vary) who:

• Is usually a CPN or social worker.

• Co-ordinates and administers treatment.

• Knows about local resources and how to access them.

• Liaises with the GP and other agencies.

• Assists in planning and monitoring of the care package, as part of the care programme approach (CPA; see below).

• Informs others of changes in the patient's state or needs.

The care programme approach (CPA)

The way in which adult mental health services are delivered in the community varies between countries—and even within the UK—due to differences in the structure of health and social care services, and the relationship between them. It is also increasingly subject to political policymaking and rapid changes in emphasis and terminology. The following is a brief snapshot of the current situation in England and Wales.

The specified model for community psychiatric care is the *care programme approach* (CPA). The aim of the CPA is to improve and standardize the planning and provision of care for psychiatric patients (although a recent systematic review shows that it offers minimal benefits compared to standard management).

The key aspects of the CPA are:
- It applies to all patients in psychiatric care who are not in hospital.
- It starts with a detailed assessment. This covers psychiatric, medical and social needs, and assessment of risk to self and others.
- The CPA has different levels depending on the complexity and severity of the case. The two extremes are: *Minimal CPA*, for simple cases where input from CMHT will be limited. No special documentation is needed. *Full CPA*, for difficult or severe cases, where several members of the CMHT will be involved and input is likely to be prolonged. CPA forms must be completed and amended regularly.
- A key worker is assigned.
- A *care plan* records the identified needs, how they will be tackled, and by whom. The care plan is drawn up in consultation with the patient and nearest relative. Both get a copy, as do all the professionals involved.
- Progress of the case is monitored by the key worker, who reports regularly back to the CMHT.
- All patients have a right to refuse CPA, unless detained under the Mental Health Act.

Assertive outreach is another form of community care 'package', with smaller caseloads per staff member and more intensive support than the usual CPA. It has not been shown to be superior in the UK.

Ms D is 27 and has been admitted with schizophrenia. At the ward round, Rob, a CPN from the CMHT agrees to be her key worker. Full CPA is implemented. Ms D has been made homeless and unemployed, so Rob liaises with the social worker and sorts out *financial arrangements and accommodation in a group home. After discharge, he visits weekly, giving Ms D her depot and monitoring her mental state. The psychiatrist sees Ms D every 6 months or whenever there is cause for concern. An exacerbation of her illness is managed at home with support and increased medication. Rob begins therapy with Ms D's family, who are supportive but over-involved. However, Ms D relapses and is found wandering the street in a state of neglect. She is detained under Section 3 of the Mental Health Act. When almost ready for discharge, a Section 117 meeting plans her future care.*

Psychiatry of old age (psychogeriatrics)

Most old-age psychiatrists deal with the whole range of psychiatric disorder in the elderly and not just dementia.
- Concurrent physical problems and medications affect presentation and management. For example, constipation is common in the elderly and is therefore a less useful diagnostic sign for depression; it may also produce delirium; it may limit the dose of antidepressant which can be given.
- Psychogeriatric CMHTs have close ties with geriatrics and social services. This is necessary given the prevalence and nature of dementia, and the frequency of associated physical and social problems of the elderly mentally ill.

Mr A is 75 and has become forgetful. A domiciliary visit reveals cognitive impairment and depressive symptoms. He lives with his healthy wife. A trial of antidepressants does not help, and his dementia gets worse. Routine investigations are negative and you diagnose probable Alzheimer's disease. An occupational therapist visits to assess his daily living skills. His wife can care for him with help from 'meals on wheels' and visits from a CPN. You liaise with the GP regarding Mr A's leg ulcers (which make him delirious when infected); the GP prescribes antibiotics and contacts a district nurse. Two years later Mr A is severely demented and aggressive, seemingly in response to hallucinations. His wife is not coping. The psychologist gives advice about managing his behaviour, which settles on a short course of an antipsychotic at low dose. You help his wife by organizing day care and a 2-week respite admission for him. The next year she dies. Mr A is admitted to a nursing home. A social worker sorts out the finances. Six months later Mr A breaks his hip. After discussion with his son, conservative management is agreed on. Mr A is kept comfortable in the nursing home and dies the next day.

Child and adolescent psychiatry

Children's psychiatric problems differ in important respects from those of adults, and the approach to their assessment and management is also different (Chapter 16).

- A child psychiatrist requires a detailed understanding of physical and psychological development. Some are also trained in paediatrics.
- The first contact with child psychiatric services may come from the GP, paediatrician or school educational psychologist.
- A child psychiatry team includes specialized social workers, nurses and psychologists. Some of the team may concentrate upon family therapy.
- On the rare occasions when in-patient care is needed, other members of the family may be admitted too, to help in evaluation. The in-patient team includes teachers who assess the child's problems in an educational setting, as well as continuing the child's education whilst in hospital.

Liaison psychiatry (psychological medicine)

Liaison means link, and liaison psychiatrists provide an important link between general psychiatric services and medical and surgical services. Such services are often referred to as departments of psychological medicine. They are based in general hospitals and are principally concerned with three patient groups:

- People who present to casualty having self-harmed. Some hospitals have trained counsellors to carry out screening of all self-harm patients; elsewhere it is left to the medical or nursing staff to decide when to refer to a psychiatrist.

- General hospital patients, whose doctors suspect they have a psychiatric problem (such as delirium, depression or substance misuse) contributing to, arising from, or complicating, their medical disorder.
- Patients whose somatic symptoms are unexplained by demonstrable medical disease.

Liaison psychiatrists offer specialist opinions on these patient groups; they may then offer treatment themselves, or refer on to other local psychiatric services.

You are asked to see Mr B in casualty. He is 49 and has taken an overdose. He is not suicidal but does have depressive and anxiety symptoms. You suspect he has an adjustment reaction after recent life events. You offer him an appointment next week, give him a number to call if he feels the urge to self-harm again, and phone his GP. On review, the severity of depression becomes clearer. He starts antidepressants. You discuss the case with the local CMHT who take over his care. Six months later you are called to see him on a surgical ward where he is awaiting a cholecystectomy. The houseman discovers his psychiatric history and wants your opinion on his mental state. Mr B is fine, but you note that his antidepressant (a monoamine oxidase inhibitor) may interact with analgesics. You alert the anaesthetist.

Substance abuse psychiatry

Abuse of alcohol and drugs leads to a wide range of psychiatric disorders and related problems (Chapter 14), which are dealt with by this subspecialty (also known as *community addictions service*). The workload comprises:

- Management of psychiatric disorder resulting from alcohol or drug abuse.
- Management of the psychological and social consequences of substance misuse. Many people have complex and multiple needs that both cause and result from their substance abuse.
- In-patient care for detoxification (in some units).
- Advice and support for people wanting to stop abusing drugs or alcohol.
- Advice to other doctors managing patients in whom substance abuse may be a factor.

• Public education and local health initiatives about the dangers of drug and alcohol abuse.

Counsellors and outreach workers play important roles in this speciality in addition to the CPNs and social workers. Considerable efforts are made to make contact with people with drug or alcohol problems who are unwilling to attend a medical setting. Co-operation with physicians is important because of the medical problems that often coexist.

Mr C had delirium tremens. After recovery, a liaison psychiatrist referred him to the drug and alcohol clinic. You take a history and discuss his medical condition with his GP. He is given information about alcohol and introduced to a CPN who will visit regularly to review progress and give support. A social worker investigates his benefit problems and contacts his ex-wife about access to his children. Mr C does not want medication to help him abstain. Things go well until he loses his job. He starts to drink heavily and drops out of care. He turns up later wanting admission for detoxification. Needle marks are noticed. He admits to injecting heroin and is found to be hepatitis B positive. He again cuts down his alcohol and denies taking other drugs thereafter. He gets a new job and his wife returns to him. He has had no relapse when seen a year later.

Forensic psychiatry

Forensic means 'of the courts'. All psychiatrists become involved in forensic issues for various reasons:
• Writing psychiatric court reports or attending court on behalf of a patient.
• Assessment of local offenders/prisoners with suspected psychiatric disorder. Court diversion schemes are being developed to reduce the delay such people experience before receiving psychiatric help.
• A forensic history (e.g. of assault) may affect management decisions even if not directly related to current psychiatric problems.
Forensic psychiatrists concentrate on work in three areas:
• Psychiatric assessment of persons charged with serious crimes, especially murder.

• Providing treatment for convicted prisoners with a psychiatric disorder. This includes running psychiatric care in Regional Secure Units and the Special Hospitals (e.g. Broadmoor).
• Giving advice to other psychiatrists encountering forensic issues, for example when assessing dangerousness.

In practice, the decision as to when a patient with a 'forensic history' should be transferred to the forensic psychiatric services depends on the crime, the likelihood of recurrence, and the availability of resources.

Groups with special psychiatric needs

Because of their circumstances, several groups have particular psychiatric needs, or are more likely to have needs unmet by the services.

The homeless

Difficulties:
• Multiple social and medical needs.
• High prevalence of psychiatric disorder, especially schizophrenia and substance misuse.
• Lack of a supportive network—family, friends, GP.
• Hard to engage in treatment and follow-up.
Solutions:
• Flexible CMHT care packages.
• Outreach workers.
• Realistic goals.

Ethnic minorities

Difficulties:
• Psychiatric disorder harder to diagnose because of cultural differences in presentation.
• Language barrier.
• Concerns about racial prejudice and stigmatization.
Solutions:
• Awareness of cultural differences in how psychiatric disorders present.
• Trained interpreters.
• Staff reflect ethnic make up of community.

People with psychiatric comorbidity

Difficulties:

- Worsens prognosis.
- Hampers management.
- Increases risk of violence (especially the combination of psychosis, substance misuse and personality disorder).

Solutions:

- Recognition.
- Extra resources.
- Prioritize management plans—target major and soluble problems.

Health care workers

Difficulties:

- Reluctance to admit to psychiatric problems.
- May knowingly mislead or conceal symptoms.
- Increased risk of alcohol abuse and suicide.
- Hard to maintain confidentiality.
- Blurring of boundaries between being a colleague and a patient.

Solutions:

- Confidential, publicised, accessible local arrangements.
- For UK doctors, the National Counselling Service for Sick Doctors (0870 241 0535).

Key points

- Most psychiatric patients are treated in the community. Care is delivered through the care programme approach (CPA) by community mental health teams (CMHT).
- In a CMHT, the psychiatrist works with psychiatric nurses, social workers, and other disciplines.
- Psychiatric admission is reserved for cases where there is known or suspected severe psychiatric disorder coupled with a significant risk of harm to self or others.
- A variety of subspecialty services address specific aspects of psychiatric need.
- Most psychiatric disorders are managed not in specialist care, but in general practice (Chapter 18).

Chapter 9

Mood disorders

In mood disorders there is a persistent disturbance of mood sufficiently severe to cause impairment in the activities of daily living. This alteration in mood is beyond the fluctuations we all experience. Normal mood (*euthymia*) can become lowered (*depression*) or elevated (*mania*). Figure 9.1 shows the spectrum of mood.

- The term depression, in a clinical sense, may refer either to someone's current mood, or to their underlying diagnosis. This can cause confusion, so the former is sometimes called *depressive episode* and the latter *depressive disorder*. The same applies to *mania* and *manic episode*.
- Mood is also called *affect*, hence the alternative term *affective disorders*.
- Review the relevant parts of the core assessment (p. 10) and the mood modules (p. 21) for fuller description of the key features of mood disorders and how they are elicited.

Clinical features of a depressive episode

The core features are:

- Low mood. The subjective feeling of being depressed. It may be described as feeling down, fed up or sad.
- Lack of energy (*anergia*). May be experienced as fatigue or tiredness.
- Decreased pleasure and interest in life—*anhedonia*.

- The symptoms must have been present for at least 2 weeks to meet the diagnostic criteria.

Depending on the severity of the episode, additional symptoms may also be present, described below. They include somatic (bodily) symptoms, summarized in Table 9.1.

Mild depression

The main complaint is often one of feeling stressed or tired. Anxiety symptoms frequently coexist, leading to the term *mixed anxiety-depression* (Chapter 10). Suicidal thoughts can occur but serious self-harm is unusual. The mood generally remains responsive, so that the person is cheered up by good news and pleasurable events. The patient may be able to work, but will become more tired than usual and concentration may be impaired.

- Though mild, the term is reserved for people who are more than just unhappy, based on the key features outlined above.
- Mild depression is the commonest form of depressive episode.

Moderate depression

The 'textbook' form of depressive episode seen by psychiatrists. The key features are:

- Mood is objectively as well as subjectively depressed.

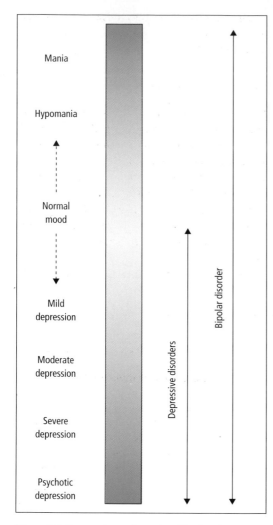

Figure 9.1 The spectrum of mood and its disorders.

Table 9.1 Somatic symptoms of depression.

Psychomotor retardation
Poor sleep with early morning waking
Diurnal variation of mood (worse in morning)
Lack of energy or tiredness
Loss of appetite
Loss of weight
Loss of libido
Constipation
Amenorrhoea

• Suicidal thoughts and intent, driven by the low mood, negative cognitions, and sense of hopelessness—these should always be asked about and taken seriously (Chapter 4).

• Social anxiety and withdrawal.

• Dysfunction becomes prominent (e.g. inability to work properly or marked social withdrawal).

Severe depression

In severe depression, the symptoms of a moderate depressive episode are magnified. A deep and pervasive sense of gloom is evident. The person no longer experiences nor is interested in the normal pleasures of life. There are many somatic symptoms. Suicidal thoughts and intentions become prominent.

Psychotic depression

Depression at its most severe becomes *psychotic depression* (also called *depressive psychosis*). Worries and perceived misdemeanours become delusional in intensity. The patient may believe she is dead or that part of her is (*Cotard's syndrome*); she may experience *auditory hallucinations* with voices cursing her or telling her that she is worthless. Suicidal risk is high.

• Psychomotor retardation can increase to the point where the person sits motionless and mute—*depressive stupor*. This often used to be fatal (from dehydration); it now calls for emergency ECT.

• Psychotic depression must be distinguished from other psychoses (Chapter 12). This is based on the presence of other depressive symptoms, and the *mood congruity* of the delusions and hallucinations.

• Somatic symptoms such as sleep and appetite disturbance are usually present (Table 9.1).

• Anhedonia and lack of motivation.

• Anergia.

• Poor concentration.

• Negative cognitions—focus on unpleasant memories, perceived failings, disappointments, and a bleak future.

• Psychomotor retardation is common, though some patients become agitated with whatever's on their mind.

• A sense of hopelessness and helplessness.

Mood disorders **Chapter 9**

How depression presents

Not all depressed patients complain of or admit to low mood. Rather, they present with the associated cognitive, behavioural or somatic symptoms (Table 9.2). Consequently, depression often surfaces in non-psychiatric settings (Chapter 18), and all doctors must be alert to its various guises.

• Somatic presentations of depression are particularly common in Asian cultures.

Clinical features of a manic episode

As with a depressive episode, there is a spectrum of severity from mild to moderate to severe (Figure 9.1). Sometimes *mania* refers to all pathological elevations of mood, but sometimes *hypomania* is used to refer to the milder or shorter-lived form. Features of mania and hypomania are compared in Table 9.3.

Mild mania (hypomania)

Hypomania is a happiness and zest for life in excess of that which is normal. The degree of functional impairment is variable. A daily routine may be just about maintained, though with less need for sleep and more nocturnal activities (e.g. spring cleaning, writing a novel). Though subjectively productivity may be increased, tasks are rarely done well nor completed. *Concentration* is impaired and *distractibility* is usual. The infectious gaiety easily switches to irritability.

• Hypomania often progresses to a full manic

Table 9.2 Ways depression presents.

Example	Depressive explanation
An old man who's become forgetful	Poor concentration
A mother unable to cope with her child	Lack of motivation and anhedonia
A student with weight loss and fatigue	Somatic symptoms
A woman worrying about having AIDS	Ruminations
A man with panic attacks	Anxiety symptoms secondary to depression
Marital conflict	About sex, due to husband's loss of libido
In casualty after failed hanging attempt	Delusions of worthlessness

Table 9.3 Symptoms of mania.

Core features
Elevation of mood
'Infectious gaiety' or irritability
Distractible
Poor concentration
Flight of ideas
Pressure of speech
Expansive or grandiose ideas
Disinhibited behaviour (e.g financial, sexual)
Increased energy
Decreased need for sleep

Features of hypomania	*Features of mania*
Present for at least 4 days	Present for at least 7 days
Core features mild or moderate	Core features marked
Mild or moderate dysfunction	Substantial dysfunction
Partial insight preserved	Minimal or absent insight
No psychotic features	Psychotic symptoms may occur

episode, especially in those with a past history of mania.

Moderate and severe mania

In moderate and severe mania the symptoms cause substantial impairment of occupational and social functioning. Thought processes become disordered and jumpy (*flight of ideas*), accompanied by *pressure of speech* (p. 25). Psychotic symptoms may emerge. These are mood congruent and *grandiose*: a patient may believe themselves blessed with special powers (e.g. that they can fly or have been sent to save the world). They may hear voices supporting these beliefs. Unfortunately, reality or gravity supervene, and people with mania do things they later regret. For example, they may suffer consequences of promiscuity or generate huge debts.

Mixed affective states

In *mixed affective states*, manic and depressive symptoms coexist within the course of a day. The disorder is not rare, but difficult to diagnose. It may be triggered by antidepressant treatment in a patient with tendency to bipolar disorder. The treatment of mixed states usually focuses initially on the manic symptoms.

Classification of mood disorders

Recognition of a depressive or manic episode is only the first part of diagnosing a mood disorder. The diagnosis also depends on the nature, severity, and course of the episodes. The classification of mood disorders is confusing; a simplified approach is shown in Figure 9.2.

First, consider the unlikely but important possibility of an organic mood disorder (i.e. one attributable directly to a medical disorder or a consequence of substance misuse; see p. 96 and Chapters 13 and 14).

The vast majority of cases of mood disorder do not come into this category and organic factors are more commonly just one component of a multifactorial aetiology (Chapter 6). In all these cases, the next diagnostic decision is between *bipolar disorder* and (unipolar) *depressive disorder* (Figures 9.1 to 9.3). This distinction is based upon the presence or absence of a history of mania. Bipolar and depressive disorders are in turn subdivided by *course* and *severity*.

Depressive disorder

ICD-10 divides depressive disorders into those with discrete episodes with recovery in between (*recurrent depressive disorder*) and those with persistent, mild symptoms (*dysthymia*). In reality, this is not always a clear cut distinction.

• If only one episode has been experienced, the ICD-10 label is just '*depressive episode*' (though in practice the terms 'depressive disorder' or just 'depression' are used loosely).

Recurrent depressive disorder is then described in terms of the severity of the episode, using the features outlined above.

• Dysthymia is longstanding but mild depression, often experienced as a lack of pleasure in life and of things being an effort; symptoms worsen at times of stress.

• Dysthymia used to be considered as depressive personality disorder. Its reclassification as a form of depressive disorder is supported by some genetic evidence, and it encourages dys-

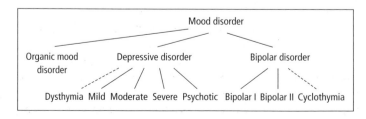

Figure 9.2 Classification of mood disorders.

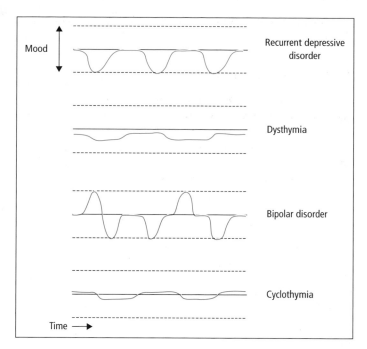

Figure **9.3** Course of mood disorders.

thymia to be seen as treatable, which to a degree it is.

Mrs J has a 6-week history of low mood, anhedonia, tearfulness, and early morning waking. She is off her food and has lost weight. Every day is a struggle and she finds it hard to concentrate or motivate herself to go to work or look after her children. However, she is just about coping and has no suicidal ideation. She had a similar episode 3 years ago. There is no evidence of an organic mood disorder. Your provisional diagnosis is that she has a recurrent depressive disorder and is currently in a depressive episode of moderate severity.

Bipolar disorder

The key feature of *bipolar disorder* is that normal mood is interspersed with both depressive and manic episodes. The frequency and magnitude of the shifts is very variable, as is the proportion of depressive to manic mood swings, although sooner or later depression almost always occurs.

- Bipolar disorder is synonymous with the older terms *manic depression* or *manic depressive psychosis*.
- Bipolar disorder in which only hypomania but

not mania has ever occurred (Table 9.3) is sometimes called *bipolar II disorder*; bipolar disorder with true mania is *bipolar I disorder*.

- For people who have only had one episode of mania and none of depression, the (temporary) diagnosis is *manic episode*.
- *Cyclothymia* is a mild, chronic bipolar variation of mood. Like dysthymia, it is sometimes viewed as a personality trait. Psychiatric help is rarely sought since the mild mood elevations are pleasant and associated with a sense of productivity and creativity.
- A history of cyclothymia, or a family history of bipolar disorder, are significant in someone presenting with a depressive episode; they increase the chances that the patient will actually turn out to have bipolar disorder. It may also increase the risk that antidepressants induce a manic episode.

Mrs J then informs you that she recalls two periods several years ago when she felt elated, slept little, became unusually gregarious, and spent money uncharacteristically. After each episode she was embarrassed and distressed by her actions, but she had not sought treatment. Your diagnosis now becomes one of bipolar (II) disorder, currently in a moderate depressive episode.

Other terms and types of mood disorder

We have already mentioned an array of mood disorder terms and types. Table 9.4 summarizes a few more which are sometimes used.

Epidemiology of mood disorders

Mood disorders are common. The risk is higher in women, and increased by a positive family history. Table 9.5 shows figures from recent population surveys. The finding of more depression in women than men is robust. Possible explanations include:

- Genetic predisposition.
- Sex hormone influences.
- Social pressures.
- Greater willingness to admit to depressive symptoms.
- Depressed men are given other diagnoses, such as alcohol abuse.

Mood disorders seem to be getting commoner and are now the fourth leading cause of worldwide disability. This rise in incidence is unexplained.

Management of depressive disorders

The first requirement is an ability to recognize depression in all its guises (Table 9.2). Depression frequently goes undiagnosed and untreated.

Table 9.4 Other mood disorder terms and types.

Atypical depression	Depression with increased sleep, increased appetite and phobic anxiety. Some evidence it responds better to MAOIs than other antidepressants.
Agitated depression	Depression with prominent anxiety, agitation, restlessness. Contrasted with *retarded depression*, a distinction of value when deciding whether to use a sedative antidepressant.
Double depression	Depressive disorder on top of dysthymia. Poor prognosis.
Endogenous depression	Depression attributed to genetic and biochemical factors. Prominent somatic symptoms, hence the term *biological depression* was applied to similar cases. Contrasted with *reactive depression*.
Melancholia	Depressive disorder with anhedonia and somatic symptoms. American term.
Mixed affective state	Simultaneous manic and depressive symptoms during the same episode of illness, even simultaneously. May respond better to valproic acid than lithium.
Rapid cycling	Bipolar disorder with >4 episodes a year. Women more than men. Hypothyroidism common. Poor response to lithium.
Reactive depression	Depression where the mood remains reactive to circumstances. Lacks somatic symptoms.
Reactive depression	See Agitated depression.
Seasonal affective disorder	Depression which recurs in autumn or winter, associated with increased sleep and carbohydrate craving. May respond to bright light therapy.

Table 9.5 Occurrence of mood disorders.

	Bipolar disorder	Depressive disorder
Lifetime risk (%)	1	15
One-month prevalence (%)	0.4	5
Sex ratio (M : F)	1 : 1	1 : 2
Mean age of onset	Early 20s	Late 20s
Risk in first-degree relatives:		
of bipolar disorder (%)	10	2
of depressive disorder (%)	15	15

• Psychiatrists only see a small percentage of people with depressive disorder, highlighting the need for GPs and all doctors to be confident about its diagnosis and first-line treatment.

Treatment depends largely on severity. Mild depressive episodes are often self limiting and antidepressant drug treatment is often not indicated. Information, advice and simple measures such as self-help guides to problem solving may be adequate. There is evidence that increased physical exercise and activity helps.

Drug treatment

The first-line treatment for a depressive episode of at least moderate severity is usually an antidepressant. However, before prescribing, consider several factors (Table 9.6). Over 60% of depressive episodes respond to an antidepressant, either TCA or SSRI (Chapter 7.1). The chances of successful treatment can be increased if simple measures are taken (Table 9.7; see also Table 7.2).

*Mr S has a moderate depressive episode. He is married and unemployed. He initially doesn't accept he's depressed and blames his problems on his own inad-*equacies. *You explain that he has a depressive disorder which would benefit from treatment. You summarize what depression is and how antidepressants work, including their possible side-effects and delayed onset of action, but also emphasize that they will help him sleep and reduce his anxiety. You recommend he takes 50mg amitriptyline tonight, and increases to 150mg/day over a week. His wife is present and agrees to supervise his tablets. You will see him in a week to review progress.*

After recovery, continue treatment at the same dose for at least 6 months. The dose is then tapered off over several weeks. Continuing treatment in this way reduces the high risk of relapse in the months after a depressive episode and tapering off reduces the risk of 'withdrawal' symptoms.

• There is no good evidence that long-term use of antidepressants is harmful.

Mr S took his tablets as prescribed. His sleep and agitation improved rapidly. The depressive symptoms responded over the next few weeks, though it was necessary to increase amitrypyline to 200mg/day for a full response. He became constipated but this improved with laxatives. He subsequently accepted that he had been ill, and conceptualized the amitriptyline

Table 9.6 Factors affecting management decisions in depression.

Question	Implication
Is there a serious suicide risk?	May need admission. Use SSRI not TCA as less toxic in overdose
Are there psychotic symptoms?	Add an antipsychotic to the antidepressant, or use ECT
What are the main symptoms?	Affects choice of drug. E.g. use sedative antidepressant if insomnia
Is there a past history?	Use the treatment which worked last time
Is there a past history of mania?	Caution with antidepressants; consider mood stabilizer
Are there medical problems?	Avoid TCAs after recent myocardial infarction
What does the patient want?	Antidepressants may be unacceptable

Table 9.7 Prescribing antidepressants effectively.

Principle	Examples
Educate patient	About efficacy, onset of effects and side-effects, and non-addictiveness
Attend to the psychosocial aspects	Restore hope; education about depression; practical advice
Give an adequate dose	Know dose ranges for specific SSRIs and TCAs
Check drug being taken	Non-adherence is common reason for non-response
Give the drug for long enough	Therapeutic trial should be 6–8 weeks, at adequate dose

as correcting a chemical imbalance which helped him solve life's problems more effectively. He no longer blamed himself for his redundancy and found a new job. His wife confirmed the improvement. On your advice, he remained on medication for a further 9 months.

Psychological treatment

CBT, IPT and probably other psychological treatments such as problem solving therapy (p. 75) are effective alternatives to antidepressants in mild and moderate depressive disorder. CBT is much more widely available than the other psychological therapies.

Psychological therapies are often preferred by patients, being seen as curing underlying problems rather than just treating symptoms. Some doctors and other health professionals feel the same. However, the shortage of trained therapists limits their use, and not all patients are able to use these therapies.

- Combining an antidepressant with a psychological treatment is a little more effective than either alone. It is a useful option in patients who have partially responded to one or other treatment.

There are no established predictors of who will benefit from psychological rather than pharmacological treatment of depression. A few pointers suggesting good psychotherapeutic response are:

- Depression not severe (as defined in Table 9.1).
- 'Psychological mindedness' (the ability and willingness to think about psychological matters).
- Willingness to engage in therapy and carry out homework tasks.
- Preference for psychological treatment or reluctance to take medication.

Non-response to first-line treatment

In a third of cases, a depressive episode does not respond to a first-line antidepressant (or to a psychological treatment). Then:

- Check the antidepressant has been taken as prescribed. Measuring plasma levels can sometimes be useful.

- Increase to the maximum tolerated and recommended dose.
- Review the case. Is the diagnosis right? Could there be powerful perpetuating factors, such as an endocrine disorder, marital strife or alcohol misuse? Can their impact be reduced?

If the patient has still not improved there are various options to consider. The commonest option is to switch from one class of antidepressant to another (e.g. TCA to SSRI) or to try a second drug from the same class (usually SSRI to SSRI). There is some evidence in favour of either strategy. Alternative options, with at least some evidence of efficacy, are:

- Add lithium to the antidepressant if depression is severe.
- Add tri-iodothyronine to the antidepressant if depression is severe.
- Cognitive–behavioural therapy (CBT) or other psychological treatment.
- Switch to an MAOI, especially in atypical depression (Table 9.4). Remember MAOI cautions (p. 61).
- Add an antipsychotic if there are psychotic symptoms.
- Try one of the newer antidepressants, e.g. venlafaxine.
- Psychiatric referral, if not already occurred (see below).
- Consider ECT for severe and drug-resistant depression (p. 69).

Psychiatric referral for depression

Referral for psychiatric assessment or ongoing care of depressive disorder is appropriate when:

- The case is unresponsive or problematic.
- A second opinion on diagnosis or treatment is required.
- Combinations of drugs or rarely-used agents are being considered.
- To access psychological services, occupational therapy, etc.
- Psychiatric admission (e.g. because of suicide risk or need for ECT) is being considered.

Prevention of relapse

Continuation of antidepressant drugs cuts relapse rates by 50% in patients with recurrent depressive disorder. Psychological treatments such as CBT may also be effective, by a long-term reduction in negative cognitions or by teaching strategies for recognizing and treating re-emergent symptoms.

• In people who do relapse, reinstitute the treatment that worked the first time but continue it for longer. Some patients appear to benefit from prolonged antidepressant treatment.

Management of bipolar disorder

Treatment of mania and mixed episodes

Patients with mild mania can be successfully treated as out-patients, if the patient has insight that they need treatment. More severe mania, especially if psychotic, usually requires admission, often compulsorily.

• Atypical antipsychotics (e.g. risperidone, olanzapine), or a mood stabilizer (e.g. valproate, lithium) are effective. Antipsychotics are probably slightly more effective than mood stabilizers, but cause more adverse effects. Benzodiazepines are used, as required, for sedation.

• The choice of drug is influenced by the patient's existing medication—they may already be on a mood stabilizer. If they are on an antidepressant, stop it. If the patient is on lithium, check the blood level to assess recent adherence.

• Some patients learn to recognize prodromal symptoms of mania (e.g. initial insomnia, increased energy). If so, a short course of antipsychotic or valproate may abort the episode.

• ECT can be highly effective in patients with severe mania that does not respond to drug treatment.

Mania can last for months if untreated. Death from 'manic exhaustion' was well recognized before treatments became available.

Treatment of depressive episodes in bipolar disorder

Depressive episodes and symptoms in bipolar disorder ('*bipolar depression*') can cause severe dysfunction and can be difficult to treat.

• Antidepressants are effective, but they should be used in combination with an effective antimanic drug (see above) because antidepressants used alone can precipitate mania.

• Lamotrigine, an antiepileptic drug, is a useful alternative.

• For severe depression, antipsychotics, ECT, and psychiatric admission may all be necessary.

Prevention of relapse

Long-term lithium treatment is the standard prophylaxis for bipolar disorder. It reduces the risk of manic relapse by about 30% and may also reduce the risk of depressive relapse. Valproic acid and olanzapine also reduce the risk of manic relapse, and are increasingly used. Lamotrigine may reduce the risk of depressive relapse.

Conventionally, long-term treatment is not offered until a patient has had at least two manic episodes, or one manic and one depressive episode. However, the effective early treatment of bipolar disorder may improve its long-term outcome and increasingly, the trend is to start long-term treatment after one serious episode, especially when there is a family history of bipolar disorder.

• The decision is an important one and the patient should be given sufficient information and time to make a properly informed choice. Furthermore, long-term lithium treatment should not be initiated unless both patient and doctor intend to continue it for at least 2 years.

• Counselling and various tests are needed before lithium is given (p. 62). Patient education may also increase adherence.

• Relapses in bipolar disorder are often heralded by non-specific symptoms (e.g. deteriorating sleep), as mentioned above. Some patients become adept at recognizing and responding to these warning signs. Based on this principle, CBT may help in preventing relapses.

Prognosis of mood disorders

Depressive disorders

Over 50% of people who have had one depressive episode will have another. The more severe the depression, the worse the prognosis; most people with psychotic depression suffer multiple episodes, and 10% never recover fully.

• The proportion with severe, recurrent and chronic illness is higher in psychiatric care than general practice.

• The risk of suicide is increased at least 10-fold in people with depressive disorder. About 4% of patients who have had depression will die by suicide, rising to 15% in those ill enough to have required psychiatric admission at some stage.

• Mortality is also increased from natural causes, notably cardiovascular disease, accidents and substance misuse.

Bipolar disorder

Bipolar disorder runs a remitting and relapsing course in 90%. After one episode, the annual average risk of relapse is about 20%. After more than three episodes, the annual average risk of relapse is about 40%. The prognosis is worse in young onset cases, rapid cycling bipolar disorder (Table 9.4), and women.

• Suicide and mortality rates are similar to depressive disorder.

• The disruption caused by the illness, especially the manic phases, often leads to problems maintaining relationships, employment and accommodation.

Aetiology of mood disorders

Organic mood disorders

As mentioned, occasionally mood disorders are so closely related to a specific 'organic' cause that they are referred to as organic mood disorder. Recognized causes of organic mood disorder are summarized in Table 9.8. See also Chapter 13.

• Even when an organic diagnosis is made, psy-

Table 9.8 Causes of organic mood disorder.

Usually depression	Usually mania
Cushing's disease	Hyperthyroidism
Addison's disease	Steroids
Hypothyroidism	Amphetamine (acute)
Hypercalcaemia	L-DOPA
Diabetes mellitus	Antidepressants
Carcinomas	Bromocriptine
Beta-blockers	Isoniazid
Digoxin	
Amphetamine (chronic)	

Either depression or mania
Multiple sclerosis
Cerebrovascular disease
Systemic lupus erythematosus
Epilepsy
Brain tumours

chological and social factors may still be relevant to course and treatment.

A 65-year-old man presented with insomnia, anorexia, back pain and weight loss. He also felt fed up and irritable. The provisional diagnosis was depression with somatic symptoms. However, physical examination revealed bony tenderness over his lumbar spine and a hard nodular prostate. Blood tests showed hypercalcaemia and anaemia. He had metastatic carcinoma of the prostate. His depressive symptoms resolved as the hypercalcaemia was treated, along with an antidepressant.

Depressive disorders

For all other mood disorders, a mixture of genetic, biological, psychological and social factors contribute to varying degrees (as in the rolling vignette in Chapter 6). There is a moderate genetic predisposition to depression (heritability 40–50%), more so in early-onset cases. The predisposition is shared between the various types of depressive disorder and overlaps with those associated with anxiety disorders, but not bipolar disorder. The number and identity of genes are unknown.

Environmental influences contribute substantially to depressive disorders (Table 9.9) and are discussed in Chapter 6.

Table 9.9 Aetiological factors in depressive disorders.

Biological
  Genes
  Medical conditions (organic mood disorder)
  Neurochemical changes
    Monoamine abnormalities
    Altered HPA axis function

Psychological
  Childhood environment
    Emotional deprivation
    Parental loss
  Abnormal cognitions
  Learned helplessness
  Personality factors—neuroticism

Social
  Life events
  Unemployment

● Hypofunction of monoamine neurotransmitter systems (5-HT and noradrenaline), in conjunction with altered hypothalamo–pituitary–adrenal axis (HPA) regulation is implicated. However, though these systems are all altered in depression, their causal role and inter-relationships remain unclear.
● Psychological models centre on the role of abnormal ways of thinking with a tendency to think negatively about the self, the future and the world (the cognitive theory of depression). The personality attributes of *'neuroticism'* (anxiety, obsessionality, poor coping with stress) and low self-esteem are also associated with depressive disorder.
● Psychosocially, adverse experiences in childhood, recent life events and lack of social support are major risk factors.
● Focal lesions of the subcortical white matter, visible on MRI scans, are a risk factor for late onset depressive disorder and are associated with a poor prognosis.
● Other structural brain changes reported in depressive disorder include a reduction of glial cells in the prefrontal cortex, and hippocampal atrophy. It is not known if these changes are cause, consequence or coincidental.

Bipolar disorder

Bipolar disorder is strongly heritable (80%). MZ : DZ twin concordance is 75% : 25%. Relatives of someone with bipolar disorder have an increased incidence of both bipolar and unipolar depressive disorder (Table 9.5).
● Loci on several chromosomes (including X, 18 and 22) are implicated, and the genes overlap with those for schizophrenia. There is some evidence for inheritance down the maternal line.
  No childhood risk factors are known. Life events can precipitate the initial episodes; once the disorder is established, its course is increasingly immune to environmental circumstances.
● Most of the neurobiological abnormalities described for depressive disorder (Table 9.9) are also implicated in bipolar disorder. However, much less is known—in part because bipolar disorder is by its nature difficult to study.
● Always consider drug-induced mania (an example of organic mood disorder) in young people with no family history of bipolar disorder. In someone first presenting in middle age, exclude cerebrovascular disease, tumours and medication side-effects (Table 9.8).

Other aspects of mood disorders

Puerperal (postpartum) disorders

The postnatal period (puerperium) is a hormonally, and often psychologically, turbulent time. It is traditional to group psychiatric disorders that occur at this time together (as puerperal disorders), partly because their clinical picture and management differ somewhat from similar disorders occurring at other times.

Maternity blues

The 'blues' refer to a tearful, irritable labile mood that affects over 50% of mothers on the third or fourth postnatal day. Symptoms resolve within days without treatment, though explanation and reassurance are appropriate. There is no association of the blues with mood disorder.

• Maternity blues may be due to the precipitous fall in sex steroids after delivery, as well as to the impact of childbirth and concerns about mothering.

Postnatal depression

Postnatal depression tends to start within a month of delivery; 1 in 7 mothers are affected. The symptoms are unremarkable, with the negative thoughts tending to focus on her failings as a mother or on her baby's wellbeing. Physical exhaustion exacerbates matters.

• As well as the standard mood and risk assessments, remember to consider the mother–baby relationship. Postnatal depression may put the baby at short-term risk and if untreated may lead to problems with bonding and child development.

• Most cases are managed at home. Use supportive measures, including explanation and reassurance. Mobilize resources (e.g. the local mothers' group), and liaise with the GP, midwife and health visitor. Many cases resolve within a few weeks, but antidepressants or psychological treatment should be considered if the disorder is moderate or severe. If admission is necessary, it should ideally be to a mother-and-baby unit, to maintain and observe their relationship.

• Before prescribing antidepressants, check whether the mother is breastfeeding (p. 69).

• Postnatal depression is commoner in women with a history of psychiatric disorder and in those lacking support. A postnatal change in sensitivity of the dopaminergic system is implicated.

Puerperal psychosis

Puerperal psychosis was formerly due mainly to sepsis; i.e. it was an organic disorder. Now, it is more often a psychotic mood disorder or schizoaffective disorder. The disorder can be severe. Perplexity and a delirium-like state are characteristic. Onset is usually in the second postnatal week. About 1 in 500 women are affected.

• Risk factors include a past or family history of psychosis and being a primigravida.

• The baby is at potential risk because of the mother's delusions, or because she is so preoccupied by her symptoms that he is neglected. The assessment should specifically address these issues.

• Admission is usually necessary. Treatment is with antipsychotics and antidepressants, and with a low threshold for ECT—which often produces a dramatic response. Full recovery is usual, but there is a 25% relapse rate after the next delivery and a 50% lifetime risk.

Premenstrual syndrome

Up to 80% of women suffer from symptoms in the days before their period: irritability, depression, abdominal bloating and breast tenderness. However, a specific premenstrual syndrome has proved difficult to validate (and is not included in ICD-10). The term *premenstrual dysphoric disorder* is sometimes used for women with prominent psychological premenstrual symptoms.

• If a woman complains of premenstrual syndrome, establish the symptoms and their relationship with the menstrual cycle. Ask her to keep a diary—it may transpire that the symptoms are present at other times too.

• There is some evidence for the efficacy of SSRIs, oestrogens, gonadotrophin agonists, danazol and CBT. There is no good evidence for progestogens or primrose oil. There is a high placebo response rate.

Other psychiatric issues specific to women

Abortion, sterilization, hysterectomy and the menopause have all been said to cause psychiatric distress, especially mood and anxiety disorders. There is no good evidence for any of these claims. Each of these events may, however, act as stressors that are relevant to the understanding, presentation, or treatment, of a disorder occurring soon afterwards.

Grief

If you know you are dying, or you have been bereaved, emotional pain and turmoil are to be expected. Many of the features overlap with those of depression. Psychiatrists and other doctors are asked to assess or support people during these times, so it is necessary to know:

- The characteristic psychological reactions to impending death and to bereavement.
- The features which distinguish these from depressive disorder.

Normal grief

People may grieve a death (*bereavement*) or other major loss, or may grieve an impending event (*anticipatory grief*). The responses are forms of adjustment reaction (p. 106). Three stages have been described:

- *Shock and disbelief.* On being told of the event there is an initial numbness that usually lasts a day or two. Behaviour may be acutely disturbed.
- *Preoccupation.* This central phase involves a preoccupation with the deceased. In the early stages anger is common, and may be directed at doctors, God, or other target of blame. Uncontrollable crying, low mood, social withdrawal and somatic symptoms akin to those of depression may be pronounced. The voice or image of the deceased may be vividly perceived, though usually with an 'as if' quality rather than being truly hallucinatory.
- *Acceptance and resolution.* With time, the person comes to term with the event, symptoms subside, and life begins to return to normal. This phase may take several months to start, and several more to be completed. Recurrence of grief is common around anniversaries.

In uncomplicated grief, *bereavement counselling* and support (e.g. from Cruse) may be useful. Such grief should not be labelled as a disorder but viewed as a natural though painful process. The therapist should, however, be on the look out for signs of abnormal grief or depressive disorder.

Abnormal (pathological) grief

Grief can be abnormal in three ways:

1. *Absent or delayed grief.* There may appear to be no outward signs of grief despite an event of grief-inducing proportions (absent grief). Grief usually begins a few weeks later (delayed grief).
2. *Prolonged grief.* A term used if there are prominent symptoms more than 6–12 months later. At this time, actively consider a developing depressive disorder and the need for treatment.
3. *Excessive grief.* The intensity of grief is unusually great—this may reflect the person's closeness to the deceased, their personality or a depressive disorder.

Grief and depression

A depressive disorder occurs in 1 in 3 grieving people, and is severe in 1 in 5. As the foregoing sections show, it is not easy to decide when the threshold from grief to depression is crossed. The distinction is made largely on the basis of excessive intensity or duration of symptoms, but other features may also help (Table 9.10). The person may need persuading that their suffering is no longer just the pain of normal grief but is now a depressive disorder meriting treatment.

Table 9.10 A comparison of depression and grief.

	Depression	Grief
Suicidal thoughts	Common, driven by low mood	Transient, driven by wish to be with deceased
Blame for situation	Self	Other people or fate
Psychomotor retardation	Yes	No
Psychotic features	In severe cases; mood congruent	No, but may imagine seeing or hearing deceased
Symptom course	Pervasive	Fluctuating

Key points

- Mood disorders involve excessive deviations or fluctuations of mood. They affect 1 in 6 people at some stage in their lives. Unipolar depressive disorders are much commoner than bipolar disorder.
- The core features of depression are low mood, lack of energy, and anhedonia. Many other psychological and somatic symptoms also occur.
- Depression may present with somatic symptoms such as fatigue and weight loss and should always be considered in the differential diagnosis of these symptoms.

- Suicidal risk needs detailed and regular assessment in everyone with mood disorder.
- Antidepressants are the usual first line treatment for depression. Give an adequate dose and continue for at least 6 months after recovery. CBT is as effective as antidepressants for mild and moderate depression but is not widely available. ECT is reserved for severe, resistant cases.
- Mania is treated with antipsychotics and/or mood stabilizers. Long-term treatment with the latter reduces the risk of relapse.

Chapter 10

Neurotic, stress-related and somatoform disorders

General characteristics of neurosis

Neurotic symptoms and syndromes

We all experience anxiety and worries. Sometimes these become excessive or inappropriate, just as normal feelings of depression can become so severe and persistent that they are appropriately regarded as an illness. *Neurosis* ('to do with the nerves') or *neurotic disorder* is the traditional term for those symptoms that are associated with emotion and that are not due to a medical disease or to a personality disorder. The disorders include emotional, cognitive, behavioural and somatic symptoms, and are often but not always associated with an external stressor.

- Anxiety is the primary emotion affected in all these disorders, although degrees of depressed mood are often present.
- The associated cognitions are worries, fears and concerns that are inappropriate or excessive, but (by definition) are not delusional.
- Associated behaviour includes avoidance and other strategies intended to reduce the worries such as repeated checking.
- Somatic ('physical') symptoms, not adequately explained by a medical disease are common.
- Neurotic disorders often present because of the associated cognitions (e.g. recurrent thoughts about illness), behaviour (e.g. the agoraphobic who cannot leave her house), or somatic symp-

toms (e.g. palpitations), not because of the emotional disturbance.
- Neurosis is common in primary care and general hospitals and easily missed (Chapter 18).
- Neuroses are not always minor illnesses and can be chronic and disabling.
- For an introduction to the clinical features of neurosis, review the module (p. 27).

The individual *neurotic disorders* (Table 10.1) differ according to the balance between these elements. Mild cases can rarely be readily placed into any one of these categories, and a useful term is *undifferentiated neurosis* or *minor emotional disorder*.

- Depressive symptoms are very common in patients with neurosis, and neurotic symptoms are very common in patients with depressive disorders. Indeed, in many patients seen in primary care, anxiety and depressive symptoms coexist in similar proportions. The diagnosis of *mixed anxiety–depression* is appropriate for such cases.
- Culture-specific variants of neurosis occur. These include *amok* (dissociative disorder in Indonesia), *koro* (severe anxiety about penis shrinkage in Chinese men) and *dhat* (semen-loss anxiety in Asian men).

Stress-related and somatoform disorders

The term 'neurosis' has a long and chequered history. In the past, it included syndromes with predominantly somatic as well as psychological

Table 10.1 Classification of neurotic, stress-related and somatoform disorders.

Neurotic disorders (Neuroses)
  Anxiety disorders
    Phobic anxiety
    Panic disorder
    Generalized anxiety
  Obsessive compulsive disorder (OCD)
  Dissociative disorders
  Neurasthenia (chronic fatigue syndrome)
  Depersonalization–derealization syndrome

Stress-related disorders
  Acute stress reaction
  Adjustment disorders
  Post-traumatic stress disorder

Somatoform disorders
  Hypochondriasis
  Dysmorphophobia
  Somatization disorder
  Other somatoform disorders

symptoms; it has also been used to mean that the disorder was caused by stress. In current classifications (Table 10.1), these forms of disorder have been given their own categories, though still grouped together with the neurotic disorders:

• If there is a major external stressor that appears to explain the presentation, a *stress-related disorder* may be diagnosed.

• In *somatoform disorders*, somatic symptoms (e.g. palpitations, pain) that are not adequately explained by a medical disease dominate the syndrome. This category is controversial (see below) because of its assumption that such somatic complaints are better regarded as a psychiatric than as a medical condition (an assumption resented by some patients, largely because of the associated stigma).

• Review the somatoform disorders module (p. 28).

Diagnosing neurosis

If a patient presents with symptoms suggestive of a neurotic disorder, ask two questions:

First, do the symptoms warrant any diagnosis?

• Gauge whether the symptoms are diagnostically significant from their intensity, number and pervasiveness, and from the resulting *dysfunction*—are they interfering with the person's life?—and do they need treatment (e.g. see social phobia)?

Second, is an alternative diagnosis more appropriate?

• Neurotic symptoms can occur as part of another psychiatric or medical condition, especially depression but also substance misuse, psychosis, eating disorders and certain organic conditions (e.g. anxiety due to thyrotoxicosis). Life-long symptoms may be better regarded as a personality disorder.

Epidemiology of neurosis

If mixed anxiety–depression is included, neurosis is very common indeed, afflicting about 15% of the population at any one time (Chapter 18). Most of the neurotic disorders are about twice as common in women. The onset is generally between early adulthood and middle age, though children suffer from neurotic disorders too (Chapter 16).

Management of neurosis

Management should be biopsychosocial. Neuroses share a common responsiveness to certain drugs and psychological treatments, though, as outlined below, there is also some evidence of specificity with individual neurotic disorders responding better to certain types of treatment:

• Antidepressants and anxiolytics are both effective, though anxiolytics are now less commonly used because of problems of dependence (p. 63). Antidepressants are effective even when there are few, if any, depressive symptoms—they could be called 'antineurotics'.

• Psychological therapies, especially CBT, are at least as effective as medication for most neuroses and especially effective for some (e.g. panic disorder). The specifics of CBT differ somewhat between neurotic disorders. As well as specialist therapies, the principles of explanation and reassurance are always important in the management of neurotic disorders.

• Social interventions such as removal of stressor

and improvement of social support can be a key part of management.

Prognosis of neurosis

In the community, the majority of neurotic disorders are acute and transient. Prognosis is better when: there is no personality disorder; the patient is strongly motivated to get better; and duration of illness is short. Psychiatrists tend to see the small proportion of cases that are severe, chronic or disabling.

Aetiology of neurosis

Neuroses have a multifactorial aetiology that is best considered from a biopsychosocial perspective.
• Neurotic disorders, and the personality trait of neuroticism (Chapter 15) are moderately heritable.
• Alterations in the 5-HT, noradrenergic, and associated brain systems probably mediate anxiety and somatic symptoms.
• Though neuroses are traditionally thought of as psychological disorders, neuroimaging studies have demonstrated abnormal metabolic activity and even altered brain structure (e.g. hippocampal atrophy in post-traumatic stress disorder). The interpretation of these biological findings is not clear.
• Cognitive factors and behavioural conditioning (Chapter 6) are important, especially in phobias and panic disorder.
• The social factors of poor coping with stressors, and abnormal illness behaviour (Chapter 6) are also relevant in some cases.
The precise combination of these factors in an individual patient in predisposing, precipitating and perpetuating a neurosis can be described in an aetiological formulation (Chapter 5).

The specific disorders

So far, this Chapter has considered the factors common to neurotic syndromes as a whole, since their similarities are greater than their differences. However, the latter are important too, and the rest of the chapter considers the main features that are, to some degree, specific to the individual disorders listed in Table 10.1.

Anxiety disorders

As the name suggests, these are neuroses dominated by the emotion of anxiety, anxious thoughts, avoidance behaviour and the somatic symptoms of sympathetic arousal that accompany it (Table 10.2). Anxiety disorders are divided into three main subtypes: *phobic, paroxysmal (panic) and generalized* (Table 10.3).
• The nature and prominence of the somatic symptoms (e.g. chest pain) often leads the patient to present initially to medical services (Chapter 18).

Phobic anxiety

In a phobia, the anxiety is *situational*, and largely restricted to the experience or anticipation of the phobic stimulus. This stimulus may be a specific concern (e.g. heights, spiders) or a more general one (e.g. agoraphobia). As a result, there is marked *avoidance* of those situations associated with the stimulus (e.g. a severe mouse phobic may avoid old

Table 10.2 Common symptoms of anxiety.

Component	Prominent features
Emotion/mood	Anxiety, irritability
Cognitions	Exaggerated worries and fears
Behaviour	Avoidance of feared situations, checking, seeking reassurance
Somatic symptoms	Tight chest
	Short of breath
	Palpitations
	'Butterflies'
	Tremor
	Tingling of fingers (due to hyperventilation)
	Aches and pains
	Poor sleep
	Frequent desire to pass urine and defecate

Table 10.3 Features distinguishing the three types of anxiety disorder.

	Phobic anxiety	**Panic disorder**	**Generalized**
Occurrence of anxiety	Situational	Paroxysmal	Persistent
Associated behaviour	Avoidance	Escape	Agitation
Associated cognitions	Fear of situation	Fear of symptoms	Worry
Somatic symptoms	With exposure	Episodic	Persistent

houses or nature programmes). Although it produces immediate relief from anxiety, *avoidance behaviour* is ultimately counterproductive because it reinforces the phobia. Overcoming avoidance is a key part of psychological treatment.

- The main differential diagnosis is from the other anxiety disorders. Occasionally, phobic anxiety may arise from delusions in a psychosis. Phobia of disease is classified separately, as hypochondriasis (see below).

- Psychological treatment is based on graded exposure and desensitization (behavioural therapy). In CBT, a cognitive component is added to help the patient accurately evaluate the dangerousness of the stimulus (e.g. a flight phobic may be encouraged to find out the actual statistical risk of dying in a plane crash).

- Antidepressants and anxiolytics are also effective, but behavioural therapy may also be required.

Agoraphobia

One of the commonest phobias is *agoraphobia* (literally 'fear of the market place') (Table 10.4). Intense anxiety is provoked either by open spaces, or large spaces which are crowded and difficult to escape from (e.g. supermarket queues). Panic attacks are commonly associated and their occurrence may become what is most feared. The appropriate diagnosis is then *panic disorder with agoraphobia*.

- The associated cognitions commonly concern anticipation of fainting, dying, or other catastrophe, rather than a fear of shops or spaces *per se*.

- The condition can be severe and avoidance can lead the person to become housebound.

- Symptoms are present for over 2 years on average before a person suffering from agoraphobia seeks help. It is commonest in young women.

Table 10.4 Symptoms of agoraphobia.

Component	Prominent features
Emotion	Situational anxiety—in shops, crowded large places
Cognition	Thoughts of collapsing and being left helpless in public
Behaviour	Avoidance of panic-provoking situations
Somatic symptoms	Physical sensations of panic (see below)
Associations	Strong association with panic disorder

Table 10.5 Symptoms of social phobia.

Component	Prominent features
Emotion	Situational anxiety in social gatherings
Cognition	Being judged negatively by others
Behaviour	Avoidance of social occasions
Somatic symptoms	Blushing, trembling
Associations	Secondary alcohol misuse

- For a vignette of agoraphobia and its psychological treatment, see p. 73.

Social phobia

Social phobia (Table 10.5) must be distinguished from normal shyness, and from social withdrawal due to depression. In social phobia there is often a history of low self-esteem and a triggering incident when the person feels they made a fool of themselves. Treatment is with CBT and antidepressant drugs, particularly SSRIs.

- There has been controversy about the boundary

between normal shyness and social phobia. This reflects the debate over the 'medicalization of life' and the sometimes arbitrary boundary between neurosis and 'problems of living'.

Panic disorder

Panic attacks are episodes of severe paroxysmal anxiety with prominent somatic symptoms and unpleasant feelings of depersonalization or derealization (Table 10.6). In *panic disorder*, the attacks are recurrent over a period of at least 1 month, and with fear of the attacks themselves. The somatic symptoms may be severe and lead to a misdiagnosis of angina, epilepsy or other medical disorders.
● The differential diagnosis of panic disorder is from panic attacks that occur only in specific feared situations (i.e. phobic anxiety) or only occasional attacks in other neuroses and depressive disorder. Also, beware that medical conditions can occasionally be a cause of paroxysmal anxiety (p. 146).
● CBT is very effective. It is aimed at helping the patient to see the symptoms as the result of anxiety and not as indicators of a catastrophe (such as a heart attack). Antidepressants are also effective, although patients with panic disorder often find them hard to tolerate as they may exacerbate the panic before reducing it—a fact important to explain to the patient.
● Aetiologically, there appears to be a lowered biological threshold for anxiety. There is good evidence that cognitive factors such as catastrophic misinterpretation of somatic symptoms (e.g. the chest pain means that I am having a heart attack)

are also important (Chapter 6). Panic attacks may start during a period of stress.

Generalized anxiety disorder

Generalized anxiety is a syndrome of persistent anxiety associated with chronic uncontrollable and excessive worry (Table 10.7). It may fluctuate but is not paroxysmal (as with panic), situational (as with phobia) life-long (as with a personality disorder) or clearly stress related (as with a stress-related disorder).
● Chronic somatic symptoms such as aches and pains and bowel symptoms may lead to a medical presentation.
● Treatment is based on the same pharmacological, psychological and stress-reducing methods as for other anxiety disorders, but efficacy may be lower. There is some evidence for the effectiveness of buspirone and the antihistamine hydroxyzine.

Obsessive–compulsive disorder (OCD)

Obsessions and compulsions were defined in Chapter 2. In OCD they are the most prominent and persistent features (Table 10.8). There is often significant disability. The main differential diagnosis is from depressive disorder (in which obsessional symptoms are common), psychotic disorder (since obsessions and delusions can be hard to distinguish), and anankastic personality disorder.
● Reassure the patient that their condition is one that does not progress to 'madness'.

Table 10.6 Symptoms of a panic attack.

Component	Prominent features
Emotion	Severe, incapacitating anxiety
Cognition	Of dying, going mad or otherwise losing control
Behaviour	Escape
Somatic symptoms	Prominent symptoms of sympathetic arousal (Table 10.2)
Associations	Depression, agoraphobia

Table 10.7 Symptoms of generalized anxiety disorder.

Component	Prominent features
Emotion	Anxiety
Cognition	Excessive, disproportionate uncontrollable worry
Behaviour	Easily startled, on edge
Somatic symptoms	Multiple chronic aches, tension, sweating, headache
Associations	Depression

Table 10.8 Symptoms of obsessive–compulsive disorder (OCD).

Component	Predominant features
Emotion	Anxiety about the topic of the obsessional thought
Cognition	Preoccupation with obsession(s)
Behaviour	Compulsions
Somatic symptoms	Tension, especially if prevented from doing compulsive act
Associations	Depression
	Anankastic personality disorder (Table 15.1)
	Tourette syndrome (p. 177)

Table 10.9 Symptoms of acute stress reaction.

Component	Predominant features
Emotion	'Dazed'
Cognition	Amnesia or denial of event
Behaviour	Overactivity or withdrawal
Somatic symptoms	Many autonomic symptoms
Association	Acute stressor

Table 10.10 Symptoms of adjustment disorders.

Component	Prominent features
Emotion	Depression, anxiety, poor concentration, irritability
Cognition	Preoccupation with event
Behaviour	Angry outbursts
Somatic symptoms	Moderate autonomic symptoms
Associations	Chronic stressor

- 5-HT-predominant antidepressants (SSRIs, clomipramine) are both effective, as is behavioural therapy. The combination may be needed.
- The prognosis untreated is poor. Because of the chronicity of the condition, patients with OCD are frequently used as cases in psychiatry exams.
- Aetiological factors include a genetic vulnerability, an anankastic personality, and social stressors. The condition is perpetuated by the avoidance of situations that trigger the obsessions, and by the performance of the compulsions; both of which stop the anxiety habituating.
- OCD is unusual amongst neuroses in being equally common in men and women.

Stress-related disorders

In some cases presenting with neurotic symptoms, the stressor appears to be of such overwhelming importance in causing the symptoms that they are classified as 'reactions to stress'. The whole range of neurotic symptoms may occur, commonly in a diffuse picture of distress, anxiety and depression.

The subtypes of stress-related disorders are:
- *Acute stress reaction*—beginning and ending within hours or days of the stressor.
- *Adjustment disorder*—beginning less acutely and lasting several months.
- *Post-traumatic stress disorder* (*PTSD*)—a delayed response to an extreme stress associated with particular symptoms and especially the re-experiencing of the trauma in dreams or imagination.

Acute stress reactions

These are transient, but severe, emotional reactions immediately following an exceptional stressor (e.g. rape). These states are colloquially referred to as 'nervous shock' (Table 10.9). The differential diagnosis includes the initial stages of other neuroses, acute psychosis (when behaviour can be very odd and out of character), and delirium. Management is by removal of the stressor (if possible), reassurance and providing support. A short course of benzodiazepines may be used.
- Trials show that early 'debriefing' (requiring that the patient tells a therapist about the stressful incident soon after it has occurred) is unhelpful and may even worsen outcome.

Adjustment disorders

Also called *adjustment reactions*, these are more prolonged reactions to stress. The symptoms typically begin within a month of the stress and do not last longer than 6 months (Table 10.10).
- Grief reactions (p. 98) and psychological reactions to medical conditions (Chapter 18) are types of adjustment reaction.

Management includes helping the patient to

address continuing stressor more effectively (perhaps by problem-solving therapy), supportive psychotherapy, and by treating significant depressive or anxiety symptoms as necessary.

Post-traumatic stress disorder (PTSD)

PTSD is a delayed response to an exceptionally severe event (e.g. serious road accident, major disaster, severe assault). It was initially described in Vietnam War veterans and more recently it has been recognized in UK law as a basis for personal compensation claims. The onset may be months or years after the original trauma. A central feature is an involuntary re-experiencing of the traumatic event in dreams or as intrusive 'day dreams', often triggered by reminders of the trauma (Table 10.11).

Management includes treating comorbid psychiatric disorder or substance misuse, and encouraging a return to normal activities. Antidepressants are modestly effective and there is good evidence for paroxetine and sertraline. There is evidence for the effectiveness of CBT as a treatment and form of prevention.

• Eye movement desensitization and reprocessing (EMDR), a treatment in which the patients is asked to think about an image of the traumatic event whilst moving their eyes from side-to-side is also moderately effective, although there is controversy about how it works.

• The prognosis for PTSD is generally good with a gradual resolution in most cases although a minority become chronic, and associated alcohol misuse and depression is very common.

Dissociative and conversion disorders

In dissociative disorder, also called *conversion disorder*, there is a medically inexplicable loss of function (Table 10.12). Both terms have Freudian origins.

• They were called *dissociative* because they were thought to represent a loss of the normal association between different mental processes such as personal identity and memories, sensory and motor function.

• The term *conversion* was used because of the unsubstantiated and outmoded theory that feelings and anxieties get converted into symptoms: resolving the mental conflict (so-called *primary gain*) or providing practical benefits such as the attention of others (so-called *secondary gain*) (see Chapter 6).

• Dissociative disorders were previously known as *hysteria*; this archaic term (suggesting causation by a wandering uterus) has now been abandoned.

Presentations include loss of psychological function such as memory (psychogenic amnesia), wandering in a trance (fugue), motor function (paralysis, pseudoseizures), or sensory function (glove and stocking anaesthesia).

Understandably, dissociative disorders often cause difficulties in diagnosis and management. When the possibility of a dissociative disorder is raised, consider the following:

Table 10.11 Symptoms of post-traumatic stress disorder (PTSD).

Component	Prominent features
Emotion	Anxiety and irritability; numb and detached
Cognition	Repeated reliving of the event in images ('flashbacks') and nightmares
Behaviour	Avoidance of situations associated with the trauma
Somatic symptoms	Exaggerated startle response
Associations	Substance misuse, depression Severe previous stressor

Table 10.12 Symptoms of dissociative disorder.

Component	Prominent features
Emotion	May be suppressed, deny anxiety
Cognition	Denial of psychological impact of stressors
Behaviour	Loss of function
Somatic symptoms	Loss of function e.g. paralysis
Associations	Acute stressors, depression

- Organic causes for the loss of function must be excluded. This may require extensive investigation.
- Dissociative disorders (which are regarded as originating in unconscious processes) must be distinguished from the consciously motivated symptoms. The latter in turn are divided into *factitious disorder*, in which symptoms are produced deliberately to obtain medical care, and *malingering* behaviour designed to achieve personal gain (see below). Deciding if someone is feigning illness is difficult and may require evidence of marked inconsistency (e.g. limping into the consulting room and then running for a bus). The other main differential is somatoform disorder.
- The diagnostic criteria require that there should be a plausible 'psychogenic' explanation for the symptoms, in terms of severe internal conflicts or a traumatic life event; this may be difficult to establish in practice.
- The person is said to often be surprisingly unconcerned about their disability (*la belle indifference*) although this phenomenon also occurs in patients with organic disease and may not be specific to dissociation.
- There have been very few randomized treatment trials. Clinical experience suggests that important components of management are: (a) accept the reality of the patient's symptoms but to explain that they are potentially reversible; (b) encourage a gradual return to normal function; (c) treat coexisting depression; (d) psychotherapy may be of value in some cases; (e) physical rehabilitation may be useful for chronic disorders affecting motor function.

Somatoform disorders

The somatoform disorders category was created to accommodate those patients who present with predominantly somatic complaints where neither depression, anxiety, nor a medical condition provides a better explanation (Table 10.13). It includes many subcategories. There are two main groups:
- Conditions in which the main feature is con-

Table 10.13 Symptoms of somatoform disorders.

Component	Prominent features
Emotion	Anxiety and depression usually present (but not predominant)
Cognition	Concern with physical symptoms and/or disease or deformity
Behaviour	Medical help seeking
Bodily symptoms	Prominent
Associations	Depressive and anxiety disorders latrogenic harm from inappropriate medical care

cern that the symptoms are evidence of disease (*hypochondriasis*) or deformity (*dysmorphophobia*).
- Conditions in which the main feature is concern about somatic symptoms themselves (*somatization disorder, persistent autonomic dysfunction, persistent somatoform pain disorder and undifferentiated somatoform disorder*).

To make the diagnosis of a somatoform disorder (see module in Chapter 3):
- The concerns and/or symptoms must be medically unjustified or disproportionate, and severe enough to cause distress, and to have persisted for at least 6 months.
- Any depressive and anxiety symptoms are insufficient to justify a diagnosis of depressive or anxiety disorder.
- The symptoms are not delusional (e.g. distinguish from a psychotic disorder with somatic hallucinations).
- The symptoms are not deliberately manufactured (cf. factitious disorder, malingering), nor is there prominent loss of a specific function (cf. dissociative and conversion disorder).
- Aetiologically, childhood deprivation or abuse are risk factors. A predisposition to health anxiety and serious (and perhaps mismanaged) illness in a relative are also common.
- A complementary perspective on diagnosis of unexplained medical symptoms is discussed in Chapter 18 and shown in Figure 18.2.

Assessment and management of somatoform disorders

The principles of management of the neuroses also apply to somatoform disorders. However, since such patients (and sometimes their doctors) often believe their symptoms are a sign of medical disease rather than of a psychiatric condition, they seek and receive medical rather than psychiatric care. Patients are often hostile to the idea that their symptoms are 'psychogenic' or that they will benefit from psychiatric treatment. The effective management of somatoform disorder therefore requires a close liaison between GP, physician and psychiatrist. The principles are:

• Take the patient's somatic concerns seriously. Neither dismiss them as 'just psychological', nor collude with unfounded beliefs about unproven medical causes for them.

• Medical investigations should be determined by the doctor's interpretation of the symptoms, not by the patient's demands. People with somatoform disorder are no more likely to die of undiagnosed organic disease than the general population, although they are at risk of harm from unnecessary medical tests and treatments. It is worth remembering that (perhaps counter-intuitively) the more somatic symptoms a patient has, the less likely are they to have a medical disease.

• Ensure a clear and consistent explanation for the symptoms is given by all doctors involved.

• Treat any coexisting depression and anxiety in the usual way.

• Antidepressants are beneficial in most somatoform disorders, even when there is no good evidence of depression. However, their use needs careful explanation if they are not to be rejected as inappropriately 'psychiatric'.

• CBT is of value but must be adapted to be consistent with the patient's predominantly somatic focus.

• Identify and help the patient to deal with major social stressors.

• Encourage a return to normal functioning and a decrease in illness behaviour.

Hypochondriasis and dysmorphophobia

The characteristic feature of these somatoform disorders is a preoccupation with the possibility of having a serious physical disease or deformity.

• The main differential diagnoses are depressive disorder (hypochondriacal worries and concerns about appearance are common) and psychotic disorders (with hypochondriacal delusions or somatic hallucinations).

Hypochondriasis

Patients with hypochondriasis are preoccupied with the idea that they have a serious medical condition when they do not. It may also be regarded as a form of anxiety disorder or of OCD. Patients repeatedly seek medical reassurance and investigation, but are not reassured by either.

• Repeated requests for investigation may be the presenting feature.

• Both antidepressants and CBT are effective. It may be necessary to help the patients to restrict their tendency to seek reassurance or check their bodies as this perpetuates the condition.

• The prognosis is variable: transient hypochondriasis is common (e.g. in medical students), but once established the condition can last many years and lead to extensive medical investigations.

Dysmorphophobia

Also called *body dysmorphic disorder*, the preoccupation is with a subjectively abnormal physical appearance (e.g. perceived ugliness or deformity) that is not objectively present and often associated with avoidance of social interaction.

• Management follows the principles described for somatoform disorder in general. Patients often request cosmetic surgery which may sometimes be helpful but which can lead also lead to further dissatisfaction. Specialist assessment is advisable before surgery is performed.

Somatic symptom disorders (somatization disorder and associated diagnoses)

Somatic symptoms such as fatigue and pain that are not associated with medical disease are common. When these are persistent and associated with disability and or distress they may appropriately be regarded as illnesses and consequently require a diagnosis. Such patients comprise about a third of all attenders in medical out-patient clinics, and so are clinically important (Chapter 18).

Confusingly, medicine and psychiatry have developed parallel diagnostic systems for these problems. Medicine uses diagnoses of functional disorders describing the symptoms in terms of the bodily system they relate to (see below). Psychiatry uses somatoform diagnoses based mainly on the number of symptoms and their duration. The current psychiatric classification is as follows, but note that it remains unclear how useful it is to differentiate between the diagnostic subtypes. They probably lie on a continuum.

Somatization disorder (Briquet's syndrome)

Patients, almost always women, present with multiple medically unexplained symptoms over many years. They have often had all removable abdominal organs surgically removed, an observation which highlights the risk of iatrogenic harm. They have been described as adopting 'illness as a way of life'. Recurrent major depression and personality disorder are common associations—indeed some regard the condition as a personality disorder.
• Management emphasizes 'damage limitation' and containment by long-term follow up rather than cure. There is no specific treatment but active treatment of associated recurrent depression and anxiety may be helpful.
• Prognosis is very poor. Iatrogenic problems, such as drug reactions and abdominal adhesions, may result from the many medical interventions.
• *Undifferentiated somatoform disorder* is used instead of somatization disorder when the patient has fewer symptoms.

Persistent somatoform pain disorder

This diagnosis is used when the main symptom is pain that is inadequately explained by a medical disease. Antidepressants are useful; TCAs and reboxetine are more effective than SSRIs.

Somatoform autonomic dysfunction

This is a rarely-used diagnosis for cases where the symptoms are thought to be clearly explicable in terms of autonomic arousal and associated overbreathing (e.g. breathlessness, chest pain, flushing, diarrhoea and tremor).

Functional somatic syndromes and their relation to somatoform disorders

The medical classification of functional somatic symptoms (Table 10.14) is parallel to the psychiatric classification of somatoform disorders. However, it should be noted that more than half of patients with a functional somatic syndrome satisfy criteria for depressive or anxiety disorder. Clearly if the right questions are not asked, this will not be diagnosed or treated, and the person may continue to be investigated unnecessarily. Of the patients with a functional somatic syndrome who do *not* have a depressive or anxiety disorder, most can be given a somatoform diagnosis (see Figure 18.2). Because the diagnostic systems overlap, but emphasize different aspects of the presentation, a combined diagnosis is preferred; for example irritable bowel syndrome and generalized

Table 10.14 Common functional somatic syndrome diagnoses.

Medically unexplained pain syndromes
Non-cardiac chest pain
Facial pain
Pelvic pain
Back pain
Irritable bowel syndrome
Muscular pain and fibromyalgia
Medically unexplained chronic fatigue
Chronic fatigue syndrome

anxiety disorder or chronic fatigue syndrome and somatization disorder.

- See the vignettes in Chapter 18.

Neurasthenia (chronic fatigue syndrome, CFS)

The term neurasthenia is now rarely used in the UK or USA but it remains in common usage in China and some other countries. There is substantial overlap with the functional syndrome of chronic fatigue syndrome (CFS). Although classified separately, it has much in common with somatoform disorders, in that physical complaints predominate, no definite medical disease has so far been identified, and the presentation is usually to non-psychiatric services. The main feature is persistent, disabling mental and physical fatigue, together with pain and other symptoms (Table 10.15).

The differential diagnosis is from fatigue associated with medical disorders and from depressive and anxiety disorders.

- There is evidence for the efficacy of CBT and graded increases in activity, but less for antidepressants.
- The prognosis is often poor with a tendency to chronicity. Avoidance of physical activity and excessive concern about its causation are associated with a worse outcome.
- The aetiology is very controversial. Both biological and psychological factors are probably involved. There is evidence for disturbed cerebral

Table 10.15 Symptoms of neurasthenia (chronic fatigue syndrome).

Component	Prominent features
Emotion	Exhaustion, tiredness, irritability
Cognitions	Concern about fatigue and its causes, poor concentration
Behaviour	Avoids physical exertion
Bodily symptoms	Physical and/or mental fatigue after minor exertion
	Muscular pain (myalgia)
	Headache
	Patchy sleep
Associations	Depression

5-HT function, social stress and inactivity. Although many patients report onset after a viral infection, and patients with documented EBV infection can develop a fatigue syndrome, the aetiological role of viruses in the majority of cases remains uncertain.

- A similar constellation of symptoms is also referred to as *myalgic encephalomyelitis (ME)*. This condition is thought by some to be better regarded as a neurological disorder and distinct from CFS, although this remains very controversial too.

Factitious disorders and malingering

The relationship between bodily symptoms and psychiatric disorder is complicated further by a final group of patients: those who consciously elaborate or even fabricate their symptoms. These conditions are not neuroses but are included here because of their importance in the differential diagnosis of patients presenting with somatic symptoms that are unexplained by medical disease. For example, someone may inject herself with insulin to produce hypoglycaemia, or collapse and claim they have chest pain radiating down their left arm.

- If the behaviour appears to be aimed principally at receiving medical treatment it is called *factitious disorder*. People with persistent, severe factitious disorder who travel from one hospital to another have been described as having *Munchausen's syndrome* (after Baron von Munchausen who told stories of fantastic exploits). The degree of conscious manipulation is often unclear. Little is known about the condition, which is usually viewed as a personality disorder.
- If such behaviour is for fraudulent purposes (e.g. to avoid legal proceedings or military conscription) it is referred to as *malingering*. Factitious disorder is regarded as a psychiatric disorder, but malingering is not.

If there is suspicion that symptoms are being manufactured, discrete but determined efforts to verify the person's details and history should be made. Once a factitious disorder has been confirmed, the patient should be gently confronted with the evidence. However sympathetically handled, a common response is verbal abuse and self-discharge. People with factitious disorder make doctors feel angry and manipulated—most doctors have been 'fooled' by a patient with Munchausen's syndrome. Take care not to generalize these negative feelings to the much larger group of patients who have medical problems the doctor cannot explain, yet in whom there is no evidence for simulation or exaggeration.

Depersonalization–derealization syndrome

Depersonalization and derealization (pp. 27 and 28) are symptoms of all neuroses. Occasionally they are the predominant feature, in which case this rarely used diagnostic category applies. The differential diagnosis is from a depressive or anxiety disorder, psychosis, and from organic causes, especially complex partial epilepsy. The usual guidelines for managing neurosis apply. Antidepressants may help, but the prognosis for established cases is said to be poor.

Key points
• The neuroses are syndromes of emotional, cognitive behavioural and somatic symptoms that are not secondary to another disorder. Neurotic symptoms occur commonly in other psychiatric disorders.
• Neuroses afflict 15% of the population, women more than men. They may become chronic and disabling. The main subtypes are anxiety disorders and somatoform disorders.
• Stress-related disorders are neuroses in which there is a clear relation to a major psychological stressor.
• Somatoform disorders encompass medically unexplained symptoms (somatization) and fears about having physical disease (hypochondriasis) and are closely related to neuroses. They are usually seen in non-psychiatric medical settings.
• Neuroses, stress-related disorders, and somatoform disorders can all be treated psychologically (especially with CBT) or with antidepressants. Anxiolytics can be useful in the short-term.

Chapter 11

Eating, sleep and sexual disorders

Disorders of eating, sleeping and sex are grouped together as they are syndromes associated with a disturbance in basic behaviours.

- Assessment of eating disorders was covered in a module (p. 30); assessment of sexual functioning is dealt with later in this chapter.

Eating disorders

All eating disorders share the same core features:
- A preoccupation and over-emphasis on body shape and weight. These thoughts are overvalued ideas, rather than delusions or obsessions.
- The use of extreme dietary restriction, often with other weight control behaviours (e.g. exercise, vomiting, laxatives).
- There is a significant impairment of physical health or psychosocial functioning.
- The problems are not secondary to a general medical disorder or other psychiatric condition.
- They occur mainly in young women.

Eating disorders are conventionally separated into *anorexia nervosa* and *bulimia nervosa*, as described below. However, bear two clinical realities in mind when reading the following sections:
- Many patients do not meet all the criteria for either disorder, or have some features of both. They are labelled *atypical eating disorder* (or *eating disorder not otherwise specified*) (Figure 11.1). This does not mean their disorder is any less severe.

- Many patients move from one category to another over time (Figure 11.2).

Anorexia nervosa

Clinical features

As well as the core features above, the key elements of anorexia nervosa are:
- *Deliberate weight loss*, induced primarily by restriction of food intake.
- *Weight ≥ 15% below normal* (BMI < 17.5).
- *Amenorrhoea* (if postmenarche and not on

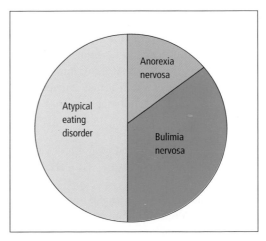

Figure 11.1 Relative prevalence of eating disorders in community samples.

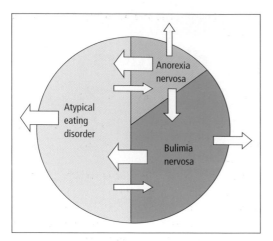

Figure 11.2 Patients move with time from one eating disorder to another. Size of arrows shows likelihood of movement; arrows outside circle indicate recovery.

Table 11.1 Physical features and medical complications of anorexia nervosa.

Physical symptoms
  Sensitivity to cold
  Gastrointestinal symptoms—constipation,
    bloatedness
  Dizziness
  Amenorrhoea
  Poor sleep

Physical signs
  Emaciation
  Cold extremities
  Dry skin, sometimes orange (hypercarotinaemia)
  Downy hair ('lanugo') on back, forearms, and cheeks
  Poorly developed or atrophic secondary sexual
    characteristics
  Bradycardia, postural hypotension, arrythmias
  Peripheral oedema
  Proximal myopathy

Abnormalities on investigation
  Low LH, FSH, oestradiol, T3
  Increased cortisol, growth hormone
  Hypoglycaemia
  Hypokalaemia, hyponatraemia, metabolic alkalosis
  ECG: prolonged QT interval (serious)
  Hypercholesterolaemia
  Osteopaenia and osteoporosis
  Delayed gastric emptying
  Acute gastric dilatation (due to over-rapid refeeding)

the pill). Part of a wider endocrine disturbance that includes elevated cortisol and growth hormone levels.

Additional features include:

• A range of bodily symptoms and signs, which get more pronounced as weight loss progresses (Table 11.1). The medical complications can be serious and life threatening, especially if the effects of starvation are exacerbated by the metabolic consequences of vomiting, or diuretic or laxative abuse.

• The core psychological features (e.g. 'fear of fatness') become paradoxically worse as weight is lost (maybe because it increases the 5-HT dysfunction which is thought to contribute to the disturbance). The disorder thus tends to be self-perpetuating—reinforced by the fact that achieving a lower weight has certain rewards: it may enhance feelings of self-control, result in approval from peers, avoid sexual development, or gain parental attention.

• Depressive and obsessional symptoms.

• If the onset is before puberty, secondary sexual development is delayed.

• Depression, fatigue and irritability, especially as weight loss becomes pronounced.

• Social withdrawal and narrowing of interests.

• Use of diuretics, laxatives, excess exercise or self-induced vomiting to enhance weight loss.

Miss T, 14, was noticed to be losing weight although this was partially disguised by baggy clothing. She enjoyed cooking for the family and took up regular aerobics. She became vegetarian and avoided all fattening foods. When the issue of her weight was raised, Miss T became upset, insisting that she was fat. She had a history of obesity. The GP found she was underweight (BMI = 14) and suspected anorexia nervosa.

Epidemiology and aetiology

Anorexia mainly affects females (sex ratio 10:1). The average age of onset is 15–16 years. The prevalence in Western societies, including the UK, is about 1% in females aged 12–18. Social pressure to be thin has been blamed. The other risk factors are summarized in Table 11.2.

- Note that most risk factors are shared with bulimia nervosa.
- The familial risk of anorexia nervosa does not seem to be genetic in origin (in contrast to most other psychiatric disorders).

Differential diagnosis

The classic picture of anorexia nervosa is unmistakeable. In the early stages it must be distinguished from other causes of weight loss. The psychiatric differential diagnosis includes depressive disorder, substance misuse, OCD and body dysmorphic disorder. The medical disorders include inflammatory bowel disease, malabsorption syndromes, hypopituitarism and cancer. The distinction is made by:

- Detecting the core psychological symptoms of anorexia nervosa.

Table 11.2 Risk factors for eating disorders.

General factors
   Female (sex ratio ~10 : 1)
   Adolescence and early adulthood
   Living in a Western society

Family history
   Eating disorder
   Depression
   Substance misuse (bulimia nervosa)
   Obesity (bulimia nervosa)

Premorbid experiences
   Adverse parenting—low contact, high expectations, arguments
   Sexual abuse
   Family dieting
   Critical comments about eating, weight or shape
   Pressure to be slim

Premorbid characteristics
   Low self-esteem
   Perfectionism (anorexia nervosa)
   Anxiety
   Obesity (bulimia nervosa)
   Early menarche (bulimia nervosa)

- Excluding physical and other psychiatric causes of weight loss.

Management

The objectives of treatment of anorexia nervosa are:

- Altering the person's attitude to weight and body shape via psychological treatments.
- Helping them increase weight.
- Detecting and treating medical complications.

The second and third components can be achieved reasonably successfully, at least in the short term; the first component is difficult as the core beliefs are often resistant to treatment. Some principles of management are:

- Establish a good therapeutic relationship—many patients are reluctant to accept treatment. Help them to see they need help, and maintain motivation thereafter. Agree some goals: what weight is the person prepared to work towards? At what rate? How much exercise is appropriate?
- Encourage early weight gain to break the cycle and to overcome the problem that starvation interferes with psychological treatments. Weight gain is promoted by behavioural strategies, e.g. contingent rewards.
- The key element of therapy is to change attitudes towards weight and shape, and the person's preoccupation with them. Family therapy may be useful for younger patients. A tailored form of CBT has been developed, and is being trialled. Previously, psychodynamic approaches were used. No therapy has been proven to be effective.
- Drugs (antidepressants or antipsychotics) do not have an established role in management, though they are sometimes used to promote or maintain weight gain, or treat depressive symptoms.
- Monitor physical condition. Serum potassium should be checked regularly.

In-patient treatment

In-patient care is indicated if weight loss is intractable and severe (e.g. weight <65% of normal), or if there is a serious risk of death from suicide or medical complications. Admission is preferably to a specialist unit. It usually lasts 8–12 weeks. The purposes are to:

- Manage medical complications.
- Actively encourage re-feeding—ensuring a balanced diet of 3000 calories per day.
- Allow intensive psychological treatments. Compulsory admission is rarely used, and considered only if life is in immediate danger. Forced re-feeding is also used occasionally and controversially.

Miss T is now 15 and has collapsed. For the past year, despite denials to her parents, she had eaten less than 1000 calories/day. She weighed 27 kg (BMI = 12), was hypothermic and had a low blood potassium. After medical stabilization she passively accepted admission to an eating disorder unit. She began a behavioural programme with a target to gain 0.5 kg/week for 2 months. A psychiatrist and nurse therapist explored eating and weight issues in individual and family sessions. Her potassium was monitored regularly. Ten weeks later her BMI was 15 and she became an out-patient.

Prognosis

The outcome of anorexia nervosa is variable. About 20% have a good outcome, with a short-lived disorder and full recovery. Another 10–20% develop a chronic and intractable disorder. The rest progress to another eating disorder, have a relapsing illness, or have residual features (Figure 11.2).

- The mortality rate is increased 10-fold in the first 10 years of illness, with 10–20% death rate in long-term follow-up studies. Death is usually from complications of starvation, sometimes from suicide.
- Poor outcome is associated with: long duration prior to presentation; onset in adulthood; severe weight loss; vomiting.

Miss T is now 27 and a beautician. She has a BMI of ~16 and has occasional scanty menstrual periods. She continues to be preoccupied with her appearance, and gains self-esteem from her control over eating and weight. She diets continually and works out twice a day. Now and then she has a large binge followed by self-induced vomiting and extra gym sessions. She avoids doctors.

Bulimia nervosa

Bulimia refers to uncontrolled eating binges. Many people binge and feel bad about it, but in bulimia nervosa it is excessive, repetitive, and associated with self-induced vomiting and other means to negate the calorific effect of the binges. It punctuates an otherwise anorexia nervosa-like pattern of dietary restriction.

Clinical features

In addition to the core features of eating disorder:

- Recurrent binge eating (more than twice a week); 1000–4000 kcal (4–8 MJ) are typically consumed in a binge.
- 'Loss of control' during binges.
- Attempts to counteract the binges by vomiting, or by using other means such as laxatives, enemas, diuretics or excessive exercise.
- Does not meet diagnostic criteria for anorexia nervosa.
- The combination of dieting and bingeing means body weight is usually unremarkable—the most obvious difference from anorexia nervosa.
- A small proportion of bulimia nervosa occurs in women with borderline personality disorder who self-harm (often by cutting) and misuse alcohol or drugs. This is a much rarer combination than sometimes believed.

If body weight is decreased, some of the physical features and complications of anorexia nervosa may be present (Table 11.1). Otherwise, fewer abnormalities are seen in bulimia nervosa. Those which are reflect the self-induced vomiting, or abuse of laxatives or diuretics:

- Repeated vomiting may produce pitted teeth (eroded by gastric acid), calluses on knuckles (from putting fingers down throat), hoarse voice, salivary gland enlargement, metabolic disturbances (Table 11.1).
- Diuretic use: electrolyte disturbances and renal dysfunction.
- Laxatives: electrolyte disturbances and colonic motility problems.

Epidemiology and aetiology

Bulimia nervosa occurs in 2% of women aged 16–35 years but is otherwise rare. Only 10% of cases ever present for help. Many of the risk factors are shared with anorexia nervosa (Table 11.2). There is a genetic predisposition, which overlaps with that for anxiety disorders.
• The genetic contribution to bulimia nervosa is controversial. Some studies suggest a surprisingly large heritability—over 80%.

> Miss V is 23. She has several episodes of bingeing and vomiting each week. In an hour she can eat 10 packets of crisps, 10 chocolate bars and a couple of loaves of bread washed down with a bottle of wine. She then makes herself sick. She is preoccupied with her weight and shape and feels fat (though her BMI is normal). She has a history of taking overdoses when particularly distressed. She was obese as a child, and sexually abused by an uncle. There is a family history of obesity and depression.

Differential diagnosis

• Anorexia nervosa with bulimic features (anorexia trumps bulimia, diagnostically).
• Sporadic bingeing in other psychiatric disorders (e.g. atypical depression).
• Medical causes of vomiting.
• Binge eating disorder—a controversial (American) category. Recurrent binges occur but without extreme weight control behaviour. Strongly associated with obesity. Compared to bulimia nervosa, is more common in men (a third of cases) and in middle age.

Management

Treatments are markedly more effective (and better evaluated) than in anorexia nervosa. Take a 'stepped care' approach, depending on the severity of the problem and the patient's wishes.
• Self-help manuals are a cost-effective and increasingly used first-line treatment.
• A modified form of CBT is effective in 60–70% of patients, with the majority remaining well 5 years later. CBT aims to help the patient: (a) understand the links between bingeing, vomiting and dieting; (b) regulate their diet and break the vicious cycle between the three behaviours; and (c) decrease their preoccupation with body shape.
• Interpersonal therapy (IPT) also works, but takes longer. IPT emphasizes the role of relationship problems in the disorder.
• Antidepressants reduce the frequency of bingeing and vomiting. The best evidence is for fluoxetine. High doses (60–80 mg/day) may be required and the disorder often relapses on stopping.

Prognosis

The prognosis of bulimia nervosa is probably better than that of anorexia nervosa (the mortality rate is certainly lower), though there are few good data.
• People have had bulimia nervosa for an average of 5 years at presentation; 30–50% still have an eating disorder (bulimia nervosa or atypical eating disorder) 5–10 years later.
• Poor prognostic factors include: childhood obesity, low self esteem, personality disturbance.

Sleep disorders

Sleep problems are usually secondary to a psychiatric or medical disorder, but sometimes a sleep disorder is the primary diagnosis.

Insomnia

Assessment

Insomnia describes a persistently unsatisfactory quantity or quality of sleep. A quarter of adults complain of it. It causes much distress and is a risk factor for premature death; 80% of cases of insomnia are related to anxiety and depressive disorders. Most of the rest are secondary to medical disease, chronic pain and substance misuse. The remaining fraction (<10%) are *primary insomnia*. To distinguish these cases, exclude the presence of an underlying psychiatric or medical disorder (e.g. restless legs syndrome, lymphoma). Ask about other factors that affect sleep such as shift working, medication, alcohol, caffeine, etc. A sleep diary and corroboration from the sleeping partner are helpful.

Treatment

Treat any associated disorder (e.g. use a sedative antidepressant if insomnia is due to depression). Interventions for insomnia include:

- *Stimulus control.* An effective method to restore a good sleep routine. The person should go to bed only when sleepy, put the light out straight away, get up if awake for more than 20 minutes, get up at a regular time and avoid daytime naps.
- *Sleep hygiene*—this approach pays attention to health practices (e.g. use of caffeine and alcohol) and stimuli (e.g. noise, light) that affect sleep.
- *Relaxation therapy*—behavioural, cognitive and biofeedback routines to reduce arousal. The person should wind down 90 minutes before bedtime and to practice relaxation when in bed.
- *Hypnotics*—short-acting benzodiazepines and related drugs (p. 63). Effective in the short-term and widely used, but may cause daytime drowsiness and long-term use should be avoided because of dependence.

Hypersomnia

Hypersomnia is excessive daytime sleepiness, or having a prolonged time in the twilight zone between sleep and wakefulness. The term excludes cases secondary to insomnia or where there are clear reasons for such behaviour (e.g. shift working). Causes are shown in Table 11.3.

- In *narcolepsy* there are repeated attacks of daytime somnolence usually leading irresistibly to sleep. It usually begins in the second decade and is associated with *cataplexy* (abrupt loss of muscle tone), *hypnagogic hallucinations* (p. 12), and *sleep paralysis* (the patient wakes but is unable to move); 98% have the DR15 variant of HLA-DR2. Stimulants (amphetamines or modafinil) are the main treatment; clomipramine is also used for the cataplexy.

Table 11.3 Causes of hypersomnia.

Psychiatric disorders
  Depressive disorder
  Neuraesthenia (chronic fatigue syndrome)

Medical disorders
  Narcolepsy
  Klein–Levin syndrome
  Sleep apnoea syndrome
  Chronic physical disease

Other
  Side-effects of drugs (prescribed or illicit)

Parasomnias

Parasomnias are abnormal episodic events during sleep—sleepwalking, nightmares, etc. They are part of normal development in children; in adults they usually reflect emotional stress.

- Distinguish parasomnias from other causes of odd nocturnal behaviour, such as epilepsy.

Sexual problems

An understanding of sexual problems and how to assess them is important in psychiatry because:

- Sexual dysfunction is a common consequence of psychiatric disorders or their treatment. For example, loss of libido in depression; ejaculatory failure due to antipsychotics.
- Sexual dysfunction may contribute to psychiatric disorder. For example, an anxiety disorder may be exacerbated by a man worrying about his impotence.
- Disorders of sexual function, preference and identity are specific mental disorders.

Sexual dysfunction

Each of the components of sex—desire, physiological arousal, and orgasm—can go awry (Table 11.4). Each type of dysfunction may be due to psychological or medical causes or both.

- Painful intercourse, loss of sexual desire and impaired orgasm are commoner in women; the main problems for men are impotence and premature ejaculation.

Table 11.4 Types of sexual dysfunction.

Sexual desire disorders
   Lack of
   Excess

Failure of genital response
   Erectile dysfunction (impotence)
   Vaginal dryness

Orgasmic dysfunction
   Premature ejaculation
   Anorgasmia

Other
   Vaginismus (involuntary spasm of vaginal
      musculature)
   Dyspareunia

- Sexual dysfunction is associated with sexual inexperience, anxiety and relationship problems.

Assessment of sexual dysfunction

Asking about sex is the topic, along with suicide, which most health professionals feel least confident and most embarrassed about. This is unnecessary. Many patients are glad to be asked, since sexual problems are common and it may be their first opportunity to seek reassurance or treatment.

- Know when to introduce the subject—try and respond to cues. For example, if a depressed patient tells you he gets no pleasure from life, it is a good moment to ask whether this has also affected his interest in sex. If no cue presents itself, preface the assessment with a comment such as: 'I need to ask you some questions about your sex life, to help me understand X . . . Is this alright?'.
- Use terminology appropriate to the person's age and culture.

Assessment of sexual function covers several areas (Table 11.5). Some of the questions will be used regularly, others rarely. Below are further details of two common sexual disorders to illustrate the general approaches to assessment and treatment of sexual dysfunction.

Erectile dysfunction

Erectile dysfunction is the inability to reach erection or to sustain an erection long enough for intercourse. Most erectile dysfunction is secondary—that is, full erection was possible at one time, but is now difficult to achieve. Primary erectile dysfunction is rare and usually has a neurological or circulatory basis.

Common causes of impotence include:
- Anxiety about sexual performance.
- Alcohol.
- Unwanted effects of prescription medicines.
- Diabetes.
- Vascular disease.

Treatment is usually with combined psychological and physical approaches. Underlying disorders should be treated. Psychological treatment is outlined below. Drug treatment with sildenafil (Viagra) and related drugs is increasingly popular and has largely replaced injections and devices.

- Prescribing of sildenafil for 'psychological' impotence is possible on the NHS but restricted.
- Sildenafil works by inhibiting phosphodiesterase type V.

Dyspareunia

Dyspareunia is pain on intercourse. It may result from impaired lubrication with vaginal secretions (due to anxiety or inadequate arousal) or from physical scarring (e.g. after childbirth). Pain on penetration may be due to pelvic pathology.

- When dyspareunia is secondary to psychological factors, sexual therapy techniques can be used (see below).

Psychological treatment of sexual dysfunction

Sexual problems may respond to reassurance or use of self-help manuals. Others require sex therapy, which is provided by some psychiatrists and by private therapists. Sex therapy uses behavioural methods, and is effective (assuming no underlying medical cause for the dysfunction). The principles are:

Table 11.5 Assessment of sexual function.

Questions	Comments
Current sexual functioning	
What is the nature and frequency of sex?	
Is there a particular problem?	Get a history of each difficulty
How much interest do you have in sex? Has this changed recently?	Increased libido is rarely complained of; occurs in mania
In men	
Erectile function:	
Any problems getting or keeping an erection?	
Do you get erections in the morning?	Loss of morning erections or when masturbating suggests medical cause
Do you worry about your sexual performance?	Impotence is often associated with performance anxiety
Ejaculatory function:	
Do you come too quickly? How long after penetration?	Common in inexperienced, anxious men
Do you feel anxious about this?	
In women	
Do you have pain on intercourse? When? Where?	Dyspareunia and vaginal dryness have psychological and gynaecological causes
Do you feel anxious or tense about sex?	Extreme anxiety can lead to vaginismus
Sexual development	
Estimate age of puberty	
When did your voice break? Periods start?	Problems or delays in sexual development may lead to psychological effects or indicate an abnormality (e.g. Turner's syndrome)
When did you first masturbate? First intercourse?	Affected by cultural and individual differences
Sexual orientation and preferences	
What is their sexual orientation?	
Does he have particular sexual preferences or fetishes? If so, what?	Detailed questioning indicated if the patient views it as a problem, or in a forensic context
Have they ever got you into trouble?	
Other issues	
Current psychiatric disorder?	Most psychiatric disorders, especially depression, are associated with sexual dysfunction
General health?	Medical disorders (e.g. diabetes, vascular disease) affect sexual functioning; do physical exam
Current medication?	Many drugs have sexual side-effects

- Treat the couple together.
- Educate about sex and the factors affecting it.
- Encourage open discussion of feelings and decrease anxiety and embarrassment.
- Use graded exposure (p. 73). The couple gradually rebuild their sexual relationship, setting aside time and commitment to follow a series of steps—starting with non-genital 'sensate focus', then moving on via genital focus before finally returning to full intercourse. Additional methods are used for specific forms of dysfunction. For example, dilators for vaginismus, the squeeze technique for premature ejaculation.
- Lack of sexual desire has the worst prognosis.

Other sexual disorders

In these disorders the problem is not sex itself but the object of sexual desire—at least to the extent that it conflicts with society or causes harm. The person may or may not agree with this view. In ICD-10, these disorders are grouped with personality disorders.

- Forensic psychiatrists may be asked to report on the psychiatric status of sex offenders.
- Homosexuality used to be classified as a psychiatric disorder.

Gender identity disorders

- In *transsexualism* the person, usually male, wishes to live as a member of the opposite sex. They seek hormonal or surgical treatment to match their body to their subjective gender. Sexual orientation is variable and sexual desire often low. Transsexuals may suffer great distress, and depression is common.
- *Transvestism* is the urge to dress in clothes of the opposite sex. If accompanied by sexual arousal it is called *fetishistic* transvestism. There is no desire to change sex. Transvestites are often married and cross dress secretly. There is no specific treatment.

Disorders of sexual preference (paraphilias)

Sexual desire can centre on a wide range of animate and inanimate objects. Such pleasures only constitute a disorder if the activity is illegal (e.g. paedophilia) or if sex becomes dysfunctional and over-dependent on an object such as shoes (e.g. fetishism). Paraphilia is almost exclusively a male disorder.

- In *paedophilia*, sexual interest or activity centres on prepubescent children. The prevalence is unknown, though there is a considerable demand for child pornography. Psychological treatments have been used to reduce reoffending rates; cyproterone acetate, an antiandrogen, has been used to suppress libido. The effectiveness of these treatments is uncertain.
- *Exhibitionism* is the exposing of the genitals to strangers. Two groups are recognized: (1) inhibited men who struggle against the urge, feel guilty and expose a flaccid penis (type 1); (2) aggressive men who expose an erect penis and masturbate then or later (type 2). The latter shows an association with actual sexual assaults. Behavioural treatments may be beneficial.

Key points

- The core psychopathology of all eating disorders is an over-emphasis on body shape and weight, with extreme methods to control weight—notably dietary restriction. They occur mainly but not exclusively in young women.
- Anorexia nervosa is characterized additionally by a low body weight (BMI < 17.5), extreme dietary restriction, and amenorrhoea in women.
- Bulimia nervosa is distinguished by recurrent binge eating and self-induced vomiting.
- Half of patients with an eating disorder do not meet criteria for anorexia or bulimia nervosa.
- Bulimia nervosa responds well to CBT. No effective treatments are proven for anorexia nervosa.
- Sleep disorders comprise insomnia, hypersomnia, and parasomnias (disturbances during sleep). Many are secondary to other psychiatric or medical disorders. They may be treated psychologically or pharmacologically.
- Sexual dysfunction is common and can affect the desire, the mechanics, or the orgasm. Assessment of sexual function is important. Sex therapy is effective for many of the problems.

Chapter 12

Schizophrenia

Historically, schizophrenia has been at the heart of psychiatry and is closest to the public conception of madness. Although by no means the commonest disorder, it accounts for a significant proportion of psychiatric morbidity and the workload of psychiatric services.

- Patients with schizophrenia occupy 25% of psychiatric beds, and account for 50% of admissions.
- Direct U.K. health costs in 1996 were £2.6 billion.
- It is in the top ten causes of worldwide disability.

Clinical features

Schizophrenia is a psychosis, typically presenting in young adults. It is distinguished from other psychoses by:

- The presence of specific types of delusions, hallucinations, and thought disorder.
- The absence of a mood disorder or organic psychosis.
- The clinical course.

The clinical picture of schizophrenia is complex. Here, the acute and the chronic stages of the disorders are described in turn—though in practice there is a continuum of features.

- Before proceeding, review the relevant parts of the core assessment (p. 10) and the psychosis module (p. 18). These earlier sections include definitions of the cardinal symptoms.

Clinical features of acute schizophrenia

The diagnostic features are shown in Table 12.1. Particular weight is placed on the presence of the first-rank symptoms (Table 3.2). The diagnosis does not require a certain number of features being present, but the more there are, the more likely schizophrenia becomes.

- The predominant features vary from case to case. At one extreme, a person may present with bizarre behaviour, a full house of first-rank symptoms, and florid thought disorder. At the other, the most notable symptoms may be insidious social withdrawal and academic decline, with psychotic symptoms only becoming apparent after direct questioning or observation.
- The duration criterion is to exclude transient schizophrenia-like syndromes that have a better prognosis, and maybe a different aetiology. If the features of schizophrenia are present but for less than a month, the (temporary) label is *schizophreniform disorder*.
- Schizophrenia beginning after age 45 used to be considered a separate disorder, *paraphrenia*.
- Delusions, hallucinations and thought disorder in schizophrenia are grouped together as *positive symptoms* (in contrast to *negative symptoms*, described below).

Clinical subtypes of schizophrenia

Because of the clinical heterogeneity, schizophrenia has classically been divided into several subsyndromes, based upon the pattern of symptoms (Table 12.2).

- The catatonic subtype is rarer than it used to be. This could reflect a change in the nature or treatment of the disease, or the past occurrence of organic disorders mistaken for schizophrenia (particularly a postviral condition called encephalitis lethargica).

Table 12.1 Clinical features of acute schizophrenia.

Characteristic symptoms
  First-rank symptoms
    Thought insertion, echo, withdrawal or
      broadcasting
    Third person auditory hallucinations
    Running commentary
    Passivity of thought, feelings or action
    Delusional perception
  Bizarre delusions
  Odd behaviour
  Thought disorder
  Lack of insight (reality distortion)
  Prodromal period of decline in performance and
    social withdrawal

Duration criterion
  Symptoms present for at least 1 month

Major exclusion criteria
  Not secondary to mood disorder
  No demonstrable organic cause (e.g. amphetamines,
    temporal lobe epilepsy)

- The disorganized subtype is also called hebephrenic schizophrenia.

Mr J is a 20-year-old student found having a conversation with imaginary demons. His room was covered in black paper to stop them interfering with his thoughts. His work had deteriorated markedly in the past term, and he had isolated himself. He was convinced he was part of a sinister plot and was being told what to do by unknown people whom he could hear talking about him. There was no evidence of substance misuse or mood disorder. A provisional diagnosis of paranoid schizophrenia was made.

Clinical features of chronic schizophrenia

In patients who progress to chronic schizophrenia, the acute symptoms have often largely resolved (with or without treatment). The characteristic picture becomes one of a 'burnt out' disease (Table 12.3). These features are called *negative symptoms*.

- The positive–acute/negative–chronic distinction is not absolute. Positive symptoms regularly persist or re-emerge in chronic cases and some patients have negative symptoms in their first episode.
- Prominent, enduring negative symptoms are sometimes called *deficit syndrome*.
- *Residual schizophrenia* is a transitional state between acute and chronic schizophrenia. It describes patients with positive symptoms within the past year who have also developed negative symptoms.
- Research has shown that the symptoms of chronic schizophrenia fall more clearly into three

Table 12.2 Subtypes of acute schizophrenia.

Subtype	Predominant symptoms	Other features
Paranoid	Persecutory, systematized delusions	Commonest form
	Hallucinations, usually auditory	Personality relatively preserved
Disorganized	Thought disorder	Early onset
	Odd behaviour	Poor prognosis
	Fleeting, bizarre delusions	Premorbid schizoid or schizotypal personality
	Labile or inappropriate mood	
Catatonic	Motor signs	Now rare in developed countries
Undifferentiated	A mixture of the above	

Table 12.3 Features of chronic schizophrenia.

Negative symptoms
Flattened (blunted) mood
Apathy and loss of drive (avolition)
Social isolation
Poverty of speech
Poor self-care

Other features
Positive symptoms persist or recur at times of stress
Mild cognitive impairment is common

clusters, rather than the two implied by the positive–negative distinction. The three are *reality distortion* (delusions and hallucinations), *disorganization* (thought disorder) and *psychomotor poverty* (similar to negative symptoms).

> *Mr J is now 45. He has had multiple admissions. Between episodes, he never regained his previous level of functioning; by 35 he was living in a group home. He spends most of his time in his room or walking the streets, often mumbling to himself. He has no specific complaints or desires. His last admission was a year ago when hallucinations recurred following a fellow resident's suicide.*

Cognitive impairment in schizophrenia

Memory problems are a neglected aspect of schizophrenia. The profile is, as with everything about schizophrenia, complex.
• The most affected domains are attention, working memory and semantic memory. These deficits are superimposed on a generalized intellectual deficit averaging about one standard deviation — though there is a wide range, and many patients score above normal.
• The impairments are, like the negative symptoms, basically stable and independent of the positive symptoms. However, the details are controversial. Some decline probably occurs well before the onset of illness, with a further decline around the first episode. There is then a long period of stability, before deterioration in later life such that a significant minority of elderly patients with schizophrenia have moderate to severe de-

mentia (which is not explained by any known neuropathological process).

The neuropsychological deficits of schizophrenia are thought to be central to the syndrome, and important for three reasons:
• They are a major determinant of poor functional outcome, along with negative symptoms.
• They may underlie the psychotic symptoms. By this view, psychosis is the 'fever' of schizophrenia — a problem which requires treatment, but which is non-specific and downstream of the disease process.
• They are potential targets for treatment.

Differential diagnosis

Acute schizophrenia

Acute schizophrenia must be distinguished from other psychotic disorders (Table 12.4).
• Drug-induced psychoses (Chapter 14) pose a particular problem. At least a third of people with schizophrenia misuse alcohol or drugs, and it can be difficult, and sometimes arbitrary, deciding whether these constitute the 'cause' of their symptoms. Judgement is based on the timing, quantity and type of substances taken.
• The organic disorders which can produce an acute schizophrenic picture (sometimes called *symptomatic schizophrenia)* are collectively common enough — about 1 in 20 cases — to require a high index of suspicion, especially if aspects of the case are atypical.

Chronic schizophrenia

In chronic schizophrenia the diagnosis itself is rarely in doubt, though occasionally neurological syndromes (e.g. a leukodystrophy) can mimic the clinical picture.
• A more common problem is to distinguish negative symptoms from depression or from the sedative and parkinsonian effects of antipsychotics (p. 64)

Investigations in schizophrenia

Schizophrenia is a clinical diagnosis. Physical

Table 12.4 Differential diagnosis of acute schizophrenia.

Category of disorder	Distinguishing features/examples
Other non-organic disorders	
Delusional disorders	Absence of specific features of schizophrenia; preserved personality
Psychotic depression	Prominent depressive symptoms
Manic episode	Prominent manic symptoms
Schizoaffective disorder	Mood and schizophrenia symptoms both prominent
Schizotypal disorder	Nature of symptoms; chronic history
Puerperal psychosis	Acute onset after childbirth
Organic disorders	
Drug-induced psychosis	History of drug or alcohol misuse
Side-effects of therapeutic drugs	Levodopa, methyldopa, steroids, antimalarial drugs
Complex partial epilepsy	Other evidence of seizures
Delirium	Acute onset; clouding of consciousness
Dementia	Age; established cognitive impairment
Huntington's disease	Family history; choreiform movements; dementia
Systemic lupus erythematosus	Skin and renal involvement
Syphilis	Other evidence of infection

investigations are mainly used to rule out the organic disorders in Table 12.4, and are chosen according to the features elicited in the history and examination.

• Brain imaging is not routine. It should be considered if there are neurological symptoms or signs.

Management of schizophrenia

The management of schizophrenia is considered according to the stage of the illness (acute *vs.* chronic) and then by the intervention (physical, psychological, social).

Management of acute schizophrenia

The key elements are summarized in Table 12.5.

• Admission for assessment is usual. Compulsory admission may be needed, since patients are at risk from neglect or dangerous acts. Ideally, there should be several days of drug-free observation; this is rarely feasible due to shortage of beds or because the behaviour is too disturbed.

• Antipsychotics are effective against positive symptoms in a majority of patients over 2–3 weeks. Their onset is gradual; in the early stages, if behaviour is difficult to manage or the patient is very distressed, add a benzodiazepine.

• Investigate the context of the disorder, as it may give clues as to its development and prognosis. For example, comorbid substance misuse worsens outcome and may require intervention.

• Involve the family. Relatives need support and explanation, and they may be directly involved in therapy.

• First admissions can last many weeks depending on progress and external factors (e.g. finding accommodation). Future management is planned at predischarge CPA meetings (p. 82).

• Following an acute episode, *postschizophrenic depression* is common, and may require treatment with antidepressants.

Early intervention programmes

There is a trend to try and intervene earlier in

Table 12.5 Components in the management of acute schizophrenia.

Intervention	Rationale
Admission	For diagnosis, investigation, and starting treatment
Antipsychotic drugs	Treatment of positive symptoms
Benzodiazepines	For sedation
Establish context of disorder	
Evaluate current personal circumstances	} To guide management—accommodation, work, etc.
Assessment of needs and of risk	
Education of patient and family	Improve understanding and treatment adherence

Table 12.6 Components in the management of chronic schizophrenia.

Intervention	Rationale
Coordinated community care	Ensure medical and social needs are met
Maintenance of antipsychotic medication	Prevent relapse
Readmission during severe relapses	Stabilize mental state and review management
Family therapy for high expressed emotion	Prevent relapse
Social skills training	Improve social functioning
CBT	Reduce residual symptoms
Compliance therapy	Improve medication compliance
Supported employment	Financial, social and self-esteem benefits
Deal with drug or alcohol problems	Improve outcome
Illness management skills training	Help coping with chronic illness
General medical care	High risk of poor physical health

schizophrenia—before symptoms become severe, and even during the prodrome before unequivocal psychotic symptoms have emerged. Early intervention services are being set up to identify, engage and treat individuals at these times. The rationale is that longer duration of untreated psychosis predicts poor outcome, and thus earlier intervention may improve it. Though preliminary, there is some evidence that early intervention, either with cognitive therapy or antipsychotics, may decrease the transition to 'full' psychosis.

The management of chronic schizophrenia

After a first episode of schizophrenia, the aims are to prevent relapse, and to optimize level of func-

tioning. To do this, a combination of pharmacological, psychological and social methods is used (Table 12.6).

• The amount of support and treatments needed varies markedly depending on the course and severity of the disorder—and, in practice, whether the intervention is available. The emphasis here is on cases where full recovery has not occurred after the first episode.

• The most important specific intervention is antipsychotic medication, which reduces the rate of relapse in the 2 years after an episode from 70% to 50%. Even the benefits of psychological and family interventions operate partly by improving treatment adherence. Equally, however, a sustained relationship must be established with the patient and due attention paid to their 'problems of living'. Without this commitment, the patient is unlikely to adhere to the management plan—bear in mind that over 50% of patients do not take their antipsychotics regularly.

- The value of a multidisciplinary approach is apparent from the range of patients' needs—benefits, accommodation, employment, physical health, etc. The nature of the disorder, especially the effect of negative symptoms, makes people with chronic schizophrenia vulnerable in all these areas.

- Patients with schizophrenia have high risks of type II diabetes and cardiovascular disease, contributing to their excess mortality. The reasons are unclear, but probably include genetic predisposition, medication, poor diet and lack of exercise. Regular medical review and investigations (e.g. for diabetes, lipids, blood pressure) should be an integral part of management.

Modes of treatment

Antipsychotic drugs

After a single episode of schizophrenia, continue antipsychotic medication for 12–24 months. If the person remains well it should then be tailed off because there is little evidence that further medication is beneficial and because of the risk of tardive dyskinesia and other long-term side-effects. Patients who have had multiple episodes or persistent symptoms usually remain on medication for many years, though the need for it (and the effect of cautious reductions in dose) should remain under regular review. Medication is often given in depot form because of the poor adherence.

- See p. 64 for detailed coverage of antipsychotics.
- Clozapine has an important role in patients poorly responsive to, or intolerant of, other antipsychotics. It may also decrease risk of suicide.
- Avoid routine coadministration of anticholinergic agents.
- Persistent negative symptoms are not improved by antipsychotics, even clozapine. Conversely, it is a myth that the drugs cause them. Similarly, medication has little overall effect, for better or worse, on the cognitive symptoms, although atypical antipsychotics may produce small improvements.

Other physical treatments

- Benzodiazepines are useful for short-term sedation.
- Antidepressants should be used in the normal fashion for depression occurring in schizophrenia.
- ECT is not effective, except for catatonic stupor.

Psychological treatments

Table 12.6 includes a range of psychological treatments. The two most widely used specific interventions are a form of family therapy, and CBT for residual symptoms. In addition to these specific interventions, remember that a supportive psychotherapeutic relationship is an integral part of management (as with every chronic illness).

The family approach arose from the finding that patients living with families who have *high expressed emotion* (EE) had a much higher chance of relapse than those exposed to low EE. EE is the intensity and amount of emotional involvement by the family with the patient. It was then found that high EE families could be taught to lower EE, and relapse rates fell. Family therapy focuses on education about the illness and by changing the behaviour of the family. A recent systematic review confirms its (modest) effectiveness, but it has been difficult to implement widely because of practical and financial constraints (e.g. relatives are often out at work).

- The converse of high EE—a lack of stimulation—is also harmful as it exacerbates the apathy and withdrawal of chronic schizophrenia. This was first documented in institutionalized patients (and contributed to the drive to close the asylums).

CBT has some efficacy against auditory hallucinations and delusions, and is being adopted as an integral component of schizophrenia management, especially for the treatment of residual symptoms. However, it effect is rather small, the proven benefits are only short-term, and not all patients are able or willing to engage in treatment.

● Hallucinations can also benefit from simple practical manoeuvres—e.g. use of ear plugs or personal stereos.

Social interventions

The nature of chronic schizophrenia means that many patients have problems with daily living. These needs should be identified and met by the multidisciplinary team working through the care programme approach (Table 12.6). Assertive outreach teams (p. 83) are intended to maintain close contact with patients. The reality is, however, that some patients slip through the net, with occasionally tragic consequences.

● Some patients cannot live alone or with their family. *Group homes* are houses where several patients live together, supported by their key worker and the group homes organization.

Ms C is a 28 year old factory worker who has had one episode of schizophrenia. She was discharged home under the care of her CMHT on a depot. A CPN visited to monitor progress, give medication, and advise the parents about how best to interact with Ms C. After discussion with her employers, Ms C returned to work part-time but 3 months later she refused medication and began smoking cannabis. She relapsed, lost her job, and her behaviour became unmanageable. She was readmitted. Once her condition had settled, a meeting was held between Ms C, her parents and the CMHT. Ms C was offered a place in a group home. She agreed to take medication regularly. She was found sheltered employment in a charity shop. The CMHT social worker helped sort out Ms C's financial problems and ensured that she got her benefits.

Prognosis

Accurate estimates for the long-term outcome of schizophrenia are surprisingly hard to obtain, because the diagnostic criteria have changed over time and because they depend on how recovery is defined. For example, some patients have persistent symptoms but live a reasonably normal life; others are functionally impaired despite minimal symptoms. Taking both symptoms and functioning into account, only about a third of cases have the stereotyped chronic, deteriorating course; a quarter have a very good outcome; and the remaining half have a relapsing, remitting illness (Figure 12.1).

● At least 1 in 20 commit suicide. Previous estimates were higher. The risk is higher after an acute episode, when the patient may have realized the nature of his disorder and its implications, and may have developed a depressive disorder.

● There is an increased mortality from natural causes too, especially cardiovascular disease, though rates of some cancers are lower than expected.

Poor outcome factors are shown in Table 12.7. However they are only weak predictors and it is impossible to foresee which category in Figure 12.1 someone presenting with schizophrenia will end up in.

● First-rank symptoms have no prognostic significance.

● The outcome of schizophrenia is better in developing than developed countries. The explanation is unknown, but probably reflects the importance of the social environment.

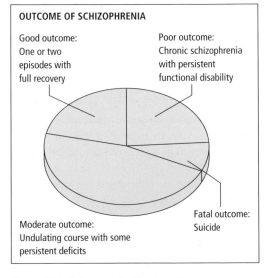

OUTCOME OF SCHIZOPHRENIA

Good outcome:
One or two
episodes with
full recovery

Poor outcome:
Chronic schizophrenia
with persistent
functional disability

Moderate outcome:
Undulating course with some
persistent deficits

Fatal outcome:
Suicide

Figure 12.1 Outcomes of schizophrenia.

Table 12.7 Factors associated with poor outcome in schizophrenia.

Demographic characteristics
Young age at onset (e.g. under 25)
Male
Isolated, unmarried
Poor work record
Premorbid personality disorder
Substance misuse

Illness characteristics
Insidious onset
Prolonged untreated psychosis
Disorganized subtype
No mood disturbance
Early negative symptoms
Non-compliance with medication

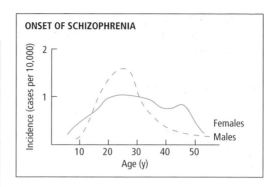

Figure 12.2 Schizophrenia: age at onset.

Epidemiology

The lifetime risk for schizophrenia is about 0.8%, with an annual incidence of 0.3 per 1000 and a point prevalence of about 5 per 1000. The onset peaks in early adulthood, though the prodromal symptoms are often in adolescence.

• The sex ratio is equal, but there are some sex differences. Women have a later and different age of onset profile (Figure 12.2). Men tend to have a more severe illness and worse prognosis. Oestrogen's regulation of dopamine receptor sensitivity may explain these gender differences.

• There is an increased frequency (relative risk ~5) of schizophrenia in the children of Afro-Caribbeans who came to Britain in the 1950s, and in some other migrant groups. Its explanation is controversial, with biological (genetic, viral) and sociological (racial prejudice, social deprivation) theories.

• Suggestions of a fall in incidence of schizophrenia over the past 30 years are probably the result of changing diagnostic practice and service provision, not a true decline.

Aetiology of schizophrenia

There have been many and diverse views of schizophrenia: as a brain disease, as a psychological disorder with no organic basis, and as a myth. Over the past 20 years, its original conception as a genetically-influenced neurodevelopmental disorder again prevails.

Genetic factors

There is an increased risk of schizophrenia in people with a family history of the condition (Figure 12.3). Twin studies show that this is due almost entirely to genetic factors and that the heritability is about 80% (Chapter 6). Adoption studies support this conclusion, in that children of a schizophrenic parent who are adopted by parents without schizophrenia retain their increased (10–12%) risk of illness.

• These studies also show that the genetic predisposition to schizophrenia overlaps with schizotypal disorder and perhaps delusional disorder. These conditions are therefore sometimes grouped together as *schizophrenia spectrum disorders*.

• The mode of inheritance is not clear, but probably involves many susceptibility genes, each of small effect, interacting with each other and with the environmental influences mentioned below.

• Several probable schizophrenia susceptibility genes have now been identified. They may all influence synaptic plasticity in the cerebral cortex (Table 12.8).

• About a quarter of people with velocardio-facial syndrome (VCFS), caused by a deletion of chromosome 22q11, develop schizophrenia,

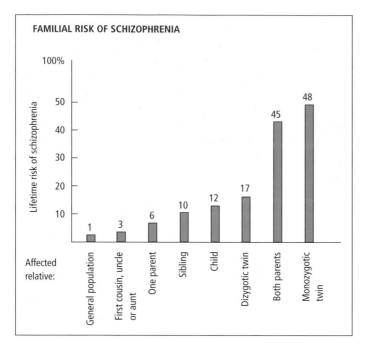

FAMILIAL RISK OF SCHIZOPHRENIA

Figure 12.3 Familial risk of schizophrenia.

Table 12.8 Schizophrenia susceptibility genes.

Gene name	Chromosomal locus	Evidence
Neuregulin-1	8p	Strong
Dysbindin	6p	Strong
G72	13q	Moderate
COMT	22q	Moderate
DISC 1	1q	Moderate
RGS-4	1q	Moderate

Table 12.9 Risk factors for schizophrenia.

Family history (genes)

Social
Urban birth
Some migrant groups
Low social class

Pre- and perinatal
Obstetric complications
Winter birth
Maternal influenza
Maternal malnutrition
Rhesus incompatibility

Postnatal
Early childhood CNS infection
Epilepsy
Learning disability
Delayed milestones
Poor child peer relationships
Ambiguous handedness
Early cannabis use
Life events (precipitate onset)

maybe because of the location of COMT (Table 12.8) and other susceptibility genes in this region.

Environmental factors

Although the most important factor, genes are not the sole cause of schizophrenia. There are many known and suspected environmental risk factors, both biological and social (Table 12.9). However, these are mostly of minor effect compared to the genetic contribution, and their independence and interpretation are unclear. Taken together this information supports the view that schizophrenia has its roots in early development.

• *Obstetric complications*. The risk of developing schizophrenia in people with a history of obstetric complications is increased about four-fold. Complications associated with foetal hypoxia are particularly implicated. However, it is not known if the relationship is causal, or a sign of a pre-existing foetal abnormality, or a consequence of the mother's antenatal behaviour or physiology.

• *Excess of winter births* (February and March). This is a true seasonal effect, being reversed in Australia (and absent near the Equator). It may be a correlate of viral infections during pregnancy being commoner in early winter, or of reproductive behaviour (i.e. conceiving in the summer), or (in one theory) a reflection of perinatal weather and vitamin D deficiency.

• *Urban birth and upbringing*. This is a dose-dependent relationship (risk increased about three-fold for a large town compared to a rural area). Its cause is unknown—e.g. pollution, noise, overcrowding, infectious agents, etc.

• *Early cannabis use* (pre-teens) is a risk factor, but studies have not fully controlled for use of other drugs.

• There is an increased seropositivity for several viruses in schizophrenia (e.g. herpes simplex type 2), but it is unclear when exposure to the virus occurred, and what causal role they played.

The brain in schizophrenia

The dopamine hypothesis

The dopamine hypothesis has been the leading biochemical explanation for schizophrenia for over 30 years. It proposes that there is an excess of dopamine transmission ('hyperdopaminergia') in schizophrenia (whether due to too much dopamine, too many receptors, etc.). It was based on three main lines of evidence:

• Antipsychotic drugs are, without exception, dopamine D_2 receptor antagonists.

• Dopamine agonists (e.g. amphetamines, L-DOPA) can produce a paranoid psychosis.

• Some CSF and brain studies of schizophrenia indicate abnormal levels of dopamine, its metabolites, enzymes or receptors.

Advancing or refuting the dopamine hypothesis has proved difficult. However, the past few years have seen considerable progress, mostly through functional imaging studies. Dopamine does indeed appear to be closely linked to the symptoms of schizophrenia, but in a much more subtle way than originally proposed:

• The dopamine system is unlikely to be the primary abnormality. Much evidence suggests that the dopamine changes are downstream of alterations in glutamate transmission.

• There is good evidence that hyperdopaminergia occurs during acute schizophrenia, in the basal ganglia (striatum). The more 'overheated' the dopamine system, the better the subsequent response to antipsychotics (which is logical, since they are dopamine receptor antagonists).

• As well as the hyperdopaminergia during acute schizophrenia in the striatum, there is probably insufficient dopaminergic activity in the prefrontal cortex in patients with chronic schizophrenia, which contributes to the cognitive and negative symptoms.

• The NMDA subtype of glutamate receptor, is also implicated in schizophrenia, both by the genetic discoveries, and the fact that NMDA receptor antagonists (ketamine, phencyclidine) produce a schizophrenia-like syndrome (p. 158).

Functional imaging studies

Abnormalities in regional cerebral blood flow and metabolism occur in schizophrenia, related to particular situations and neuropsychological tests. Such differences support the idea that particular neuronal circuits are impaired in schizophrenia, especially those involving the frontal cortex, hippopcampus, thalamus and cerebellum. For example, patients show:

• Failure to activate the prefrontal cortex when performing tasks requiring its use (*hypofrontality*).

• Greater activation in order to complete a task successfully, due to less efficient processing.

• Abnormal blood flow responses to dopaminergic drugs.

• Characteristic metabolic patterns depending on the predominant symptoms.

Structural brain changes

The most robust finding is enlargement of the lateral ventricles and a slight decrease in brain size. There may be a preferential involvement of the temporal lobe and a loss of normal cerebral asymmetries.

• The structural brain changes are statistically robust, but not diagnostically useful since there is much overlap with controls and the same findings can also occur in other disorders.

• The histological basis of schizophrenia is unknown, though the cytoarchitecture of the cerebral cortex—its neuronal and synaptic organization—appears altered. The white matter and its myelination may also be affected. There is no gliosis, suggesting an absence of neurodegenerative processes.

Psychological and social theories

The earlier psychological and social theories of the causation of schizophrenia lack convincing supporting evidence. However, psychological and social factors are clearly important in its outcome, exemplified by the effect on the patient of the emotion expressed by family members. These factors may also precipitate schizophrenia, since there is an excess of life events in the months preceding the first episode.

• Psychological interest is now directed mainly at the neuropsychological mechanisms. For example, one theory views schizophrenia as affecting the ability to distinguish actions generated by internal events (thoughts, feelings) and external stimuli (sensations).

The neurodevelopmental model

Putting the various findings together, most researchers now view schizophrenia as a neurodevelopmental disorder. That is, it is caused by abnormalities of brain development, largely driven by genetic predisposition and early environmental factors (Figure 12.4).

• Different versions of the model emphasize the prenatal environment ('doomed from the womb'), adolescence, or a combination of both.

• Ongoing factors throughout life may well contribute as well, since a pure developmental model does not explain well the age of onset, the fluctuating clinical course, or cases beginning later in life. One notion is that the developmental abnormalities render the brain less able to undergo 'plasticity'—its normal adaptive response to changing environmental demands and stressors.

• Though psychosocial and family factors are neglected in the model, their influence should not be ignored, as mentioned above. These are likely to be mediated via stress and its effects upon the brain.

The evidence in favour of the neurodevelopmental model includes:

• The fact that the neuropathological findings (e.g. ventricular enlargement) are present before the onset of symptoms.

• The lack of gliosis and cytoarchitectural abnormalities suggest a prenatal origin.

• Most of the robust environmental risk factors (Table 12.9) act *in utero* or early childhood.

• Children destined as adults to get schizophrenia have impaired behavioural, intellectual and motor development, demonstrable from infancy onwards.

• People with schizophrenia have increased rates of minor physical anomalies and abnormal dermatoglyphics, both of which point to prenatal developmental disturbance.

Disorders related to schizophrenia

Several other disorders are grouped together with schizophrenia, because:

• They are also psychoses which are not secondary to a mood disorder or organic disorder (in the case of schizoaffective disorder and delusional disorders), or

• They are thought to be causally related (in the case of schizotypal disorder), and

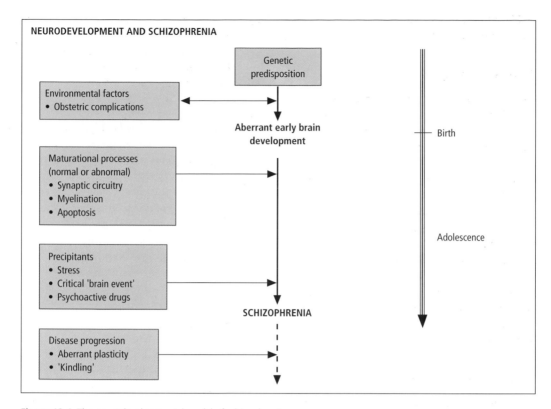

Figure 12.4 The neurodevelopmental model of schizophrenia.

- They do not meet the criteria for diagnosis of schizophrenia (Table 12.1).

Schizoaffective disorder

Clinical features

The distinction of schizophrenia from bipolar disorder originated in the belief that these were two discrete disorders. It is reflected in the classification of bipolar disorder as a mood disorder separate from schizophrenia. However, this view may well be wrong. Certainly, many patients have features of both conditions, hence *schizoaffective disorder*.

- Use the diagnosis only for patients who satisfy criteria for schizophrenia *and* mood disorder *during the same episode*. Otherwise, diagnose the predominant syndrome (or neither). For example, one first-rank symptom in mania does not warrant a label of schizoaffective disorder (let alone schizophrenia). Similarly, labile mood is common in acute schizophrenia.
- Overuse of the diagnosis is a common mistake—and often seized upon by examiners.

Management and prognosis

Mood symptoms and schizophrenic symptoms are treated on their merits. Mood stabilizers and antipsychotics are often used in combination.

- The prognosis is intermediate between schizophrenia and mood disorder. It is better in those whose predominant mood disturbance is manic rather than depressive.

Delusional disorders (paranoid psychoses)

Many patients have a psychosis without an underlying mood disturbance or organic disorder but do not satisfy the criteria for schizophrenia. Persecutory delusions are the main feature. Hallucinations are rare. Personality remains intact. These disorders are divided into acute and chronic types.

● The disorders in this 'residual' category of psychosis have had a variety of names. The preferred collective term is now *delusional disorder*, though *paranoid psychosis* is still commonly used.

Acute delusional disorder

These conditions are characterized by their acute onset, clinical features and rapid resolution. There are multiple, transient persecutory delusions, a sense of perplexity or suspicion, and a labile mood.

● They may be caused by drugs (in which case they are diagnosed as such) or follow extreme stresses, hence the older terms *psychogenic psychosis* and *brief reactive psychosis*. There is also an evocative French term, *bouffée delirante* (a 'puff of madness').

● Some cases will, of course, turn out to be more persistent psychotic disorders.

Persistent delusional disorder

A *persistent delusional disorder* is one lasting more than 3 months. *Chronic paranoid psychosis* and *paranoia* describe similar disorders.

● The delusions are usually *systematized* (i.e. stable and combined into a complex system). They often centre upon alleged (and plausible) injustices. The person may embark on litigation, or occasionally retribution, so it is important to ask about thoughts of aggression and hostility.

● The delusions are often *encapsulated*. The rest of the mental state can be unremarkable to the point that, if the delusional system is not detected, no abnormal features are elicited. Because of this, the disorder can go unrecognized for years, becoming hard to distinguish from paranoid personality disorder (Chapter 15)—though in the latter the paranoid ideas are not truly delusional.

● The appropriate diagnosis may change to one of mood disorder or schizophrenia.

● Onset is usually in middle age. Social isolation, deafness and paranoid personality traits are risk factors.

A 50-year-old librarian, Mr Y, was arrested for threatening his boss, having been made redundant after 30 years. He had no psychiatric history. Mr Y was convinced that the boss had plotted against him. His diary revealed an increasing preoccupation with these ideas and included allegations and events known to be false. Hallucinations, thought disorder, mood disorder and substance misuse were excluded. Mr Y was single, without close friends, and had a lifelong interest in spying. He reluctantly agreed to take haloperidol, which gradually resolved the delusions and he stopped pestering his ex-boss. However, the beliefs remained in attenuated form, and he continued to suspect various conspiracies were going on.

Specific variants of persistent delusional disorders

The following variants of persistent delusional disorder are mentioned either because of their clinical importance or because they have a memorable eponym and are beloved by examiners.

● *Morbid (pathological) jealousy* is not uncommon and is potentially dangerous. The patient, usually male, has the delusional belief that his partner is unfaithful. He may go to elaborate lengths to prove this and remains unconvinced by evidence to the contrary. He may threaten and finally attack his partner or the alleged third party. Usually morbid jealousy is a symptom of psychotic depression, schizophrenia, alcoholic psychosis or dementia, but it can be seen in isolation. The risks posed by morbid jealousy (and other psychoses with persecutory delusions with potential for violent acts) sometimes overrule patient confidentiality so the intended victim can be warned. Full risk assessment is mandatory.

● *Monosymptomatic hypochondriacal psychosis (somatic delusional disorder)* is the delusional belief that the person has an illness or deformity. It can lead to a prolonged search for inappropriate medical or surgical treatments. It must be distinguished from hypochondriasis and dysmorphophobia.

• In *De Clèrambault's syndrome (erotomania)*, the patient, usually female, has a delusion that a man of high standing (a pop star, even a psychiatrist) is in love with her. Some stalkers have this disorder.

• In *folie à deux*, two people, often isolated sisters, share the same delusions. One is genuinely psychotic, the other is 'induced' to become so and is said to recover spontaneously when they are separated.

• *Capgras' delusion (illusion des soisies)* is the belief that someone close by has been replaced by an impostor or double. *Fregoli's delusion* is the belief that someone close to them is impersonating other people. Both have been called syndromes, but they are really symptoms (delusional misinterpretations). Both are very rare. They occur in schizophrenia, dementia, and after right hemisphere damage.

Management and prognosis of delusional disorders

Delusional disorders, like all psychoses, usually respond to antipsychotic drugs.

• Acute delusional disorders often resolve within days, especially if the triggering stressor is removed. Full recovery is the rule although relapses may occur. Continue medication for a few months.

• Persistent delusional disorders can be resistant to treatment (or go untreated) and continue for years. Unlike schizophrenia, negative symptoms rarely occur. It has been claimed that pimozide is more effective than other antipsychotics, but without good evidence. SSRIs can also be useful.

Schizotypal disorder

Schizotypal disorder is like a chronic, attenuated form of schizophrenia, in which the beliefs stop short of being delusional, and the sensory experiences are not quite hallucinatory. The key features are:

• An aloof and suspicious manner.
• Eccentric behaviour.
• Avoidance of social contact.
• Odd beliefs and magical thinking.
• Vague, rambling or metaphorical speech.
• Tendency to odd ideas and sensory experiences.
• At least three of the above present for more than 2 years.

Schizotypal disorder is diagnosed infrequently, partly because people rarely come into psychiatric contact, and partly because it overlaps with paranoid and schizoid personality disorders.

• Schizotypal disorder appears to have a similar genetic background as schizophrenia.
• There are no specific treatments.

Key points

• Schizophrenia is a psychosis characterized by specific types of delusions, hallucinations and thought disorder, called first-rank symptoms. By definition, schizophrenia is not secondary to a mood or organic disorder and the symptoms must have lasted more than a month.

• Some patients progress to a chronic state where social isolation, apathy and poverty of speech predominate. These are called negative symptoms, in contrast to the positive symptoms which characterize the acute episodes. Cognitive deficits also occur and contribute to poor functional outcome.

• Antipsychotic drugs are effective for positive symptoms but they do not prevent or treat negative symptoms. Clozapine is an atypical antipsychotic effective in some otherwise treatment-resistant cases.

• Most patients with schizophrenia need long-term, multidisciplinary support. Psychological and social interventions are an integral part of management.

• Schizophrenia is a neurodevelopmental disorder caused primarily by genetic factors. Many susceptibility genes exist and contribute to the risk. Obstetric complications and urban birth are important environmental risk factors.

Chapter 13

Organic psychiatric disorders

Organic psychiatric disorders are those with demonstrable pathology or aetiology, or which arise directly from a medical disorder. They are thereby distinguished from all other psychiatric disorders, which are traditionally called *functional*. This distinction is an oversimplification and conceptually flawed as all disorders have biological, psychological and social contributions (Chapter 1). The term causes both practical and semantic problems, but remains in widespread use and so is used here:

• The major organic disorders, *dementia* and *delirium*, are defined, like other psychiatric syndromes, by their characteristic clinical features. However, unlike other syndromes they are known to arise from different diseases with various aetiologies and pathologies. A complete diagnosis requires the disease as well as the dementia syndrome to be identified.

• Other organic disorders are simply psychiatric disorders of any type that appear, in a particular case, to be caused by an identifiable medical condition. Sometimes it is the psychiatric symptoms that first bring the person to medical attention.

• Substance misuse disorders are organic, in that there is a specific pharmacological cause. By convention they are classified separately (Chapter 14).

• Psychiatric disorders which are considered *psychological reactions* to illness—such as becoming depressed after being told you have cancer—are excluded from the organic category.

Dementia

Clinical features of dementia

• Review the core and module approach to assessment of dementia (Chapter 2 and 3).

Dementia is also known as *chronic brain syndrome*. Its cardinal feature is memory impairment (short-term worse than long-term) without impaired consciousness (cf. delirium). The overall clinical profile differs depending on the specific type of dementia, as outlined below, but other common features of dementia are:

• Symptoms present for 6 months, of sufficient severity to impair functioning.

• Personality and behavioural change—e.g. wandering, aggression, disinhibition.

• Dysphasias, dyspraxias and focal neurological signs may be present.

• Psychotic symptoms in half of cases at some stage.

• Unawareness of deficits (except early on).

• Nearly always progressive (though this is not a diagnostic criterion).

The incidence of dementia rises rapidly with age, affecting <5% of 65 year olds and 20% of 80 year olds. (Exact figures depend on severity threshold.) The risk of dementia is doubled in those with an affected first-degree relative. Other risk factors depend on the type of dementia concerned.

- The rapid rise with age is typified by Alzheimer's disease (Figure 13.1).
- Dementia in the under 65 s is termed *presenile dementia*.

Differential diagnosis of dementia

Established dementia is usually unmistakeable, but mild dementia can be confused with (or coexist with) other conditions:

- *Depression*. Poor concentration and impaired memory are common in depression in the elderly, hence *pseudodementia*. Two factors which help distinguish depression from dementia are: Did low mood or poor memory come first? Is the failure to answer questions due to lack of ability or lack of motivation?
- *Delirium*. See next section.
- *Deafness*. Check the person can hear.
- *Dysphasia*. Check they can understand and speak.
- *Amnesic syndrome*. A purer short-term memory defect (see below).

- *Late-onset schizophrenia* (paraphrenia). Check for prominent symptoms of psychosis.

The causes of dementia

The common dementias are listed in Table 13.1. Alzheimer's disease accounts for over half of all cases, with the majority of the rest explained by vascular dementia and Lewy body dementia.

- The syndromes are not mutually exclusive, and the common ones often coexist.
- In presenile dementia, a higher percentage of cases are due to rare genetic disorders or severe head injury.

Clinical features differentiating the dementias

Careful clinical evaluation identifies the specific dementia in more than 80% of cases (Table 13.2).

- A distinction is sometimes made clinically between *cortical dementia* (e.g. Alzheimer's disease) and *subocortical dementia* (e.g. Huntington's

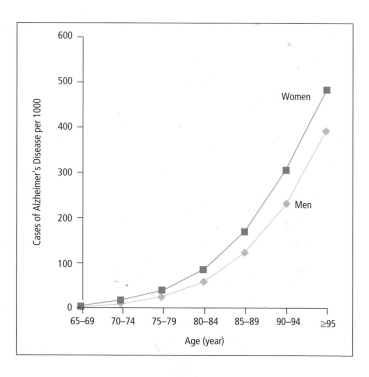

Figure 13.1 The prevalence of Alzheimer's disease with ageing. Adapted from Nussbaum RL, Ellis CE. *New Engl J Med* 2003, **348**, 1356–64.

Table 13.1 Causes of dementia.

Alzheimer's disease (50–60% of cases)
Vascular dementia (20–25%)
Dementia with Lewy bodies (10–15%)
Other causes (<10%)
Degenerative disorders
Frontotemporal dementia
Pick's disease
Huntington's disease
Prion disease
Progressive supranuclear palsy
Metabolic disorders
Alcoholic dementia
Vitamin B12 deficiency
Infections
HIV
Syphilis
Other causes
Normal pressure hydrocephalus
Intracranial tumours
Subdural haematoma
Head injury

disease) (Table 13.3). However, it is better to try and make a specific diagnosis (and the terms are misleading as most dementias affect both brain regions).

• The disorders themselves are discussed in the next section.

Assessment of dementia

In the history and examination, look for clues pointing towards one of the diagnoses in Table 13.2. For example, a history of a fall (?subdural haematoma) or incontinence (?normal pressure hydrocephalus), rapid fluctuations (?dementia with Lewy bodies); on examination you might find hypertension and a carotid bruit (?vascular dementia). Table 13.4 shows the baseline and specialized tests used in the investigation of dementia.

• Only the baseline blood tests would routinely be ordered, with further investigation depending on the age of the patient and the suggestion of a treatable aetiology (for example, a scan to exclude a subdural haematoma). In the absence of such

clues, further tests in an elderly person rarely change the diagnosis, let alone reveal a reversible cause.

• Conversely, in a young person, every effort is made to make a diagnosis—not only in case it is treatable and to inform prognosis, but because the dementia may well be inherited and genetic testing available for the family. Presenile dementia is usually referred to neurologists.

Management of dementia

Occasionally, dementia is potentially reversible (e.g. space occupying lesion; B12 deficiency) and responds to appropriate treatment. Specific interventions to treat symptoms in Alzheimer's disease are also now available, as discussed below. However, the management of dementia generally has more modest goals, the main one being to optimize quality of life for patient and carer. Whatever the cause of the dementia, the following principles and strategies are important:

• Think about the patient, their environment, and their carers as potential targets for intervention.

• Characterize and treat the non-cognitive abnormalities. Simple interventions can improve problems such as wandering (e.g. by regular exercise or raising the door handle) and incontinence (e.g. by a toiletting routine). Non-pharmacological methods should always be employed first.

• Psychotic symptoms respond to low-dose antipsychotics. They should be used sparingly and for brief periods only, because psychosis in dementia is usually transient, and because they are associated with more rapid cognitive decline and with sudden death, especially in Lewy body dementia. Atypical antipsychotics may also increase risk of stroke.

• Antipsychotics should *not* be used for non-specific behavioural problems or to sedate people with dementia.

• Treat depression. SSRIs are better tolerated than tricyclics.

• A range of other interventions are also sometimes used, including reality orientation, lavender oil aromatherapy, carbamazepine, reminiscence therapy, music therapy, art therapy, and memory

Table 13.2 Clinical features distinguishing between the dementias.

	Prominent symptoms and signs	Other clinical features
Alzheimer's disease	Memory loss, especially short-term	Relentlessly progressive
	Dysphasia and dyspraxia	Survival 5–8 years
	Sense of smell impaired early	
	Behavioural changes, e.g. wandering	
	Psychotic symptoms at some stage	
Vascular dementia	Personality change	Stepwise progression
	Labile mood	Signs of cerebrovascular disease
	Preserved insight	History of hypertension
		Commoner in men, smokers
Dementia with Lewy bodies	Fluctuating dementia	Antipsychotics worsen condition
	Delirium-like phases	
	Parkinsonism	
	Visual hallucinations	
Frontotemporal dementia	Stereotyped behaviours	Slowly progressive
	Personality change	Family history common
	Early loss of insight	Commoner in women
	Expressive dysphasia	Onset usually before age 70
	Memory relatively preserved	
	Early primitive reflexes	
Huntington's disease	Schizophrenia-like psychosis	Presents in the 20s–40s
	Abnormal movements (choreiform)	Strong family history
	Depression and irritability	
	Dementia occurs later	
Normal pressure hydrocephalus	Mental slowing, apathy, inattention	Commonest in 50–70 year olds
	Urinary incontinence	Commonest reversible dementia
	Problems walking (gait apraxia)	
Prion disease	Myoclonic jerks	Often presenile
	Seizures	Rapid onset and progression
	Cerebellar ataxia	Death within a year

Table 13.3 Clinical features of subcortical versus cortical dementias.

	Subcortical dementia	Cortical dementia
Memory loss	Moderate	Severe, early
Language	Normal	Affected (Dysphasia)
Personality	Apathetic, inert	Indifferent
Mood	Flat, depressed	Normal
Co-ordination	Impaired	Normal
Motor speed	Slowed	Normal

training. There is some evidence that the first three may be beneficial for behavioural problems.

• Social interventions such as meals-on-wheels, day care and respite admissions help carers cope.

• Investigate any sudden deterioration. It may be due to a treatable cause (e.g. superimposed delirium due to a UTI).

• In advanced dementia, palliative rather than active treatment is often indicated. Next-of-kin should be fully involved in these decisions (see vignette pp. 83–4). Advanced directives are becoming popular and should be respected.

Prognosis of dementia

Most dementias progress inexorably. Life expec-

Table 13.4 Investigation of dementia.

Test	What the test may show
Blood tests	
Full blood count	Macrocytosis, anaemia
Electrolytes	Hypercalcaemia, renal disease
Liver function tests	Alcoholic liver disease
Thyroid function	Hypothyroidism
Vitamin B12 and folate levels	Deficiencies can produce dementia
Syphilis serology	Now rare, but overlooked
HIV test	Dementia common in AIDS
Radiography	
Chest X-ray	Bronchial carcinoma with ?cerebral metastases
Brain imaging (CT or MRI)	Tumour; infarcts; haematoma; temporal lobe atrophy suggests Alzheimer's
EEG	Characteristic abnormality in prion disease (3 Hz 'spike and wave')
Other tests	
Lumbar puncture	Normal pressure hydrocephalus; herpes encephalitis
Cerebral blood flow studies	Parietal hypometabolism suggests Alzheimer's
Neuropsychological testing	Assess severity; profile of deficits may point to brain region most affected
Genetic testing	Available for some familial dementias—an area of rapid developments
Brain biopsy	Very rarely done; mainly for suspected prion disease

tancy is decreased, though the reasons are not clear. Death is usually within 5 to 8 years of onset, with some dementias, notably prion disease, progressing much more rapidly. Younger cases and those with focal neurological signs or psychotic symptoms have a worse prognosis.

• People with dementia should not be blood or tissue donors in view of the risk of transmission of prion disease.

Specific dementing disorders

This section summarizes the aetiological, pathological and therapeutic factors for the important dementias.

• Their main distinguishing clinical features are summarized in Table 13.2.

Alzheimer's disease

As the commonest dementia, it is fortunate that substantial progress has been made recently in understanding Alzheimer's disease, and the first specific treatments are now available.

It is a neuropathological diagnosis. The cardinal features are neurofibrillary tangles and senile (amyloid) plaques in the hippocampus and cerebral cortex. Loss of synapses is also important. Neurochemically, the main abnormality is a loss of acetylcholine due to degeneration of the cholinergic neurons of the basal forebrain. The cholinergic deficits and synaptic loss are proportional to the severity of the dementia.

A considerable amount is now known about the causes of the disease (Table 13.5).

• The major risk factor, apart from age, is the E4 (epsilon4) variant of the apolipoprotein E (apoE) gene. Three polymorphisms exist, apoE2, apoE3 and apoE4: 20% of the population carry one copy of apoE4 and have twice the risk of Alzheimer's disease; the 3% who are apoE4 homozygotes (i.e. two copies of apoE4) are at several-fold increased risk. Conversely, the risk is ~40% lower in people without an apoE4 allele, and those with apoE2 alleles may be at lower risk still. The effect of apoE4 is probably that it brings forward the age of onset of dementia, by about a decade. (Note that apoE4 is neither necessary nor sufficient for Alzheimer's disease—it is a risk factor.)

Table 13.5 Risk factors for Alzheimer's disease.

Factor	Comments
Genetic	
Apolipoprotein E (chromosome 19)	ApoE4 allele markedly increases risk
Amyloid precursor protein (chromosome 21); presenilins 1 and 2 (chromosomes 14 and 1)	Autosomal dominant mutations which cause early-onset familial Alzheimer's disease
Other genes (chromosomes 6, 10 and 11)	Identity and contribution uncertain
Down's syndrome (trisomy 21)	Alzheimer's disease occurs in middle age
Other risk factors	
Increasing age	Predominant risk factor (Fig. 13.1)
Females	Slightly higher risk than men (Fig. 13.1)
Homocysteinaemia	High plasma homocysteine doubles risk
Head injury	Doubles risk of Alzheimer's disease
Latent herpes simplex infection	In people with an apoE4 allele
History of depression	Risk of dementia may be increased
Aluminium exposure	Controversial
Environmental—protective factors	
High educational level	'Cerebral reserve'
Physically and mentally active lifestyle	'Use it or lose it'
Non-steroidal anti-inflammatories	?Retard a chronic brain inflammatory process
Statins	?Decrease atherosclerotic risk factors
Hormone replacement therapy	?Oestrogens are neuroprotective (but see text)

• Presenile Alzheimer's disease is often familial and (unlike most cases) caused by an autosomal dominant mutation. Three genes have been found so far, with several different mutations in each: amyloid precursor protein (APP), and presenilin (PS) 1 and 2. Though extremely rare, these cases helped identify the pathways involved in Alzheimer's disease generally (see below).

• A history of treatment with NSAIDs, HRT or statins has been associated with a lower risk of developing dementia and Alzheimer's disease. Plausible mechanisms exist to explain these effects. However, it is unclear if the association is genuine, or reflects other factors (e.g. women given HRT tend to be healthier and better educated).

• Prospective studies show that plasma homocysteine is an independent, graded risk factor for developing Alzheimer's disease several years later. This may be due to its role in atherosclerotic processes.

The key process leading to Alzheimer's disease is abnormal metabolism of β-amyloid, the main constituent of senile plaques, and a fragment of the amyloid precursor protein. The abnormality results in formation of insoluble forms of β-amyloid which accumulate and trigger a range of other harmful biochemical events. This 'amyloid cascade' is promoted in various ways by the causal factors mentioned (Figure 13.2). For example, NSAIDs and apoE4 both affect β-amyloid trafficking or processing.

• The central role of β-amyloid is supported by findings in transgenic mice with Alzheimer's disease-causing mutations in amyloid precursor protein gene. They become demented and get senile plaques, a fate which does not afflict normal rodents.

• Abnormalities in tau protein (which forms neurofibrillary tangles), oxidative stress and inflammatory processes may also be important. Their connection to β-amyloid is unclear.

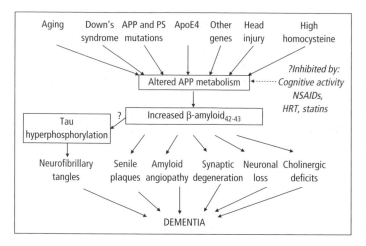

Figure 13.2 The pathogenesis of Alzheimer's disease.

Treatment of Alzheimer's disease

The first specific treatments for Alzheimer's disease are now available, and many more are in development.

• Cholinesterase inhibitors (e.g. donepezil) are licensed for mild and moderate Alzheimer's disease. They have modest effects against cognitive symptoms, global outcome and activities of daily living. The effect is roughly equivalent to a 6-month delay in cognitive decline. They may also have benefit for behavioural symptoms. In the UK, they must be prescribed by a specialist according to specified diagnostic and severity criteria.

• Memantine is an NMDA glutamate receptor antagonist. It has some efficacy in more severe Alzheimer's disease. Its therapeutic value in practice is not yet established.

• Various treatments directed at β-amyloid and its metabolism are being tested. These include the surprising finding that active and passive immunization against β-amyloid may be effective.

• Treatment trials with NSAIDs and folic acid (to lower homocysteine) are underway. Trials of HRT have been negative.

• CSF and MRI markers of the disease and its progression are being developed and may soon become useful either for diagnosis or for monitoring response to treatment.

• Any potential preventative or disease-retarding intervention must take into account the fact that

the pathology begins in earnest at least a decade before the first symptoms.

Vascular dementia

An umbrella term for dementia thought to be vascular in origin. One type is caused by multiple small infarcts (hence the earlier name of *multi-infarct dementia*). Others include 'small vessel disease' and Binswanger's disease. It is associated with risk factors for atherosclerosis and cerebrovascular disease.

• There is no specific treatment, other than to attend to the cerebrovascular risk factors (e.g. aspirin, smoking).

• Vascular impairment acts synergistically with Alzheimer's disease to produce dementia.

Dementia with Lewy bodies

Also called *Lewy body disease*, it is the third commonest form of dementia. The overlap with Parkinson's disease reflects their common pathology, viz. Lewy bodies (intracellular inclusions made of α-synuclein), but in dementia with Lewy bodies these occur in the cerebral cortex. Its aetiology is unknown, and no genes have been identified.

• Cholinesterase inhibitors are valuable (and more effective than in Alzheimer's disease).

• Antipsychotics should be avoided because of

the risk of sensitivity reactions and increased mortality.

Parkinson's disease dementia

Dementia with Lewy bodies merges into *Parkinson's disease dementia*. The convention is that the latter category is used for dementia occurring more than 12 months after onset of parkinsonism. By this definition, dementia occurs in about 40% of cases of Parkinson's disease, especially later onset cases.
- L-DOPA does not improve the dementia; cholinesterase inhibitors may.
- Clozapine is useful for psychotic symptoms.

Frontotemporal dementia

A spectrum of conditions affecting the frontal and temporal lobes, including *Pick's disease* (characterized by Pick bodies and Pick cells), and dementias associated with motor neuron disease. Causes about ~5% of dementia, more so in younger subjects.
- The diseases are all thought to involve abnormalities in tau protein (see Alzheimer's disease). A few cases are caused by mutations in the tau gene on chromosome 17.
- There is no specific treatment. Patients are very sensitive to many psychotropic drugs, which should be used with caution to treat depressive or psychotic symptoms.

Huntington's disease

Also called *Huntington's chorea*. Unlike most psychiatric disorders, it is entirely genetic. It is autosomal dominant, caused by a trinucleotide repeat expansion ('molecular stutter') in the huntington gene on chromosome 4. Pathologically, there is marked atrophy of the caudate nucleus, and later in the frontal lobe. The abnormal huntingtin protein is though to be neurotoxic. Genetic testing is possible.
- The psychosis and depression can be treated symptomatically, but the dementia, and the disease itself, remain untreatable.

Normal pressure hydrocephalus

Accounts for up to 5% of dementia, and the commonest potentially reversible type. The term is a misnomer as CSF pressure is often increased. The clinical triad (Table 13.2) is characteristic, and MRI or CT scanning may help diagnostically.
- Treatment is by ventricular shunting; 50% respond well.

Prion disease

Includes *Creutzfeldt–Jakob disease (CJD)*. Prion disease is caused by an abnormal form of a protein called prion protein. The abnormality can be inherited or acquired, because abnormal prion protein is transmissible, via blood, diet and contaminated surgical instruments. Prion disease is exceedingly rare but notable, especially in the UK, because of 'variant CJD (vCJD)', acquired from cows with bovine spongiform encephalopathy (BSE)—prion disease in cattle.
- About 150 cases of vCJD have been reported (November 2004), and the current best predictions are for hundreds or thousands more. Unlike typical CJD, these have occurred in young adults and present with prominent psychiatric symptoms, especially depression and personality change.
- Any suspected case of prion disease should be referred to the National Surveillance Unit in Edinburgh.

Alcoholic dementia

True alcoholic dementia is rare. Visuospatial deficits are often prominent. It is associated with atrophy of the white matter and frontal lobes.
- Dementia in those with alcohol dependence is more often due to Alzheimer's disease or vascular dementia.
- Alcoholic dementia does not usually improve with abstinence.
- Alcohol dependence also causes amnesic syndrome (see below).

Delirium

Also known as *acute confusional state* or *acute brain syndrome*. It is common on medical and surgical wards—a third of elderly patients in hospital have an episode of delirium—so all doctors should be able to recognize and manage it.

- Review the unresponsive patient and cognition modules (Chapter 3).

Clinical features of delirium

Clouding of consciousness is the most important diagnostic sign. It refers to drowsiness, decreased awareness of surroundings, disorientation in time and place, and distractibility. At its most severe the patient may be unresponsive, but more commonly the impaired consciousness is quite subtle.

- Minor degrees of impaired consciousness can be detected by problems estimating the passage of time (e.g. how long the interview has been going on), and with concentration tasks (e.g. counting from 20 down to 1).

Because clouding of consciousness may not be apparent, the first clue to the presence of delirium is often one of its other features:

- Fluctuating course, worse at night.
- Visual hallucinations.
- Transient persecutory delusions.
- Irritability and agitation, or somnolence and decreased activity.
- Impaired concentration and memory.

The differential diagnosis includes dementia (Table 13.6), acute psychosis, and depression. Usually the clinical picture (especially the acute onset and rapid fluctuations), and its context, is sufficiently characteristic to make delirium a relatively simple diagnosis. However, differentiating delirium from Lewy body dementia can be difficult without a good history.

Aetiology of delirium

Recognition of delirium is followed by an urgent search for its cause (Table 13.7).

- Medication is implicated in a third of cases,

Table 13.6 Delirium versus dementia.

	Delirium	Dementia
Onset	Acute	Insidious
Short-term course	Fluctuating	Constant
Attention	Poor	Good
Delusions and hallucinations	Common, simple, fleeting	Less common, more stable

Table 13.7 Common causes of delirium.

Prescribed drugs
Tricyclic antidepressants
Benzodiazepines and other sedatives
Digoxin
Diuretics
Lithium
Steroids
Opiates

Other drugs
Alcohol intoxication
Alcohol withdrawal and delirium tremens

Medical conditions
Postoperative hypoxia
Febrile illness
Septicaemia
Organ failure (cardiac, renal, hepatic)
Hypoglycaemia
Dehydration
Constipation
Burns
Major trauma

Neurological conditions
Epilepsy (postictal)
Head injury
Space occupying lesion
Encephalitis

mostly drugs with anticholinergic effects (e.g. tricyclics) or sedatives.

Several demographic factors predict those who are at high risk of developing delirium (Table 13.8). In these individuals, delirium can follow relatively trivial precipitants (e.g. constipation).

Table 13.8 Predisposing factors for delirium.

Elderly
Male
Pre-existing dementia
Pre-existing frailty or immobility
Previous episode of delirium
Sensory impairment

Table 13.9 Management of delirium.

Environmental components
Quiet surroundings (side room), constant lighting,
   clock, calendar
Regular routine
Clear simple communications
Limit numbers of staff (e.g. key nurse)
Involve family

Medical components
Monitor vital signs
Investigate and treat underlying cause (e.g. antibiotics,
   oxygen, stop drug)
Control agitation or psychotic symptoms with
   antipsychotics

Management of delirium

Delirium is managed where it occurs—usually in general hospitals. Psychiatrists may be asked to assess the patient, make the diagnosis and give advice. Treatment is directed both at the symptoms and at the cause, and includes both medical and environmental interventions (Table 13.9).

- In practice (and in an exam), emphasize both the need to search for a cause and for environmental steps whilst this is ongoing. The latter may avoid the need for medication, which can complicate the problem, and should only be used when necessary.
- Antipsychotics are the first-line pharmacological treatment. Haloperidol is often used, by intramuscular injection if it cannot be taken orally. It can be given intravenously but this is rarely required.
- The exception is for alcohol- or seizure-related delirium, when a benzodizaepine (e.g. lorazepam) is indicated (because of the epileptogenic potential of antipsychotics).

- A delirious person may occasionally be a risk to self, other patients, or staff. Call for help, ensure safety, and use physical restraint if essential (e.g. to allow drug to be administered).
- Patients with delirium are often incapable of giving informed consent. Treatment is therefore given under the common law. If continuing interventions without consent are anticipated, the Mental Health Act may be required.

Prognosis of delirium

Prognosis depends on the cause. Within a week the patient is usually better or has died. A quarter have died by 3 months. There is no good evidence that delirium progresses to dementia (although pre-existing dementia is a risk factor for delirium).

A 75-year-old lady was found lying on the floor and taken to hospital. She is drowsy, disorientated in time and place, distractible, and unable to give any history. She thinks you are trying to kill her. She is febrile and hypotensive, but has no neurological signs or injuries. Blood tests and X-rays are performed. She is given oxygen, and antibiotics for the clinical suspicion of septicaemia. Her agitation worsens but settles with haloperidol. The GP tells you that there is no past history of note. Blood cultures grow an organism sensitive to the antibiotic. Her condition improves over 72 hours. The haloperidol is tailed off and her cognitive function returns to normal.

Other organic disorders

Dementia and delirium have been described in detail because they are common. As mentioned at the start of the Chapter, there are many other 'organic' conditions which can together present with the whole range of psychiatric disorders. The important principles, and some specific examples, are summarized here.

Organic psychiatric disorders

The diagnostic rule is to preface the psychiatric label with 'organic' and state the aetiology (Table

Table 13.10 Organic psychiatric disorders.

Syndrome	Example of cause
Organic brain syndromes	Dementia, delirium, amnesic syndrome
Organic delusional (psychotic) disorders	Systemic lupus erythematosus
Organic mood disorders	Multiple sclerosis
Organic anxiety disorders	Thryotoxicosis
Organic personality disorders	Head injury

13.10). For example, 'Organic anxiety disorder due to thyrotoxicosis'.

Each organic syndrome is very rare compared to its 'functional' counterpart. In areas with good primary care, psychiatrists rarely see undiagnosed organic psychiatric disorders. However, when an organic syndrome does occur it is essential to recognize it. Detecting an organic disorder requires that you:

- Consider the possibility, with every patient. If this is done, it is easier not to forget to take a brief medical history and conduct a relevant physical examination and order investigations.
- Always include an organic disorder on your list of differential diagnoses in an exam situation.
- Be suspicious if aspects of the psychiatric presentation are unusual. For example, organic syndromes often produce abnormalities in unexpected functions—e.g. anosmia in depression due to a frontal meningioma.

There may or may not be an effective treatment for the organic disorder. Regardless, the psychiatric symptoms are still treated with the appropriate pharmacological, psychological and social interventions.

- As a rule, treatment response in an organic disorder is similar to that of its functional equivalent; for example, depression responds to antidepressants whether it is organic or not. The presence of the organic disorder may, however, affect the choice of drug (e.g. avoid TCAs in depression following myocardial infarction).

Amnesic syndrome

Amnesic (or *amnestic*) syndrome completes the triad of conditions (with dementia and delirium) which affect memory and which always have an organic cause. Its features are

- Selective loss of recent memory.
- Confabulation: the unconscious fabrication of recent events to cover gaps in memory.
- Time disorientation.
- Attention and immediate recall intact.
- Long-term memory and other intellectual faculties intact.

Amnesic syndrome is rare, and in practice difficult to distinguish from some dementias. It is due to damage to the mammillary bodies, hippocampus or thalamus. The usual cause is alcohol-induced thiamine deficiency (*Korsakov's syndrome*), which is treated with thiamine and abstinence. Other causes include herpes simplex encephalitis, severe hypoxia and head injury.

The memory deficits are often irreversible.

Epilepsy

There are several main types of epilepsy (Table 13.11). Epilepsy is usually managed by neurologists, but has many psychiatric aspects. Only the latter are covered here (Table 13.12).

- Consult a neurology text for general coverage of epilepsy.

Relationship of psychiatric symptoms with seizures

Complex partial epilepsy was called *psychomotor epilepsy* because of the frequency of psychiatric symptoms during seizures (Table 13.13). It has also been referred to as *temporal lobe epilepsy*, though this is not always the site of the seizure focus.

- The risk of schizophrenia is several-fold higher in people with complex partial epilepsy, more so if the focus is in the left temporal lobe, and due to an early developmental abnormality.
- The association with sexual dysfunction may be

Table 13.11 The main forms of epilepsy.

Type	Comments	Conscious level during seizure
Generalized seizures	No focal onset	
Tonic–clonic (Grand mal)	The 'classic' type of seizure	Unconscious
Absence (Petit mal)	Subtle and brief	Impaired
Partial seizures	Focal onset	
Complex partial (psychomotor)	Of most psychiatric significance	Impaired
Simple partial		Unaffected

Table 13.12 Psychiatric aspects of epilepsy.

Category	Example
Psychiatric symptoms related to seizures	
Due to shared aetiology	Temporal lobe tumour
At start of seizure	Hallucinations during aura
During seizure	Non-convulsive status presenting as a fugue state
After seizure	Postictal delirium
Between seizures	Psychosis of complex partial epilepsy
Psychiatric disorder masquerading as epilepsy	Pseudoseizures
Psychiatric disorder associated with epilepsy	
Depression	Common in people with epilepsy
Suicide	Several times more common in people with epilepsy
Psychiatric problems of treatment	
Side-effects of anticonvulsants	Depression with barbiturates
Seizures as medication side-effect	Antipsychotics and tricyclic antidepressants

due to the epilepsy, or the medication. Psychiatric presentations can occur with other epilepsies, but are much rarer.

• *Absence seizures* in children produce transient lapses in concentration or simple automatisms and can be mistaken for a behavioural disorder.

• A *generalized seizure disorder* can present to a psychiatrist if, for example, the person was found wandering in a postictal delirium.

Psychiatric disorders masquerading as epilepsy

Pseudoseizures (hysterical seizures or *non-epileptic attack disorder)* is a form of dissociative disorder (p.

107). It can be hard to distinguish clinically from a true seizure. EEG monitoring during attacks may be required to make the diagnosis. Pseudoseizures are commoner in people who also have epilepsy.

• Other conditions which can be misdiagnosed as epilepsy include panic attacks, hypoglycaemia and schizophrenia. In children, consider temper tantrums and nightmares.

Psychological problems associated with having epilepsy

Historically, epilepsy has been attributed to demonic possession and its sufferers seen as irritable, self-centred people with criminal tendencies. Although entirely false, persisting negative attitudes, acting in concert with the real disabilities, probably explain the higher incidence of psychiatric disorders and suicide in epilepsy.

- The commonest psychiatric disorders are anxiety and depressive disorders.

Table 13.13 Psychiatric symptoms of complex partial seizures.

During the seizure (ictal)
Impaired consciousness
Hallucinations and other distorted perceptions
olfactory
somatic—especially epigastric
Sense of *déjà vu*
Depersonalization and derealization
Speech and memory affected
Automatisms and stereotyped behaviour
After the seizure (Postictal, hours to days)
Transient, florid psychosis
Between seizures (interictal)
Schizophrenia-like psychosis
Depression
Sexual dysfunction and lack of libido

- The suicide risk is increased 5-fold, and more so in those with complex partial seizures.
- Anticonvulsant treatments can compound the psychiatric problems—phenobarbitone causes hyperactivity and irritability in children; phenytoin can produce ataxia and delirium.

Head injury

Head injury is a major cause of organic psychiatric syndromes in young adults. They can be difficult to treat and services are greatly under-resourced.

- The psychiatric consequences of a head injury depend partly on the nature and location of the injury, and partly on the person's premorbid characteristics. In blunt trauma, the brain suffers contusions at the point of impact, focal damage elsewhere as the brain reverberates in the skull and diffuse axonal damage due to the shearing forces.
- People with an apoE4 allele are at greater risk of persistent deficits following head injury.

A wide range of psychiatric problems can follow a head injury:

- A head injury with loss of consciousness may produce amnesia, either *anterograde* (post-traumatic), for events after the injury, or *retrograde*. Anterograde amnesia >24 hours predicts a poor

Table 13.14 Other medical disorders with psychiatric manifestations.

Medical disorder	Psychiatric manifestations
Cerebral tumour	Psychiatric symptoms in 50%, more so if tumour is in frontal or temporal lobes
Cerebral abscess	May present with psychiatric symptoms
Multiple sclerosis	Mood disturbance in 25%—bland euphoria or depression; cognitive deficits in 25%—can become severe; personality changes in 25%—apathy, irritability
Parkinson's disease	Depression in 50%, L-DOPA therapy may cause psychosis
Systemic lupus erythematosus	5% at presentation, 50% at some stage: mood disorder, psychosis, delirium and seizures
HIV	Dementia in 30% with AIDS; psychosis—prevalence uncertain
Cushing's disease	Severe depression common; occasionally psychosis and cognitive impairment
Addison's disease	Apathy and fatigue in 80%; depression in 50%; cognitive impairment in 50%; psychosis in 5%
Hyperthyroidism	Anxiety (common), depression, mania, delirium
Hypothyroidism	Mental slowing and depressive symptoms very common; rarely 'myxoedema madness'—delirium, depression, dementia; symptoms may persist despite thyroxine replacement
Hypercalcaemia	Psychosis, delirium and mood disorders in 50%; cognitive impairment in 25%

long-term outcome, including persistent cognitive deficits. The impairment ranges from a subtle slowing of thought and distractibility through to dementia. It tends to improve in the first year but thereafter deficits are likely to be permanent. There is no specific treatment.

- *Personality changes* are frequent. Typically the changes are indicative of frontal lobe damage: impaired ability to plan or persevere; emotional shallowness and lability; impulsivity and irritability. Altered sexual behaviour (in any direction) and long-winded speech also occur. Improvement is partial and slow.
- *Mood disorder, anxiety disorders* and *schizophrenia* are commoner than expected after head injury. Left- and right-sided frontal lobe damage are associated with depression and mania respectively.
- *Postconcussional syndrome* describes emotional, cognitive and bodily symptoms occurring after relatively minor head injury. The symptoms are sometimes thought to be 'psychological' or even feigned, related to hopes of compensation but may reflect subtle brain injury.

Other medical disorders associated with psychiatric disorders

Table 13.14 lists some medical disorders that often have psychiatric manifestations.

Key points

- Organic psychiatric disorders are those due to a recognized medical cause or pathology. Dementia and delirium are by definition organic disorders; all other psychiatric disorders can be. Hence consider an organic cause for every psychiatric presentation—epilepsy and endocrine disorders are classic culprits.
- Dementia is characterized by memory loss. It is usually insidious and progressive, sometimes reversible. The commonest causes are Alzheimer's disease, vascular dementia and dementia with Lewy bodies.
- Delirium is an acute, fluctuating confusional state, with clouding of consciousness. It has many causes (e.g. drugs, septicaemia). It is usually treatable.
- Treatment of organic disorders is aimed at the underlying cause *and* at the psychiatric symptoms.

Chapter 14

Substance misuse

General issues

Many substances are taken for pleasure. A substance is regarded as being *misused* (or *abused*) if it produces physical, psychological or social harm. Commonly misused substances are shown in Table 14.1. This chapter describes:

• The features of substance misuse.
• Its psychiatric consequences.
• The management of substance misuse and its associated psychiatric disorders.

Substance misuse presents in diverse ways. For example, as depression or morbid jealousy (both associated with alcohol), as an acute psychosis (amphetamines) or as haemetemesis (alcoholic cirrhosis). Its various presentations, and frequency, mean that detection of substance misuse, notably of alcohol, is part of every psychiatric assessment.

• Review the substance misuse module (p. 32).

There are no reliable prevalence figures for misuse of substances other than alcohol, since honesty about an illegal activity is unlikely. Clinic data or statistics about registered addicts give a misleading impression of what is being misused and the common health consequences. Bear this in mind when reading this chapter.

• In the USA, 1.5% of adults admit to having tried heroin, 7% amphetamines, 8% LSD, 12% cocaine and 30% cannabis. A quarter of each group were regular users.

Types of substance misuse

There are several categories of substance misuse:
• *At-risk consumption*—(alcohol) intake at a level associated with increased risk of harm.
• *Harmful use*—misuse associated with health and social consequences, but without dependence.
• *Dependence*—prolonged, regular use of some substances (especially alcohol, opioids, amphetamines) can lead to *dependence (addiction)* and *withdrawal* syndromes.
• *Intoxication* is the acute effect of the substance—being drunk (alcohol), tripping (LSD) or stoned (cannabis). Intoxication with illicit drugs may lead to an acute psychiatric presentation.

Assessment of substance misuse

The principles of assessment are similar for all substances:
• Be willing and able to ask screening questions (pp. 9 and 32).
• Know the features of misuse of alcohol and other commonly used substances.
• Be aware of the psychiatric and medical conditions associated with substance misuse.
• Drug testing can be useful. Alcohol can be measured in breath or blood; most illicit drugs or their metabolites can be detected in the urine—some briefly (e.g. amphetamines), some for weeks afterwards (cannabis).

Table 14.1 Commonly misused substances.

Alcohol
Other legal or prescribed drugs
Benzodiazepines
Nicotine
Caffeine
Cannabis
Opioids
Heroin
Morphine
Methadone
Stimulants
Amphetamines
Cocaine
Ecstasy
Hallucinogens
LSD
Phencyclidine
Solvents

Table 14.2 Identifying motivation—the 'stages of change' model.

Stage	Features
Precontemplation	Denial of problem
Contemplation	Considering problem and whether change needed
Decision	Decides to do (or not to do) something about it
Action	Chooses strategy and implements it
Maintenance	Makes progress and sustains it
Relapse	Returns to earlier behaviour

Assessment of the *motivation* of the patient to change is also important. The *stages of change model* helps assess (and encourage) motivation (Table 14.2). People may go through many cycles of this process.

Management of substance misuse

Management is also based upon a set of uniform principles:
- Identify at-risk consumption and harmful use early, and give accurate information and advice.

Table 14.3 Factors associated with substance misuse.

Genetic
Variation in metabolizing enzymes
Variation in occurrence of withdrawal phenomena
Variation in dopamine receptor and transporter genes
Neurobiological
Brain activity: trait differences in EEG patterns
Chemicals: abnormalities in dopamine, GABA, and endogenous opioid systems
Anatomical: key site is nucleus accumbens
Psychological
Personality factors
Learned behaviour
Positive reinforcement—the drugs lead to behaviours which increase their use
Socioeconomic
Price and availability
Cultural norms and acceptability
Legal
Restrictions on sale
Penalties for possession or dealing

- In dependency, facilitate withdrawal (detoxification) and abstinence.
- Help maintain abstinence following withdrawal—a form of rehabilitation.
- If abstinence not possible, minimize harm associated with continuing use.
- Treat the complications, for example drug-induced psychosis.
- Prevention—this largely involves population-level interventions such as pricing policies.

To achieve these goals, a variety of psychological, pharmacological and social treatment methods are used. See below, and vignette on p. 85.

Aetiology of substance misuse

Substance misuse has a multifactorial aetiology (Table 14.3). Together, the factors determine both the prevalence and the type of substance misused.
- Aetiology has been studied in most detail for alcohol. Similar factors confer vulnerability to

misuse of substances in general (and perhaps to other addictions such as gambling).

Alcohol

Definitions and epidemiology

Over 90% of adults in the UK drink alcohol. About a quarter drink more than the recommended limits (21 and 14 units per week for men and women respectively). About 5% of the adult population (6% of men and 3% of women) consume heavy weekly amounts of alcohol (Figure 14.1).

- UK consumption has increased over the last 50 years, mainly accounted for by wine and spirits, with no reduction in beer drinking (Figure 14.2).
- Consumption of alcohol by teenagers is increasing; 12% of 11–15 year olds are regular drinkers.

A low intake of alcohol may be beneficial: up to 2 units per day is associated with a moderate protective effect against heart disease in men aged over 40 years. As intake increases, however, there is an escalating morbidity and mortality (Table 14.4). This produces a so-called J-shaped curve when mortality is plotted against alcohol consumption. Alcohol also has many other costs (Figure 14.3). For example in the UK, per year:

- Direct health service costs: £1.7 billion.
- Crime and antisocial behaviour: £7.3 billion.
- Lost productivity: £6.4 billion.
- Specialist alcohol treatment services: £95 million.
- 22 000 premature deaths.
- 30 000 hospital admissions.
- Up to 70% of all presentations to accident and emergency departments.
- 1.2 million violent incidents.

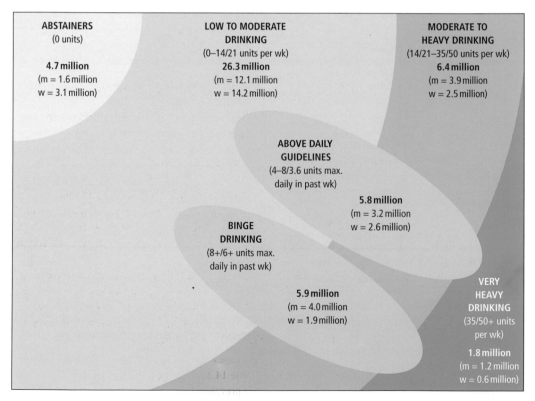

Figure 14.1 Weekly consumption of alcohol by adults in UK. One unit is 13.5 g alcohol; m = men, w = women. (Reproduced with modifications from: Prime Minister's Strategy Unit Alcohol Harm Reduction Strategy for England, 2004.)

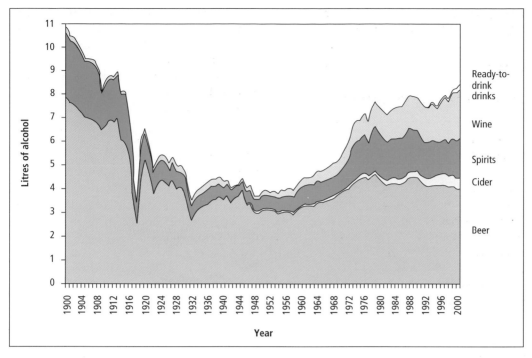

Figure 14.2 Alcohol Consumption in the UK: 1900–2000 per capita consumption of 100% alcohol. (Reproduced from: Prime Minister's Strategy Unit Alcohol Harm Reduction Strategy for England, 2004.)

Clinical features of alcohol misuse

Dependence

The concept of dependence was introduced in Chapter 3. The diagnosis of alcohol dependence (alcoholism) is made if three or more of the following are present:

- Feeling compelled to drink.
- Primacy of drinking over other activities, for example, eating, family life, work, health.
- Increased tolerance to alcohol—being able to drink quantities that would incapacitate others.
- Relief drinking—drinking to stop or prevent withdrawal symptoms.
- Stereotyped pattern of drinking.
- Reinstatement after abstinence—unable to give up alcohol for long.
- Drinking despite awareness of harmful consequences.
- Withdrawal symptoms.

Withdrawal and delirium tremens

The main features of alcohol withdrawal are:

- Tremulousness ('the shakes').
- Agitation.
- Nausea and retching.
- Sweating.
- Overwhelming desire to drink (craving).

Withdrawal symptoms are relieved by alcohol. If untreated, the symptoms may last for several days. Transient misperceptions and hallucinations may occur.

- Withdrawal symptoms often occur on waking as the blood alcohol concentration falls during sleep.

The most severe form of withdrawal (5% of cases) is *delirium tremens* (the 'DTs'), a potentially fatal condition (Table 14.5).

Wernicke's syndrome

An acute encephalopathy presenting with delirium, ataxia, nystagmus and ophthalmoplegia,

Table 14.4 Harmful effects of alcohol.

Medical
    Liver damage—hepatitis, cirrhosis
    Cardiovascular—cardiomyopathy, hypertension
    Gastrointestinal—peptic ulcer, oesophageal varices,
        pancreatitis
    Neoplasms—liver, oesophagus
    Blood—anaemia, haemochromatosis

Neurological and organic psychiatric
    Blackouts
    Epilepsy
    Neuropathy
    Delirium tremens
    Wernicke's syndrome
    Korsakov's syndrome
    Cerebellar degeneration
    Central pontine myelinosis
    Head injury (from falls)

Psychiatric
    Alcoholic hallucinosis
    Morbid jealousy
    Alcoholic dementia
    Depressive disorders
    Anxiety disorders
    Sexual dysfunction
    Suicide

Social
    Accidents
    Problems with relationships
    Domestic violence
    Employment difficulties
    Crime

occurring in the severely alcohol dependent, usually in the context of withdrawal. It is due to thiamine deficiency and requires *urgent treatment*. It may progress to Korsakov's syndrome (p. 146).

Harmful alcohol use

Defined as >50 units per week for men and >35 units per week for women. There are no specific features, since it is defined as people who have problems due to alcohol intake but who are not dependent. It may be detected in several ways, for example:
- By asking about alcohol intake during a routine medical history.

- The patient volunteers that he thinks he is drinking too much.
- Unexplained macrocytosis or abnormal liver function tests.
- Because of one of its psychiatric or social consequences (Table 14.4).

Associated medical disorders

If alcohol misuse has led to a medical disorder, then psychiatric or social impairments (Table 14.4) are also likely. These should be screened for and appropriate action taken. Conversely, if an alcohol-related psychiatric disorder is diagnosed, check for physical symptoms and signs of alcohol dependency.

Associated psychiatric disorders

Alcohol misuse is associated with an increased risk of, and worse prognosis for, most psychiatric disorders. These are covered in the respective Chapters.
- In *alcoholic hallucinosis*, a heavy drinker experiences recurrent auditory hallucinations, usually of a threatening or derogatory nature. The hallucinations occur in clear consciousness (cf. withdrawal hallucinations). The syndrome is an example of a drug-induced psychosis.
- About 10% of people who are alcohol dependent commit suicide.

Management of alcohol problems

The focus in this section is on clinical rather than on population-based interventions.
- Detection of alcohol misuse follows the principles outlined above, and the practical issues covered in the core assessment (Chapter 2) and substance misuse module (Chapter 3).

Management of at-risk consumption and harmful alcohol use

A brief intervention in primary care is usually sufficient if someone is drinking more than the safe limits but is not dependent and has no specific medical or psychiatric disorder. The components are:

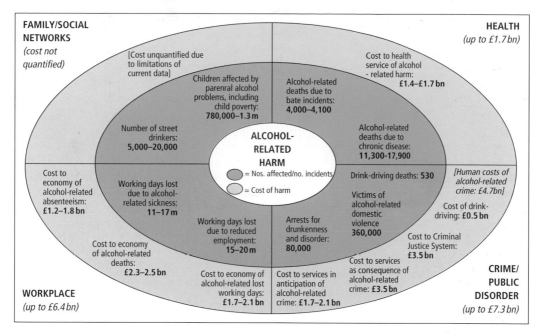

Figure 14.3 The costs of alcohol-related harm in the UK. Abbreviations: bn, billion; m, million. (Reproduced from: Prime Minister's Strategy Unit Alcohol Harm Reduction Strategy for England, 2004.)

Table 14.5 Features of delirium tremens.

Onset 24–48 hours after stopping heavy, prolonged drinking
Delirium
Visual hallucinations
Delusions, usually persecutory and transient
Fear and agitation, sometimes aggression
Coarse tremor
Seizures
Autonomic disturbance (sweating, fever, tachycardia, hypertension)
Insomnia
Dehydration and electrolyte disturbance
Lasts 3–4 days, followed by exhaustion and patchy amnesia for the episode

- Assess accurately the amount consumed (use diaries, informants).
- Assess the nature and extent of harm (e.g. liver function tests, work record).
- Ensure person is fully informed of the hazards of excess alcohol intake. Tailor advice to the individual, and reinforce with written information.

- Review progress. If problem drinking persists, give details of further resources available locally.

Treatment of alcohol dependence

The first requirement is detoxification ('detox', 'drying out'), which is controlled withdrawal, using a reducing course of a benzodiazepine in place of alcohol. This is usually undertaken in primary care. The specialist substance misuse service and admission may be required if the problem is complicated (e.g. comorbid psychiatric disorder, lack of support at home).

- A suggested regimen is chlordiazepoxide, starting at 20 mg qds and reducing daily to finish with 10 mg on day 7. Advise the patient to drink plenty of non-alcoholic liquids. Prescribe vitamins—deficiencies are common and withdrawal may precipitate Wernicke's syndrome.
- A similar strategy can be used if a patient presents in the early stages of unintentional withdrawal.
- Chlormethiazole is no longer recommended due to toxicity and misuse.

Maintaining abstinence

Various strategies are used to prevent relapse following withdrawal from alcohol. None has been shown to be very effective.
- Aim for abstinence where possible—it has a better long-term outcome than controlled drinking.
- Regular liver function tests and breath alcohol measurements help monitor progress.
- Encourage attendance at groups run by local community alcohol services or Alcoholics Anonymous.
- Consider disulfiram (Antabuse), acamprosate or opioid antagonists (p. 68).
- Psychological interventions include cognitive behavioural therapy, social skills training, problem solving and motivational interviewing (helping them make the decision to change their behaviour).
- About 50% are drinking again within 6 months of abstinence.

Treatment of associated medical disorders

Many of the medical syndromes arising from alcohol misuse can present as emergencies (e.g. Wernicke's encephalopathy, bleeding varices), and the admission provides an opportunity for psychiatric intervention. Look out for withdrawal symptoms occurring during hospitalization.

Treatment of associated psychiatric disorders

The principles are:
- Reduce intake to safe limits, since continuing alcohol misuse acts as a perpetuating factor.
- Treat the psychiatric disorder on its merits. Check for interaction of alcohol with prescribed medication (e.g. antidepressants).

Opioids

Opioids (*opiates*) cause high levels of morbidity and mortality, and are highly addictive. Heroin is the most common; others include morphine, buprenorphine, codeine and methadone. There are an estimated 100000 regular users in the UK. There are several modes of use:
- Intravenous injection ('mainlining'). It is associated with a high risk of infections, thrombosis and phlebitis. Hepatitis B and C, and HIV, should be suspected and testing performed (with informed consent and appropriate counselling) in anyone who has injected drugs.
- Inhalation—'chasing the dragon': the opiate is melted on metal foil and then inhaled as it vaporizes.
- 'Snorting'—the opioid is cut into a fine powder and then sniffed.

Clinical features

Dependence

The main effect of opioids is a feeling of euphoria and analgesia. Less pleasant features occurring in regular users include chronic malaise, anorexia, loss of libido, impotence, pinpoint pupils and constipation. Tolerance to all opioids rapidly develops. Because of this (and because of batch-to-batch variation in purity), overdose is common and frequently fatal due to respiratory depression.
- Tolerance makes pain management in an opioid user difficult as higher doses may be required.

Withdrawal

Stopping opioids leads to an extremely unpleasant withdrawal syndrome called 'cold turkey' (Table 14.6). The onset is usually within 8–12 hours of the

Table 14.6 Features of opioid withdrawal.

Craving
Restlessness and insomnia
Myalgia
Sweating
Abdominal pain, vomiting and diarrhoea
Dilated pupils, running nose and eyes
Tachycardia
Yawning
'Goose bumps'

last dose (longer after methadone), peaking 24–48 hours later and subsiding over 10 days. Though severe, opioid withdrawal is rarely life-threatening.

Management

Opioid dependence can be managed in two ways.

Rapid detoxification and abstinence

- In-patient detoxification is more effective than out-patient detoxification—probably because many opioid-dependent people live in chaotic, unsupportive environments (often with other users). Information is given about the nature and course of withdrawal symptoms.
- Prescribe reducing doses of a substitute drug, methadone linctus, which reduces the severity of the withdrawal symptoms. Clonidine and naltrexone (an opioid antagonist) are also used.
- Postwithdrawal abstinence programmes vary from specific relapse-prevention therapies to residential houses where a network of ex-users helps the recovering addict overcome the craving.
- Even when withdrawal is achieved, the relapse rate is high (40% at 6 months; the majority at a year).

Harm reduction and maintenance therapy (substitution treatment)

In maintenance therapy for opioid dependence, the priority changes from abstinence to reducing the harm from ongoing opioid use. The first aim is to make services acceptable to users in order to engage them in treatment. Then, the aims are to:
- Reduce injecting.
- Stabilize drug use and lifestyle.
- Reduce criminal behaviour by avoiding need to obtain expensive drugs.
- Reduce the death rate.

The harm reduction approach is pragmatic and includes a range of initiatives such as free needles and syringes and public education. A central feature is *substitute prescribing*. Oral methadone is prescribed to prevent the need for intravenous injections. Long-term use of the oral drug is usual.
- Substitute prescribing does not suit all opioid users. It is best targeted at those whose social functioning and health has already been seriously affected by drug use, and where abstinence is an unrealistic goal.

Stimulants

Amphetamines

Amphetamines ('speed', 'whizz') may be taken orally, snorted or injected. They produce symptoms similar to those of hypomania: elevated mood, over-talkativeness, increased energy and insomnia. Pulse and blood pressure increase, pupils dilate and mucous membranes become dry.
- *Dependence* occurs. Regular users develop depression and mood swings. The withdrawal syndrome can be severe (a 'crash'), with agitated depression, lethargy, suicidal thoughts and craving.
- Management and prognosis is similar to that for opioids. Treat intoxication or psychosis with benzodiazepines and antipsychotics; treat depression with tricyclic antidepressants.
- Prolonged use can lead to *paranoid psychosis*, which can last for months after use has ceased.
- Amphetamines are used clinically for attention deficit hyperactivity disorder and narcolepsy.
- Amphetamines are potent dopamine enhancers—they inhibit its reuptake and stimulate its release.

Cocaine

Cocaine produces similar effects to amphetamines, but the features tend to be more dramatic.
- Cocaine is either snorted, or smoked in the form of 'crack' or 'freebase' (cocaine processed to remove the hydrochloride), which increases the intensity of the effect.
- Cocaine misusers often also misuse opioids and alcohol.
- Immunization against the effects of cocaine is currently being tested.

3,4-Methylenedioxymethamphetamine (MDMA, ecstasy)

Ecstasy is a synthetic amphetamine analogue with stimulatory and hallucinogenic effects. It is widely used in Britain—30% of teenagers say they've tried it. Tolerance occurs and the best experience is said to be the first. Though safer than amphetamines or cocaine, there is concern about its harmful effects:

• Adverse reactions—hyperpyrexia and acute renal failure due to dehydration, as well as water intoxication in users who overcompensate. There are rare, but well-publicized, fatalities.

• Acute psychosis—prevalence unknown.

• The drug is neurotoxic to 5-HT fibres (at least in monkeys), and chronic users have lowered central 5-HT levels and some cognitive deficits. There is therefore concern that depression and impulsivity may be a long-term consequence.

Hallucinogens

Hallucinogens alter perception, producing *psychedelic* experiences. They are taken orally. LSD is the main synthetic hallucinogen; similar effects can be achieved using magic mushrooms. Agonism at 5-HT2 receptors is a likely common mechanism.

Lysergic acid diethylamide (LSD)

The 'trip' starts about 2 hours after consumption, lasts 8–12 hours, and consists of distorted sensory perception, alteration of the sense of time and scale, and changes in body image (e.g. out of body experiences). The effects can be very intense—and occasionally terrifying (a 'bad trip').

• Hallucinogens rarely cause dependence or withdrawal. They are associated with *flashbacks* when the sensations of a trip are re-experienced long afterwards.

• Emergency psychiatric referral may occur because of the panic or agitation associated with a bad trip. Reassurance, reorientatation and 'talking down' are necessary. Sedation as required with benzodiazepines. The person may also come to harm from responding to the hallucinations.

Cannabis

Cannabis is the most widely used illicit drug. It is derived from the hemp plant *Cannabis sativa*. The main psychoactive ingredient is δ-9-tetrahydrocannabinol, which acts on endogenous cannabinoid receptors. It is usually smoked. It has several effects including:

• Exaggeration of pre-existing mood.

• Mellowness and increased enjoyment of aesthetic experience.

• Distortion of sense of space and time.

• Reddening of eyes.

• Impairment of motor performance—for example, car driving.

Adverse reactions include anxiety and paranoid ideation—especially in first time users—and occasionally delirium. Cannabis does not cause dependence or withdrawal, though some tolerance occurs (and use may become so ingrained as to warrant the term 'psychological dependence'). Users rarely seek treatment or come to medical attention.

• The occurrence of an 'amotivational state' in chronic heavy users remains unproven.

• Early use of cannabis may be a risk factor for schizophrenia and subsequently associated with a worse treatment response.

Other substances

Phencyclidine

Phencyclidine (PCP, 'angel dust') and ketamine are volatile anaesthetics which in smaller doses produce a sense of drunkenness, hallucinations, disorientation and agitation. The picture resembles schizophrenia. Complications include nystagmus, tachycardia, hypertension and seizures.

• Usage is common in the USA but rare in the UK.

• The drugs are antagonists at NMDA glutamate receptors.

• When managing PCP intoxication or psychosis, avoid chlorpromazine. The medical complications may need treatment.

Solvents

Solvent misuse (of glue, aerosols, petrol, etc.) is mainly an adolescent male group activity. The effects are rapid in onset and short-lived—euphoria, disinhibition, blurred vision, ataxia.
• Solvent use comes to medical attention when complications arise—cardiac arrhythmias, inhalation of vomit, coma. Chronic damage to the liver and brain can occur.

Anabolic steroids

Anabolic steroids are misused mainly by male athletes and bodybuilders. They produce a range of psychiatric effects that can be severe and persistent—euphoria, depression, aggression ('roid rage') and hyperactivity. A form of dependency may result in some users. Clinical suspicion may be raised by the physical appearance.

Benzodiazepines

Benzodiazepines are taken illicitly, often as part of multiple drug misuse and as an opioid substitute. It can be difficult to decide whether symptoms and side-effects are attributable to the benzodiazepine or to the other drugs being used.
• Iatrogenic benzodiazepine dependence and its management is mentioned in Chapter 7.

Nicotine and caffeine

Both nicotine and caffeine are addictive—ask any smoker or serious coffee drinker. Each has its own acute actions and side-effects, but psychiatric problems are rare.
• Psychiatric patients smoke more than the population average—90% of people with schizophrenia do so. For unknown reasons they have a lower incidence of lung cancer than other smokers.
• Abstinence rates after nicotine dependence (30% at 6 months) are worse than for opioids, cocaine and alcohol.

Key points

• For each substance consider: What are its acute effects? Does it cause dependence and withdrawal? What are the associated psychiatric, medical and social complications?
• Dependence is a combination of physical and psychological effects. It is common in people who regularly use alcohol, opioids or stimulants. Withdrawal occurs if the substance is withheld.
• Substance misuse is widespread. Those in treatment are a small and unrepresentative fraction.
• Substance misuse is often comorbid with psychiatric disorders. Both need to be treated. The combination worsens prognosis.
• Alcohol produces a wide range of psychiatric, medical and social problems. Enquire about alcohol intake and consider a role for alcohol misuse in all patients.
• Management of substance misuse includes psychological, pharmacological and social components. The prognosis for persistent abstinence after being dependent on any substance is poor.

Chapter 15

Personality disorders

Personality and personality disorder

Personality describes the characteristic behavioural, emotional and cognitive attributes of an individual. Thus we talk about an aggressive man, a nervous lady and so on. Such traits are usually apparent by mid-adolescence and remain fairly stable thereafter. Psychiatrists are interested in personality because it forms a major part of the contextual understanding of every case (Chapter 5) and interacts with psychiatric disorders in many ways, as discussed below.

• Although long-term stability is a characteristic, personality traits are exacerbated in the short-term by stress (*'decompensation'*), and it is usually at such times that they are medically encountered.

Personality is also of interest to psychiatrists because in some individuals certain personality traits may be extreme and lead to problems for the person or others. This constitutes *personality disorder*. People with personality disorder come into contact with medical and psychiatric services either because they are concerned about themselves or, more commonly, because their actions affect others around them. For example:

• A spinster who has been too timid to ever have a close relationships takes an overdose because she is so lonely.

• A tax inspector whose obsessive need for tidiness at work leads to an industrial dispute and a psychiatric report is requested.

• A young woman who takes impulsive overdoses each time a boyfriend leaves her.

A personality disorder may also be detected during the assessment or treatment of a psychiatric disorder—though bear in mind that the person's behaviour and self-description may be modified by the illness and give a misleading impression about their 'normal' personality.

Core features of personality disorder

This section covers the features common to all personality disorders. The following section deals with the factors specific to particular personality disorders.

Diagnosis

Diagnosis of personality disorder is based on a marked deviation of one or more aspects of personality. The main effect may be on:

• Cognitions (attitudes; ways in which others' actions are interpreted).

• Mood (range, intensity, and appropriateness of emotions).

• Impulse control and gratification of needs.

• Relationships and the way interpersonal situations are handled.

In addition, other criteria must be met, which help establish that the disturbance is sufficient to merit a diagnostic label:

- The personality attributes cause distress or dysfunction for the individual or those he interacts with.
- The dysfunction occurs across a range of situations.
- The characteristics are pervasive, stable and recognizable since late adolescence.

The specific personality disorders are diagnosed according to the domain(s) of personality which are most affected, and the most prominent behaviours.

Assessment

The above features mean that a diagnosis of personality disorder requires considerable information about the patient's previous behaviour, personal history and mental state (see Chapters 2, 3 and 5).

- Use of an informant is very important to corroborate the history.
- Always describe clearly the characteristics upon which the diagnosis is being based.
- Always seek and record positive as well as negative personality attributes; the former will prove useful in management.
- Carefully examine for the presence of a psychiatric disorder—it may be a differential diagnosis or a comorbid condition.
- Do the same for substance misuse, which exacerbates many personality traits.

Classification

Personality disorder in ICD-10 is divided into ten types. However, the validity and reliability of these categories is either very poor or unknown. Most patients seem to fit several descriptions or none of them. A simpler and slightly more evidence-based option, from DSM-IV, is to use three clusters, which encompass the individual categories (Table 15.1). In practice, both clusters and categories are used by clinicians.

- Personality traits and personality disorders are, in reality, *dimensional*, i.e. they merge into each other (and into psychiatric disorders). Consequently, any categorical classification is bound to be problematic. One illustration is that several categories formerly included as personality disorders are now considered to be psychiatric disorders, e.g. schizotypal disorder (p. 135).
- Other difficulties with the concept of personality disorder are covered later in this chapter.
- The vignettes below illustrate the category and cluster approaches to personality disorder.

Miss D is 22 and has taken an impulsive overdose. She felt bored and angry with her boyfriend and various others. She has repeatedly self-harmed since early adolescence in response to minor life events— particularly when she feels abandoned. She reports having been sexually abused by her step-father. Her lifestyle is chaotic and she misuses alcohol. Previous attempts to offer help have been thwarted by her failure to keep appointments. Her one enduring pleasure in life is looking after horses. Two days later she discharges herself; her boyfriend sent her some flowers and she is planning to marry him.

Key features: Impulsivity, sensitive to rejection, emotional instability.

Positive attributes: The care of animals. Has done unpaid work for an animal charity.

Cluster: B (Dramatic)

Subtype: Emotionally unstable (borderline) personality disorder.

Dr E is a 60-year-old scientist who has accepted psychiatric referral under protest. He is unmarried and has had several brief, unsatisfactory relationships. He feels strongly that he has been denied the acclaim he deserves and is currently complaining bitterly to his head of department after unsuccessfully applying for promotion. He alleges that other workers steal his ideas. He does not mix with his colleagues and is uneasy in social gatherings.

Key features: Socially isolated, suspicious, tendency to exaggerate self-importance.

Positive attributes: His research eminence shows a high level of functioning.

Cluster: A (Eccentric)

Subtype: Paranoid personality disorder.

Table 15.1 Personality disorders.

Cluster or subtype	Main features
Cluster A (Eccentric)	**Aloof or suspicious, solitary**
Paranoid	Suspicion and distrust of others
	Sensitivity to criticism
	Bears grudges
	Self-importance
Schizoid	Emotionally cold and detached
	Introspective
	Social isolation
	Lack of *joie de vivre*
Cluster B (Dramatic)	**Emotionally labile and intense, others affected**
Dissocial (= psychopathic, antisocial)	Callous
	Unstable, transient relationships
	Low frustration threshold
	Irritable and impulsive
	Failure to learn from experience
	Failure to accept responsibility, lack of guilt
	Tend to be young men
Borderline (= emotionally unstable)	Multiple, turbulent relationships
	Impulsivity
	Recurrent emotional crises
	Variable, intense mood
	Stress-related psychotic-like symptoms
	Tend to be young women
Histrionic	Exaggerated, theatrical emotional expression
	Attention seeking
	Vain
	Suggestible
	Shallow, labile mood
	Crushes and fads
Narcissistic	Grandiose self-importance
	Exaggerates achievements and abilities
	Exploits others
	Arrogant
	Expects special praise and respect
Cluster C (Anxious)	**Timid, dependent, low self-esteem**
Anankastic (= obsessional)	Excessive orderliness
	Preoccupation with detail
	Inflexible and dogmatic
	Humourless
Anxious (= avoidant)	Persistent feelings of tension and apprehension
	Avoid personal contact
	Fear of criticism or rejection
Dependent	Encourage others to make decisions
	Excessive need to be taken care of

Management

Personality cannot be modified to any significant degree. Instead, management of personality disorder is aimed at helping the person limit excesses of behaviour, or by tailoring the surroundings and circumstances to the personality.

- Reinforce skills and positive traits.
- Help the person find a lifestyle which suits them, maximizing their strengths and minimizing the effects of their personality difficulties.
- Identify stressors that precipitate crises, and try and avoid or reduce them.
- Avoid an inconsistent or excessive reaction to crises. Admissions are rarely helpful and may reinforce the behaviour. A consistent, limited and community-based approach is better.
- Treat any coexisting substance misuse.
- Treat any coexisting psychiatric disorder.
- Some personality disorders may benefit from specific psychotherapies (see below). Very occasionally, inpatient psychotherapy (a *therapeutic community*) is used.

Prognosis

The fact that personality disorders are considered to be lifelong and stable implies that prognosis is uniformly bad. In fact, considerable fluctuations do occur, and improvement is often observed by middle age. Some clinicians distinguish:

- Mature personality disorders (equating to Cluster A), which are first recognizable in late adolescence and which remain stable or worsen with age.
- Immature personality disorders (Clusters B and C) which have an onset in childhood and which mellow with age.

Epidemiology

The estimated prevalence of personality disorders in different settings is given in Table 15.2. These estimates are from studies using different methodologies and definitions and must be interpreted cautiously. For example, the prevalence of personality disorder in some surveys is only 2%.

Aetiology

Very little is known of the aetiology of personality disorders, partly because so little is understood about the determinants of normal personality. Most current research focuses on borderline and dissocial personality disorder, largely because they cause the greatest clinical and forensic difficulties (see below).

- There is a moderate genetic contribution to personality traits (e.g. 35–50% heritability for neuroticism and extraversion) and to some personality disorders, especially anankastic and dissocial types.
- Patterns of childhood behaviour, as young as infancy, predict personality and personality disorders, albeit only weakly. Nevertheless, it emphasizes the early origins and stability of personality characteristics.
- Upbringing and childhood experiences have major influences on our personality for better and

Table 15.2 Prevalence of personality disorders in different populations.

Setting	Type of personality disorder	Prevalence (%)
General population	Any	13
	Dissocial (psychopathic)	4 (men); <1(women)
	Cluster A (eccentric)	1–3
	Cluster B (dramatic)	2–3
	Cluster C (anxious)	2–3
General practice	Any	34
Psychiatric in-patients	Any	50 (men); 40 (women)
	Emotionally unstable (borderline)	15

worse. Adverse childhood events, including sexual and physical abuse, are risk factors for personality disorder.

• Aggressive behaviour may be slightly commoner in men with sex chromosome abnormalities (especially XYY), but much less so than sometimes portrayed.

Specific personality disorders

Cluster A personality disorders

People with cluster A personality disorder (especially schizoid type) by their nature tend to avoid services, and usually present (as with Dr E in the vignette) when their suspiciousness or persecutory beliefs lead them to behave in a way which brings them to attention (e.g. making accusations or threatening retribution for a perceived wrongdoing). The key issues are:

• To distinguish the personality disorder from a psychosis, especially chronic delusional disorder (p. 134). Paranoid personality is a risk factor for development of a psychosis.

• To decide if there is a significant risk of harm to others or self as a result of the beliefs (Chapter 4).

• To decide what, if any, treatment should be given for the personality disorder. Low dose antipsychotics may be tried, with appropriate consent, but compliance is likely to be poor. Similarly, social interventions may be offered, but isolation is rarely perceived as a problem. Psychotherapy is said to be ineffective, even harmful, and is contraindicated.

Cluster B personality disorders

There is considerable overlap between the individual disorders in this cluster. In practice, the commonly used categories are borderline (for women) and dissocial (for men).

Borderline personality disorder

Miss D (see vignette above) fits the typical profile of borderline personality disorder. There may be frequent presentations for a variety of reasons:

• Following an overdose or self-cutting.

• With depressive or 'quasipsychotic' symptoms or suicidal ideation. The psychiatric presentation and subjective description is often dramatic, yet somewhat out of keeping with the objective impression.

• With a dramatic plea or demand for help of some kind (e.g. admission, medication).

Management can be difficult; clinicians may oscillate between over-reacting and failing to intervene. Base management around the following:

• Careful differential diagnosis from mood disorders and psychosis. Borderline personality disorders are lifelong, beginning in adolescence—a disorder beginning at 30 years cannot simply be a personality disorder.

• Patients need a written care plan. Ensure good communication between the agencies involved to avoid 'splitting' (disagreements between staff induced by the patient—people with these personality traits induce a range of strong feelings).

• Respond to threats consistently and do not reinforce manipulative behaviour.

• Clear boundaries should be agreed about acceptable behaviour and about the nature of the service to be provided. For example, recurrent psychiatric admission is probably not helpful. Try alternative forms of crisis intervention.

• A psychotherapeutic assessment should be considered. A very intensive and specific form of psychotherapy, *dialectical behaviour therapy*, is effective in decreasing self-harm rates. Cognitive analytical therapy is also advocated. Neither is widely available in the UK. Group therapy in *therapeutic communities* may be helpful.

• Trials of an antidepressant or a mood stabilizer may be indicated even in the absence of a clear depressive episode. Tricyclic antidepressants probably do more harm than good, but there is some evidence that SSRIs, low dose antipsychotics and mood stabilizers may be effective at reducing impulsive behaviour and mood variability. However, although good responses are seen in a few patients, long-term medication is not appropriate for many patients.

• The diagnosis is sometimes applied loosely and pejoratively, especially to young women who self harm, abuse alcohol, have eating difficulties and have chaotic lifestyles. Use the label carefully, sticking to the principles outlined here.

Borderline personality disorder is under active research investigation at present.

- The key neuropsychological deficits are thought to be *affective instability* and *impulsivity*.
- Brain imaging suggests dopamine and the frontal lobes are important.
- An emerging view is that the disorder may be a form of bipolar mood disorder.
- There is an association of borderline personality disorder with childhood sexual abuse, post-traumatic stress disorder, and bulimia nervosa. However, these associations are not as strong nor as specific as sometimes claimed.

Dissocial (psychopathic) disorder

Historically, *psychopathic disorder* (as it is still called in legal circles) has had its own status: it is grounds for detention under the Mental Health Act (Chapter 7). In practice, most general psychiatrists rarely treat people with dissocial personality disorder (with or without consent) as no interventions have been shown to be effective. Admission is usually avoided, as it is often disruptive for other patients. The main goal is to exclude other diagnoses that may be more treatable. Forensic psychiatrists, on the other hand, spend much of their time assessing and managing the disorder.

- The Mental Health Act is used to send some people with dissocial personality disorder who have committed serious crimes to secure psychiatric hospitals rather than to prison. This is a controversial decision, affected by societal and financial influences rather than by evidence of effectiveness. In hospital, prolonged psychotherapy or antipsychotic drugs may be tried.
- The problems of dissocial personality disorder are often worsened by drugs and alcohol.
- The whole range of genetic, developmental, psychological and social factors are thought to be involved in the origins of dissocial personality disorder. A few people have temporal lobe EEG abnormalities. *Minimal brain dysfunction* refers to the view that the disorder results from minor brain injury or delayed maturation.

- As with borderline personality disorder, the core neuropsychological deficits are thought to involve impulsivity and decision making, and relate to abnormalities in the regulation of frontal lobe activity by dopamine and 5-HT.

Cluster C personality disorder

This cluster rarely presents clinically, and there is little information about how to manage it. If it does, set realistic goals for treatment, try and enhance self-esteem, and avoid escalating contact which simply fosters dependency.

- The diagnosis is usually made in someone who presents with a depressive disorder or anxiety disorder. Cluster C personality disorder is a risk factor for both.

Personality disorder and psychiatric disorder

The interaction between personality and psychiatric disorder is important and manifold (Figure 15.1):

- Personality disorder can *predispose to* psychiatric disorder.
- Personality disorder can *coexist with* psychiatric disorder (a type of comorbidity). This worsens prognosis. For example, comorbidity of schizophrenia and personality disorder increases the risk of violence; the comorbidity of depression and personality disorder increases suicide risk. Additional comorbidity with substance misuse further elevates such risks.
- Personality disorder, in reality, *merges into* psychiatric disorder. As illustrated by the reclassification of cyclothymia from a personality disorder to a form of bipolar disorder.
- Personality disorder can be *mistaken for* psychiatric disorder, and *vice versa*. For example, someone with a depressive disorder may give the impression that they have a personality disorder; a person with borderline personality disorder may be misdiagnosed as having a psychotic disorder.
- Personality can be *affected by* psychiatric disorder. For example, the deterioration in personality in chronic schizophrenia.

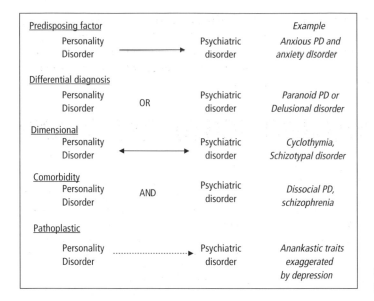

Predisposing factor			Example
Personality Disorder	→	Psychiatric disorder	*Anxious PD and anxiety disorder*
Differential diagnosis			
Personality Disorder	OR	Psychiatric disorder	*Paranoid PD or Delusional disorder*
Dimensional			
Personality Disorder	↔	Psychiatric disorder	*Cyclothymia, Schizotypal disorder*
Comorbidity			
Personality Disorder	AND	Psychiatric disorder	*Dissocial PD, schizophrenia*
Pathoplastic			
Personality Disorder	⇢	Psychiatric disorder	*Anankastic traits exaggerated by depression*

Figure 15.1 Relationships between personality and psychiatric disorders.

Table 15.3 Multiaxial classification.

Axis I	Psychiatric disorder
Axis II	Personality disorder and mental retardation
Axis III	General medical conditions
Axis IV	Psychosocial and environmental problems
Axis V	Global assessment of functioning (rated on a 1–100 scale)

- Personality can have a *pathoplastic effect* on psychiatric disorder. That is, it can modify the clinical features even if it has no direct causal role.

Multiaxial classification

These interactions have led to a *multiaxial* classification system in which psychiatric disorder and personality disorder are coded separately. Other axes record additional information (Table 15.3).
- Multiaxial classification is part of DSM-IV. In the UK it is used mainly in child psychiatry.

A 55-year-old man has lived alone all his life, usually in hostels. He has developed delusions of persecution. He has few interests, is barely literate, and has never held down a job. His mobility is limited. He improves moderately with treatment.
  Axis I: delusional disorder.

Axis II: schizoid personality disorder; mild mental retardation.
  Axis III: osteoarthritis.
  Axis IV: homelessness, illiteracy.
  Axis V: Global assessment 25 (on admission), 45 (on discharge).

Problems with the concept of personality disorder

The very concept of personality disorder has been controversial because:
- It isn't a 'disease'. It medicalizes individual differences and implies they can and should be treated by doctors.
- It is unreliable.
- One man's personality disorder is another man's virtue. Many famous people meet the criteria for personality disorder, yet the traits are either tolerated or are intrinsic to their success.
- The term is pejorative: the label is applied to patients that doctors don't like or find hard to manage, or is used as a justification to avoid trying to help.
- A current controversy is *dangerous and severe personality disorder (DPSD)*, a concept introduced by the UK government in 1999. It is intended to allow people with a severe personality disorder who are

thought to be at risk of committing serious violence to be detained—possibly indefinitely. Virtually all mental health professionals, patients' organizations and civil rights campaigners oppose it on scientific and moral grounds.

Some of these issues go well beyond the boundaries of psychiatry. Given the current state of knowledge, psychiatrists must at least ensure that the term 'personality disorder' is used as reliably and usefully as possible.

Key points

- Personality is the combination of emotional, cognitive and behavioural traits which characterize each of us. A personality is disordered if the traits cause problems for the individual or those around him.
- Personality disorders are classified pragmatically into three clusters: eccentric, dramatic and anxious. Important specific types are paranoid, dissocial (psychopathic) and borderline.
- Always be wary of diagnosing personality disorder solely on the basis of behaviour during an episode of psy-

chiatric illness. Illness can affect how personality is expressed.
- Personality disorder interacts with psychiatric disorder in several ways: predisposing factor; pathoplastic factor; prognostic factor; comorbid disorder; and as a differential diagnosis.
- Focus treatment on modifying circumstances, removing exacerbating factors and reinforcing positive behaviours. Medication has a very limited role. Specific psychotherapies may help borderline personality disorder.

Chapter 16

Childhood disorders

Principles of child psychiatry

Interviewing children

When interviewing a child, the objectives are the same as with adults: to establish rapport, make a diagnosis, understand its context and plan treatment. However, for several reasons, the nature of the interview differs, especially with young children:

- The child may not understand the question or be unable to express himself.
- The range of disorders being sought, and hence the diagnostic focus, is different.
- Parents determine when and how the child presents.
- Family factors contribute to many disorders—so more attention is paid to the family environment. Child psychiatry interviews have several features:
- Parents are present and are often interviewed alone first.
- The interviewer must be able to jump from one topic to another as led by the child.
- Assessment may start with play and gentle conversation to gain trust.
- Much information comes from the child's appearance and behaviour.
- Significant others (e.g. teachers, siblings) provide key parts of the history.
- More than one session may be needed to complete the interview.

By adopting these strategies, the interviewer aims to collect information about the topics in Table 16.1.

In addition a paediatric history and neurological examination may be indicated. To complete the assessment, background information is sought from relevant sources, such as teachers or social services.

- Get parental consent at each stage, unless abuse is suspected, in which case the duty of care to the child may override this principle.

Classification

The major childhood psychiatric disorders are shown in Table 16.2. A *multiaxial* scheme is often used to record the diagnostic information because of the importance of developmental stage, overall abilities and social circumstances:

Axis I—Psychiatric disorder(s) present.
Axis II—Developmental stage and delays.
Axis III—Intellectual level.
Axis IV—Medical problems.
Axis V—Abnormal social situations.

- Learning disability in children is covered in Chapter 17.

Epidemiology

Transient symptoms and behavioural disturbances are common in children of all ages. As in adults,

Table 16.1 Topics for the child psychiatric interview.

Presenting problem
  Onset, duration, factors affecting it
  Associated problems and symptoms
  Recent life events
  Parents' and child's explanation for it

Developmental milestones
  Motor—e.g. sitting, walking
  Social—e.g. smiling
  Emotional—e.g. attachment behaviour
  Cognitive—e.g. talking, reading
  Other—e.g. toilet training

Emotional profile
  Temperament
  Problem behaviours
  Likes and dislikes

Family
  Relationship with parents and siblings
  Problems at home
  Separations from parents
  Parental and sibling health and personalities

Schooling
  Educational record
  Attendance
  Relationship with peers

General health
  Hospital admissions
  Previous psychiatric history

Observation of child
  General appearance
  Interactions with interviewer and family members
  Attention and concentration
  Prevailing mood and range of emotions expressed
  Language and motor skills

Table 16.2 Childhood psychiatric disorders.

Emotional disorders (neuroses)
  Anxiety disorders
  Somatoform disorder
Behavioural disorders
  Conduct disorder
  Attention deficit hyperactivity disorder (ADHD)
Depressive disorder
Developmental disorders
  Pervasive (e.g. autism)
  Specific (e.g. specific reading disorder)
Miscellaneous conditions
  Enuresis
  Encopresis
  Selective mutism
  Tics

- Commonest diagnoses are emotional disorders and conduct disorders.
- Disorders are commoner in children with learning disability, epilepsy and chronic physical illnesses.

Aetiology

The same broad range of aetiological factors operate in childhood as in adulthood (Table 16.3).

- There is a genetic component to most disorders, mediated partly through its influence on temperament and intelligence.
- The major environmental factors are the family and social circumstances.
- Genes and environment are not independent factors, but interact to determine risk.

Management

Management of children with psychiatric disorders is based upon several principles:
- Take the child's developmental stage and overall level of functioning into account.
- Most problems are treated initially with advice, support and behavioural interventions.
- Involve the family.
- Avoid removal from school or home wherever possible.

making a psychiatric diagnosis requires a persistence and pervasiveness of symptoms, and evidence of dysfunction. The major epidemiological features of childhood psychiatric disorder are:

- Prevalence at age 10 is: 7% in rural areas, 13% in urban areas. At age 14 the prevalence is higher. (These numbers come from a classic, though dated, UK study).
- Boys affected twice as often as girls for most diagnoses.

Factor	Examples
Genetic	Autism
Environmental	
Family factors	
Parenting styles	Harsh, critical style associated with conduct disorder
Parental conflict	Increased risk of emotional or conduct disorder
Parental psychiatric disorder	Increased risk of eating disorder
Social factors	
Deprivation	Increased risk of conduct disorder
Bullying	School refusal
Other factors	
Prematurity	Increased risk of developmental delays and behavioural disorders
Medical disorder	Epilepsy increases risk of most disorders
Physical abuse	Increased risk of emotional and behavioural disorders

Table 16.3 Causative factors in child psychiatry.

- Medication has little or no role in most disorders (with a few notable exceptions).

Further details are discussed in the sections describing the specific disorders.

- The organization of child psychiatric services, through which treatments are delivered, was mentioned in Chapter 8.

Prognosis

Childhood psychiatric disorders have a variable outcome, in part because of the influence of the child's ongoing development and experiences. The basic pattern is summarized in Table 16.4.

Emotional disorders

Neuroses (emotional disorders) were described in Chapter 10. In children, the disorders are in many ways similar but there are important differences too:

- 'Emotional disorder' is the usual term in children.
- Some subtypes are different (e.g. separation anxiety).
- Medication is rarely if ever used.

- Equal male to female ratio (cf. 1 : 2 in adults).
- Most affected children do not become affected adults.

Anxiety disorders

Crying when mummy goes out, or becoming fearful of spiders, are anxieties which children normally experience at particular developmental stages, especially at times of stress and transition. They must be distinguished from persistent, significant symptoms warranting a diagnosis of anxiety disorder. The latter affect 5% of children at some time. As in adults, anxiety manifests with behavioural, psychological and physical symptoms (Table 16.5).

Separation anxiety

Among 5–11 year olds, 3–4% have excessive anxiety when faced with separation from parents or others they are attached to. The child clings—literally or metaphorically—to the person and tries to avoid being separated from them. Sleep disturbance and nightmares occur. Older children may describe being fearful that the person will be

Table 16.4 Prognosis of psychiatric disorders in childhood.

Category	Long-term outcome
Emotional disorders	Good, two-thirds resolve in a 4-year period
Mood disorder	Poor, half have depressive disorder in adulthood
Behavioural disorders	
Conduct disorder	Poor, often leads on to personality disorder or substance misuse
ADHD	Variable
Developmental disorders	
Autistic spectrum	Lifelong
Specific reading disorder	Moderate
Other conditions	
Enuresis	Good
Encopresis	Good
Tics	Usually transient (unless Tourette syndrome)
Selective mutism	Uncertain, may have persistent communication problems

harmed and will not return. Separation anxiety often begins at times of stress, such as after the death of the family dog. Some parents are noted to be overprotective. Management includes:

- Working with the family to explain and reassure.
- Identification and resolution of stressors.
- Ensuring the parents are not reinforcing the problem (e.g. by appearing anxious when about to leave the child).
- Use of specific interventions for secondary problems that develop, such as school refusal.

Somatoform disorder

Children readily develop somatic symptoms, especially when stressed. Non-specific abdominal pain and headaches are the commonest and may lead to a paediatric referral. As in adults, *somatoform disorder* describes bodily symptoms that are unexplained by a medical condition. The assessment of these requires:

- Exclusion of a medical disorder that fully explains the symptoms.
- Exclusion of emotional or depressive disorder.
- Identification of likely precipitating and perpetuating factors. For example, the child may be unhappy at home, is worried about a sick sibling or is using the symptoms to gain attention.

Table 16.5 Symptoms of anxiety in children.

Behavioural
  Clinging to parent (or other carer)
  Unwilling to leave house
  Unwilling to go to bed
  Actions designed to avoid feared event (e.g. hiding)

Psychological
  Feeling worried
  Nightmares

Physical
  Abdominal pain
  Headaches

Management is aimed at avoiding reinforcing the symptoms (for example by teaching the parents how not to do this inadvertently) and at tackling the underlying stresses. The prognosis is variable. Some children proceed to somatoform disorder as adults.

Other emotional disorders

Obsessive–compulsive disorder in children is rare clinically, but has a prevalence of 1 in 400 in British 5–15 year olds. It is sometimes associated with Tourette syndrome (see below). It is the only childhood emotional disorder with good evidence that antidepressants (clomipramine, fluoxetine) and psychological (cognitive behavioural) therapy are effective. Nevertheless, the prognosis in severe cases is quite poor.

Children also suffer from the other emotional disorders seen in adults (Chapter 10). For example, they can get *specific phobias* or develop emotional disorders following particular stresses (*adjustment reactions*).

- *Chronic fatigue syndrome* is also now well recognized in children. As in adults, its aetiology and management remain controversial. Pending better evidence, treatment is based on the same principles of graded return to activities and cognitive behavioural methods, with the close involvement of the family.

School refusal

School refusal is not a psychiatric disorder, but it is a common cause of referral to a child psychiatrist and is frequently attributable to an emotional disorder. Its assessment is summarized in Table 16.6. First, exclude truancy and parental behaviour as causes for the absence from school. The characteristics of school refusal and truancy are different (Table 16.7). School refusal is usually due to separation anxiety, often provoked by recent events at home or at school. In older children, school refusal may reflect bullying; it can also herald a more pervasive problem such as social phobia or depressive disorder.

Management of school refusal is aimed at a rapid return to school before avoidance is too ingrained. Sometimes a graded re-exposure is needed. Address any specific fears or stresses, and treat any associated psychiatric disorder.

The prognosis in younger children is good. In older children, the problem may become prolonged and other psychiatric problems emerge. It may recur at times of transition (e.g. moving schools). There is a slightly increased risk of anxiety disorder in adulthood.

Mood disorders

The existence of mood disorders in prepubertal

Table 16.6 Assessment of suspected school refusal.

Why is the child absent from school?
School refusal
Truancy
Parents keeping child at home
Physical illness

What does the school refusal reflect?
Reluctance to leave home (i.e. secondary to separation anxiety)
A specific 'school phobia' (e.g. of getting there, or being bullied)
A more generalized disorder (e.g. social phobia, depressive disorder)

What other factors are relevant?
Recent life events (e.g. bereavement)
Recent events at school (e.g. change of class)
Parental characteristics (e.g. overprotective)

Table 16.7 Distinguishing school refusal from truancy.

School refusal	Truancy
Younger (<11 years old)	Older (>11 years old)
Underlying emotional disorder	Underlying conduct disorder
Good academic and behavioural record	Poor school record
Good prognosis	Poor prognosis
Parents overprotective and anxious	Broken home

children used to be disputed. It is now clear that they occur, even in young children.

- Prevalence estimates are variable. They increase dramatically after puberty, when the higher rate in females first appears.
- The occurrence of bipolar mood disorder prepubertally is more controversial, but gaining acceptance (especially in the USA, where some argue it may be related to the widespread use of stimulants for ADHD).

When evaluating mood and mood disorder in a child, apply the same principles as in adults:

- Symptoms should be present for at least 2 weeks and associated with distress and dysfunction.
- If there are also symptoms of an emotional

disorder, attempt to distinguish the primary diagnosis.

- Children, especially adolescents, may present in crisis or after self-harm, with isolated or transient depressive symptoms, which (as in adults) are better viewed as an adjustment reaction than a depressive episode.
- Childhood depressive disorders are classified using the adult system (Chapter 9).
- As in adults, depression in postpubertal children carries an increased suicide risk. In severe cases, psychotic symptoms may occur.
- The main difference from adults concerns young children, who may not experience depression in the same way or be unable to articulate their feelings. Much diagnostic attention must therefore be placed on their appearance and behaviour both in the interview and elsewhere (e.g. school work, activities, sleep pattern).

The aetiology of childhood depressive disorder involves the same mixture of genes, life events and unknown influences as prevail in adult cases.

Management includes support, monitoring and reducing stressors. Neither antidepressants nor psychological treatments have been shown unequivocally to be effective.

- Despite the lack of evidence, SSRIs have been widely prescribed to children and adolescents, but their use is now very restricted because of concern that they increase suicide risk. Only fluoxetine is currently allowed (in the UK) for use in under 18 s.
- Admission may be needed for severe or psychotic depression. ECT is occasionally (and controversially) used.

The prognosis of childhood depressive disorder is often poor. The condition may become chronic, and half suffer from depressive disorder in adulthood.

Behavioural disorders

Behavioural disorders are diagnosed in children who have persistent problematic and antisocial behaviour. The main distinction is between behavioural problems that result mainly from over-activity (attention deficit hyperactivity disorder, ADHD) and those that do not (conduct disorder)—though in practice the boundary is blurred.

- Neither label should be applied unless the diagnostic criteria are met—all children are naughty and 'hyper' from time to time.

Conduct disorder

Conduct disorder is the commonest psychiatric disorder of childhood and adolescence. Prevalence estimates range from 1–15%. It occurs mainly in boys (sex ratio 5:1). Conduct is disturbed and antisocial well beyond the range of misbehaviour normally observed for that age group (Table 16.8). Diagnosis is usually made after age 7, though problems have often been apparent much earlier. The term *oppositional defiant disorder* may be used for these younger children.

- A distinction is sometimes made between *socialized conduct disorder*, where the activities occur within a peer group, and *unsocialized conduct disorder*, where the child acts in isolation.

In adolescence, conduct disorder has a strong relationship with juvenile delinquency and substance misuse. There is often repeated police contact and convictions for theft, criminal damage or assault. Conduct disorder is associated with a variety of indices of social deprivation and poor parenting (Table 16.9). Any genetic contribution is small.

Table 16.8 Clinical features of conduct disorder.

In preschool children
Aggressive behaviour
Poor concentration
In mid-childhood
Lying
Stealing
Disruptive and oppositional behaviour
Bullying
In adolescence
Stealing
Truancy
Promiscuity
Substance misuse
Vandalism
Reckless behaviour

Table 16.9 Factors associated with conduct disorder.

Family factors
  Parental personality disorder
  Paternal alcoholism
  Parental disputes and violence
  Harsh, inconsistent parenting
  Being in care early in life
  Large family size

Social factors
  Inner cities
  Deprivation and overcrowding

Individual factors
  Brain damage
  Epilepsy
  Specific reading disorder

Table 16.10 Features of attention deficit hyperactivity disorder (ADHD).

Core features
  Hyperactivity
  Poor attention and concentration
  Impulsivity
  Present for at least 6 months
  Evidence for impaired functioning in two or more
    settings
  Onset by age 9, usually by 5

Other features
  Distractibility
  Poor at planning and organizing tasks
  Learning difficulties
  Clumsiness
  Low self-esteem
  Socially disinhibited
  Unpopular with other children
  Non-localizing neurological signs
  Conduct disorder coexists in 50%

The long-term prognosis is poor; 50% of cases progress to dissocial personality disorder, and persistent substance misuse and criminality are common. Those who form stable relationships have a better outcome. There is no standard therapeutic approach, and no convincing evidence that any intervention affects outcome. In practice, a mixture of attempts to shape and reward behaviour is used:

• Family focused treatments seek to identify and remedy causes for the behaviour, improve the home environment, and includes teaching parents how to cope with the behaviour and reduce conflict ('parental training').

• 'Problem-solving skills training' is a recent approach that focuses on the child rather than the parents. It is based on evidence that children with ADHD are poor at problem solving and social skills.

• Alternative outlets for energies and behaviours (e.g. youth clubs, car workshops).

• Tackle associated problems such as truancy and substance misuse.

• Stimulant medication is increasingly being used, especially if there are coexistent ADHD features.

• Residential care is occasionally unavoidable.

Attention deficit hyperactivity disorder (ADHD)

The clinical features are shown in Table 16.10. As with conduct disorder, the diagnosis requires that the problem is both persistent and extreme. In Britain, the prevalence is 2%; three-quarters are boys. In the USA, where less stringent criteria are used, prevalence and treatment rates are correspondingly higher.

• *Hyperkinetic disorder* is sometimes used interchangeably with ADHD. Strictly, it refers to a severe subgroup of ADHD in which all three core signs (inattention, hyperactivity, impulsiveness) are present, pervasive, and with onset before age 7.

• ADHD is often comorbid with conduct disorder, anxiety, depression and tic disorders. ADHD symptoms may also be seen in pervasive developmental disorders.

The aetiology of ADHD is multifactorial:

• There is a modest genetic contribution. Families also show increased rates of depressive disorder, learning difficulties, alcoholism and dissocial personality disorder.

• A neurodevelopmental abnormality is suspected, on the basis of the soft neurological signs and learning difficulties, and from brain imaging and EEG findings.

• There is an association with social deprivation, though less striking than for conduct disorder.

- Many parents blame food allergy but this is rarely substantiated when investigated properly.

The management of ADHD involves:

- Support for the child and family.
- Specific educational approaches, including attention to associated learning difficulties.
- Firm adherence to behavioural principles (to reward good behaviour and discourage hyperactive behaviour).
- Psychostimulants (e.g. methylphenidate, atomoxetine) have an important role and are recommended in UK guidelines as part of a comprehensive treatment programme. This seemingly paradoxical treatment originated from the (incorrect) belief that there is a failure of cortical arousal in ADHD. Their main neurochemical effect is to increase dopamine in the synapse. Side-effects are insomnia, poor appetite and headaches. Concerns about addiction and growth retardation have not been noted in practice.
- Modafinil is an attention-enhancing drug also used in ADHD. Its mechanism is unknown.

ADHD has a variable prognosis. Gradual improvement occurs in adolescence and a third of cases resolve. The rest have residual hyperkinetic features, especially in those with learning difficulties or conduct disorder. Dissocial personality disorder and substance misuse commonly develop.

- There is increasing interest in the occurrence of ADHD in adults, but no consensus on its diagnostic status or management.

Developmental disorders

Developmental disorders can be *pervasive* or *specific*. The former, typified by *autism*, affect many aspects of psychological and neurobiological development; in the latter, there is impairment in only one domain (e.g. reading) relative to overall development. These seemingly diverse conditions are grouped together for three reasons:

- The child is seemingly normal until late infancy or early childhood, at which point progress stops or reverses.
- The abnormality is thought to be directly related to aberrant brain development.

- Their course lacks the fluctuations of most psychiatric disorders.

Pervasive developmental disorders

Current classification divides this category into several distinct disorders, as outlined here. However, the concept of *autistic spectrum disorders* is increasingly being used, recognizing that all share core impairments in social interactions, language and communication, and the child's range of interests and activities.

Autism

Autism is a syndrome characterized by a failure to develop normal communication, especially social and emotional communication. Autistic children have a delayed, restricted and deviant use of language. They seem oblivious to non-verbal cues and emotional expressions, with little desire to interact with others or form relationships. Instead, they demonstrate a limited range of solitary, repetitive behaviours and resist attempts to change their routine. Most also have a degree of learning disability. The features are summarized in Table 16.11.

- A very few autistic children (and adults), called *idiot savants*, have remarkable abilities in discrete areas, such as complex mental arithmetic (as in the film *Rain Man*).

The differential diagnosis of 'true' autism com-

Table 16.11 Features of autism.

1 in 2000 children
80% are boys
Age of onset <3 years
Key features (the 'autistic triad')
No emotional warmth (autistic aloneness)
Impaired language and communication
Solitary, repetitive behaviours
Associated features
Mannerisms and rituals
Epilepsy in a quarter
Learning disability in 75%
Non-specific behavioural problems

prises other disorders with autistic features such as Asperger's and Rett's syndromes (see below), and fragile X syndrome and tuberous sclerosis complex (Chapter 17). However, these other disorders account for only about 10% of autism.

• Remember other causes of a failure to develop communication which may be mistaken for autism, such as specific language disorder and deafness.

The aetiology of autism is strongly genetic, with many susceptibility genes involved. Probable loci exist on chromosomes 7 and 15 (amongst many others), but no genes have yet been identified.

• No confirmed environmental risk factors are known. Despite public concern, there is no good evidence that vaccines cause autism.

• Similarly, there has not been a genuine rise in prevalence recently, merely greater awareness and loosening of the concept of autism.

• MRI scans show increased brain size early in life in autism, suggestive of an aberrant growth trajectory. Neuropathological studies suggest cellular alterations in several brain areas, notably Purkinje cells in the cerebellum, also brain stem and hippocampus. Neurochemically, excess 5-HT (serotonin) function affecting neurodevelopment has been postulated.

The prognosis is poor. Speech eventually develops in some, but communication remains limited and the core abnormalities rarely improve. Seizures can occur later in childhood. Most autistic children need special schooling and residential care, and only a minority are ever able to live independently.

There is no specific treatment. The main components of management are to:

• Make the diagnosis and support the family in understanding autism and its implications.

• Provide appropriate education and, if required, accommodation.

• Deal with abnormal behaviours and associated medical problems (e.g. epilepsy).

Asperger's syndrome

Asperger's syndrome (also called *autistic psychopa-*

thy) is like a milder version of autism, with similar abnormalities in social communication and repetitive, isolated behaviours. The child is solitary, clumsy and eccentric. Unlike autism, intelligence and language are unremarkable, and seizures are not a feature. The prevalence is uncertain, with estimates from 1 to 50 per 10000.

• The aetiology is unknown. It may or may not be causally related to autism.

• Asperger's syndrome persists into adulthood, and sometimes first presents at that time, when it may be mistaken for schizotypal or schizoid personality disorder, or schizophrenia.

Rett's syndrome

Rett's syndrome is a rare, progressive, and severe disorder occurring almost exclusively in girls. The main features are autism, learning disability, seizures, loss of speech and movements and irregular breathing. It is usually caused by sporadic mutations in the MeCP2 gene on the X chromosome, and is fatal by early adulthood.

Specific developmental disorders

Specific developmental disorders are conditions in which there is marked delay in one area of development relative to the child's overall IQ. The commonest problem is with reading (80% of cases), but also arithmetic, language or motor skills. Though the disorders are not really 'psychiatric', they are often referred to (or detected by) child psychiatric services because of associated emotional or behavioural difficulties.

Specific reading disorder

In specific reading disorder, reading skills are significantly (>2 standard deviations) below that predicted by the child's overall performance. Visual impairment or lack of education must be excluded as the cause. It affects 2–10% of 10 year olds, and is four times commoner in boys than girls.

• It is associated with conduct disorder in a third of cases, also with ADHD, low social class and a disturbed family background. The direction of causality between these factors is unclear.

- Assessment should be by an educational psychologist using standardized tests.
- Management involves enhancing self-esteem and appropriate expert educational help.
- Nutritional supplements (fish oils) are being advocated by some researchers and families.
- Prognosis is poor, with reading abilities often remaining well below average.

Other conditions

Enuresis

Enuresis is urinary incontinence after the age at which bladder control is expected (*primary enuresis*; must be at least 5 years old) or after previous normal continence (*secondary enuresis*). It usually presents as bedwetting in the first half of the night (*nocturnal enuresis*). It affects 15% of 5 year olds, 2% of 10 year olds, and 1% of 14 year olds. Boys outnumber girls 3:1.

- Enuresis can cause great distress, affect self-esteem, interfere with normal activities (e.g. sleepovers) and can lead to bullying or intolerant parenting.

In the assessment, exclude urinary tract infection, diabetes or neurological disorder. Enuresis may be a sign of sleep apnoea. Search for recent stressors and symptoms of emotional disorder (twice as common as expected in those with enuresis). There is often a history of enuresis in male relatives.

The management of enuresis includes:

- Reassurance, explanation and limiting fluid intake in the evening.
- Treatment of associated psychiatric or medical disorder.
- Behavioural methods are the main treatment. A *star chart* is best for younger children; they are rewarded for achieving a realistic target (which may not be a 'dry bed' initially) with stars or other suitable token. An *enuresis alarm* ('pad and buzzer') is a moisture-sensitive pad worn by the child. When urine is passed, a buzzer goes off which wakes the child in time to go to the toilet to finish. He also participates in changing the sheets. An alarm is usually effective if persisted with for several weeks, especially in children over 7 years old.

- Pharmacological methods are sometimes used, though behavioural methods are preferred. Intranasal desmopressin is the usual first-line drug, with moderate success and few side-effects. The tricyclic antidepressant imipramine is licensed for enuresis from the age of 6, but is of limited efficacy, potentially dangerous and not recommended. Relapse is common with both methods.

The prognosis is good, though a few boys remain enuretic into adulthood.

Encopresis

Encopresis is the passing of faeces in an inappropriate place after age 4. As with enuresis it can be primary or secondary. Children may soil their pants, pass faeces in hidden places or occasionally smear them. At assessment, exclude physical problems (e.g. constipation, Hirschsprung's disease) and learning disability.

- There is often a history of inadequate or harsh toilet training combined with recent stresses and emotional disorder in the child.

Management is by reassurance, help with associated problems and ensuring that the parents do not become punitive. The standard behavioural manoeuvre is to toilet the child after each meal, and to reward him for staying there, for producing a motion and for not soiling. Most encopresis resolves with treatment within a year. Occasionally it persists into adolescence.

Tics

Tics are involuntary, rapid, spasmodic movements, usually repeated blinking and grimacing. They are common, especially in young boys, and may begin after an emotional upset. They are generally transient and need no specific treatment. However, some tics become severe, prolonged and incapacitating.

The main tic disorder is (*Gilles de la*) *Tourette syndrome*, in which tics are accompanied by vocal grunts and sometimes by stereotyped phrases, movements or expletives (*coprolalia*). Obsessive–compulsive and ADHD symptoms often occur. Boys are affected more than girls (3 : 1). Incidence is usually considered to be around 1 in 2000, but much higher figures exist.

Mild cases need no treatment. Troublesome tics are controlled by low-dose antipsychotics. Obsessional and hyperactivity symptoms can be treated as appropriate. Though the tics tend to diminish in adulthood, some symptoms persist.

• Tourette syndrome has a genetic basis, which overlaps with that of obsessive–compulsive disorder. Autoimmune processes may also contribute. Abnormalities in basal ganglia pathways and the dopamine system are implicated.

Selective mutism

In selective mutism (also called *elective mutism*), children refuse to speak although able to do so. Speech is usually normal in one setting (e.g. at home) but absent elsewhere. Non-verbal communication is preserved. Onset is from 4–8 years old. Affected children tend to be shy, anxious and isolated in most settings, but aggressive and disturbed at home. The disorder is rare, and unusual in being commoner in girls than boys. It is said to be associated with overprotective parents and depressed mothers.

• Selective mutism is increasingly being viewed as an anxiety disorder.
• There is no specific treatment; a range of behavioural interventions may be tried.
• Selective mutism can persist for several years, and residual social anxiety and communication problems are common.

Psychoses in childhood and adolescence

Schizophrenia may begin in adolescence, and occasionally in younger children. *Bipolar disorder* can also start in adolescence.

• The disorders are treated in a similar fashion to adult-onset cases, and are one of the few clear indications for medication in child psychiatry.

Special groups

Toddlers

Toddlers are notorious for *temper tantrums*. Reassurance that this normal, and simple advice on setting limits, are usually all that is needed. Consistency in the parents' response to the behaviour is crucial. Self-help books are available.

Sleep disturbances are common, either refusal to settle or night-time waking due to *night terrors* and *nightmares*. Use reassurance and a consistent bedtime routine. Psychiatric referral is rare, though occasionally the disturbances herald an emotional or behavioural disorder.

Teenagers

Contrary to the stereotype, neither emotional turmoil nor delinquency is normal for teenagers. Persistently withdrawn, disruptive or bizarre behaviour should be assessed to exclude psychiatric disorder. Diagnostically, adolescents get the tail end of childhood disorders and the early onset of adult disorders (Table 16.12), so the clinician must know about both, and the continuities between them. This has led to *adolescent psychiatry* as a subspecialty.

Children in institutions

Children in care, especially in children's homes, have increased rates of psychiatric disorder, notably conduct disorder, substance misuse and self-harm. This may be both a cause and a consequence of being in care.

Table 16.12 Important psychiatric disorders of adolescence.

Conduct disorder
Eating disorder
Substance misuse disorders
Depressive disorder
Anxiety disorder
Schizophrenia
Bipolar disorder
Deliberate self-harm

• Teenagers in detention facilities have extremely high rates of psychiatric disorder, with conduct disorder, substance misuse and self-harm again prominent.

Children with physical illness

Children with any chronic illness are at increased risk of psychiatric disorder. This is especially true for organic brain syndromes and epilepsy. The associations may partly reflect a common aetiology, but also the effects of physical illness on the child's intellectual, psychological and social development.

• Close co-operation between those involved in the psychiatric and medical disorders is essential.

Children with psychiatrically ill parents

If a parent has a psychiatric disorder, the child is at risk of psychiatric problems via an increased likelihood of inadequate or abnormal parenting, as well as from inheritance of a genetic predisposition. Hence the mental health (and personality) of parents is part of the child psychiatric assessment (Table 16.1). Specific parental problems associated with particular outcomes in the child include:

• Maternal substance misuse affects foetal development.

• Paternal alcoholism and development of conduct disorder.

• Maternal depression impairs infant bonding.

• Maternal eating disorder and abnormal feeding of the child.

• Factitious illness by proxy (sometimes called *Munchausen syndrome by proxy* or *Meadows' syndrome*)—the parent fabricates symptoms or signs in the child.

Abused children

Children can be abused sexually, physically or emotionally. The abuse has psychiatric as well as medical and legal repercussions. Key points concerning the psychiatric aspects of child abuse are:

• Take specialist advice whenever abuse is suspected. This may be obtained from paediatricians, child psychiatrists, and social services' child protection teams.

• Your responsibility is first and foremost to protect the child. This may override the usual duty of confidentiality.

• Children who are being abused may show physical, psychological or behavioural signs.

• Managing abused children is difficult and needs multidisciplinary input. Child psychiatrists have particular roles in identifying and treating the psychological consequences of the abuse. It is unknown whether intervention alters the long-term prognosis.

• Physical abuse (non-accidental injury) causes significant morbidity and mortality. Either the child or the abuser may need to be removed from the home. Physical abuse leads to higher rates of emotional and behavioural disorder.

• Children who are emotionally abused or neglected have delayed psychological and physical development and increased rates of emotional disturbance. In extreme cases, they may present with failure to thrive (*deprivation dwarfism*).

The effects of child abuse may continue into adulthood:

• Women who were sexually abused have double the risk of psychiatric disorder and five-times higher rates of psychiatric admission. Borderline personality disorder and possibly bulimia nervosa appear to be particularly common.

• There are no good data on the outcome of sexually abused boys, apart from their risk of becoming abusers and perpetuating the cycle.

• Emotional abuse may lead to persistent low self-esteem, relationship difficulties and personality disorder.

> ## Key points
>
> - Conduct disorder and emotional disorder are the commonest childhood psychiatric diagnoses. The former tends to do badly, the latter well.
> - The principles of child psychiatry and psychiatric assessment are the same as in adults. However, more attention must be paid to the child's developmental history, and to the home and school environment.
> - The risk of child psychiatric disorder is greater in urban areas, in boys, in those in care, and in children with learning disability or chronic illness.
> - Most disorders arise from an interaction between genetic and environmental factors.
> - Treatment is usually behavioural and, given the degree of influence the parents have on a child's behaviour, must be aimed at the family as well as at the child.
> - Medication is limited mainly to ADHD and psychosis. Antidepressants should not be used without a specialist opinion.

Chapter 17

Learning disability (mental retardation)

Principles

Definition and key features

Mental retardation, mental handicap, mental subnormality, developmental disability and *learning disability are synonyms. Mental retardation* is the ICD-10 term. *Learning disability* is usually preferred, and is used here.

Learning disability is defined as:
- IQ below 70.
- Impairment across a wide range of functions.
- Onset before 18 years old.

The features of learning disability are shown in Table 17.1. It must be distinguished from
- Lower than average intelligence but IQ > 70.
- Specific developmental disorders (Chapter 16).
- Intellectual impairment secondary to an adult organic syndrome (Chapter 13).

The incidence of learning disability has declined because of medical advances (e.g. immunization) and termination of affected pregnancies. However, the prevalence has not changed because of improved survival.

Mild learning disability represents the tail end of the normal population distribution for intelligence and, as such, results from an interaction between multiple genetic and environmental factors. A specific cause is more often identifiable for severe cases.

Clinical features

Learning disability can be *mild, moderate, severe* or *profound* depending on IQ (Table 17.2). Its cause, if known, is coded separately.

Assessment of learning disability

The presence of learning disability may be suspected:
- Before birth—from antenatal tests or pregnancy complications.
- At birth—from the physical appearance.
- In infancy or childhood—as a result of developmental delay.

Assessment of a child with suspected learning disability encompasses:
- Making the diagnosis—establish its presence, severity and likely cause. This may involve paediatricians, paediatric neurologists and clinical geneticists.
- Evaluating the level of adaptive functioning.
- Evaluating comorbid psychiatric problems.

The areas of assessment are listed in Table 17.3. The procedures necessary depend on the child's age and the circumstances of the assessment. Compared with the standard psychiatric assessment there is a special emphasis on the obstetric and neurodevelopmental history and on the physical examination.

Psychiatric aspects of learning disability

Children and adults with learning disability have high rates (about 40%) of behavioural disturbance and psychiatric disorder. The risk of these problems is higher with coexistent epilepsy, and lower in Down's syndrome.

Psychiatric disorder in learning disabled children

All the main psychiatric disorders are commoner in learning disabled children. The assessment of these follows the principles of the child psychiatric assessment, but modified according to intellectual level (Table 17.4).

Table 17.1 Features of learning disability.

Mild, moderate, severe and profound forms
Prevalence is about 2%, with a male : female ratio of 3 : 2
Usually untreatable
Often accompanied by:
Psychiatric disorder
Behavioural disturbance
Medical problems (e.g. epilepsy)
Caused by:
Genetic factors
Environmental factors
Commonest specific causes are Down's syndrome and fragile X syndrome

Psychiatric disorder in learning disabled adults

An adult with learning disability may require psychiatric assessment for a number of reasons:

• To assess the level of functioning and nature of current problems in order to help plan future management (e.g. placement).

• To investigate a suspected psychiatric disorder, such as schizophrenia and depression. These occur more commonly than in the general population. Their recognition may be difficult because of the learning disability. Various scales have been devised to help but sometimes the effect of a trial of medication may be needed.

• To assess and characterize a behavioural problem—called a *challenging behaviour*—such as shouting or inappropriate sexual activities, and to determine if it is secondary to a psychiatric diagnosis (e.g. depression).

• As part of a forensic or risk assessment. People with learning disability sometimes commit arson or other dangerous behaviours.

• To assess a decline in abilities. This may reflect the progressive nature of the condition or a superimposed disorder (e.g. depression). Also, dementia is commoner than expected in learning disability (not just in Down's syndrome).

Psychiatric diagnoses in adults with learning disability follow ICD-10 criteria, in a modified, multiaxial approach (Table 17.5).

Table 17.2 Features of mild, moderate, severe and profound learning disability.

	Mild	Moderate	Severe/profound
IQ range	69–50	49–35	<35 (Profound = <20)
Percentage of cases	85%	10%	5%
Ability to self-care	Independent	Need some help	Limited
Language	Reasonable	Limited	Basic or none
Reading and writing	Reasonable	Basic	Minimal or none
Ability to work	Semi-skilled	Unskilled, supervised	Supervised basic tasks
Social skills	Normal	Moderate	Few
Physical problems	Rare	Sometimes	Common
Aetiology discovered	Sometimes	Often	Usually

Table 17.3 Assessment of a child with learning disability.

History
Details of pregnancy
    Foetal growth
    Infections, trauma, eclampsia
    Alcohol or substance misuse
    Exposure to other drugs, toxins
Delivery
    Gestational age
    Complications
    Condition of baby
Child's development
    Milestones
    Physical difficulties
Family history
    Mental retardation
    Physical anomalies
    Consanguinity of parents

Examination
General
    Overall health
    Weight, height, head circumference
    Physical anomalies
    Skin
Neurological
    Tone, posture, power, reflexes
    Cranial nerves
    Motor skills
    Comprehension and use of language

Neuropsychological testing
    Intelligence quotient
    Language development

Laboratory investigations
    Karyotyping and genetic testing
    Biochemical studies
    Brain imaging
    EEG

Table 17.4 Psychiatric assessment in learning disability.

Background
    Overall level of functioning
    Associated physical handicaps
    Cause of learning disability

Psychiatric history
    Normal temperament and behaviours
    Recent changes in environment
    Recent changes in behaviour

Examination
    Interactions
    Attention
    Perseverance
    Mood
    Presence and nature of emotional expression
    Features of autism

Investigations
    Behavioural rating scales
    Autistic rating scales

Table 17.5 Diagnostic system for psychiatric disorders in adults with learning disabilities.

Axis I: Severity of learning disability
Axis II: Cause of learning disability
Axis III: Psychiatric disorders
    Level A: Developmental disorders
    Level B: Psychiatric illness
    Level C: Personality disorders
    Level D: Problem behaviours
    Level E: Other disorders

- Overall level of functioning.
- Ability in specific domains (e.g. communication, socialization, daily living tasks).
- Physical handicaps (including epilepsy) and motor skills.
- Coexisting psychiatric disorder.
- Prevailing temperament and behaviour.
- Support from family.

The management of learning disability is based on the approaches employed elsewhere in psychiatry:

- The majority of children with learning disability live at home. Most adults with severe learning disability live in well-supported group homes.

Management

Half of those with learning disability do not require any specific service provision, mostly because they are at the mild end of the spectrum. Their psychiatric problems tend to be managed by general psychiatry services. Amongst the rest, the nature and amount of intervention needed is determined by:

Long-stay institutional care has now virtually disappeared in the UK.

- Care is provided by multidisciplinary community learning disability teams using a framework similar to CMHTs (p. 82).
- Most local services have a few in-patient beds for the assessment and treatment of behavioural and psychiatric disorders. Forensic services for people with learning disability are provided regionally.
- Voluntary agencies play an important role.

Four principles guide the current strategy for care of people with learning disability:

- Legal and civil rights—to a decent education, to marry, to have children, to vote, etc.
- The right to independence—independence, not dependence, is the default position.
- The right to choice—in where to live, what work to do, who cares for them.
- The right to inclusion—in mainstream services and local communities.

'*Essential lifestyle planning*' is one approach by which to find out what the person thinks about these decisions, and to provide the right package of care and support to help them achieve their goals.

Conditions associated with learning disability

The main individual causes of learning disability are mentioned here. Chromosomal and genetic factors predominate. By and large, the aetiology does not markedly affect management, but it may have major implications for prognosis, and the likelihood of similar problems arising in other family members.

- A useful concept is *behavioural phenotype*. That is, the association of a certain profile of behaviours with a genetic condition, such that recognition of the profile gives useful clues as to the cause of the learning disability. For example, self-injury suggests Lesch–Nyhan syndrome, and overeating suggests Prader–Willi syndrome.

Chromosomal abnormalities

A range of chromosomal microdeletions, translocations and aneuploidies can cause mental retardation. In total they explain 5–35% of cases.

- Many of the abnormalities can be detected by routine karyotyping. Others require specialist tests, such as subtelomeric analyses, which assess the ends of chromosomes (telomeres) that are relatively common sites of abnormality (5–10% of severe learning disability).

Down's syndrome

Down's syndrome (trisomy 21) produces learning disability and characteristic physical features (Table 17.6). The diagnosis is usually made at, or before, birth. It is the commonest cause of learning disability. Its 'true' incidence is 1 in 650 live births, (though this has fallen to 1 in 1000 in the UK due to antenatal testing and pregnancy termination). The risk is strongly dependent on maternal age, rising from <1/2000 at age 20 to 1/30 at age 45.

The aetiology in 95% of cases is triplication of chromosome 21, with the syndrome presumed to result from expression of the extra copy of the genes on the chromosome. The remainder are due to a translocation involving chromosome 21 or to mosaicism (a mixture of normal and trisomic cells).

Table 17.6 Features of Down's syndrome.

Moderate or severe learning disability
Placid temperament
Physical features
Slanted eyes and epicanthic folds
Small mouth with furrowed tongue
Flat nose
Flattened occiput
Stubby hands with single transverse palmar crease
Hypotonia
Associated medical problems
Cardiac septal defects
Gastrointestinal obstruction
Atlantoaxial instability
Susceptibility to infection
Increased risk of leukaemia, hypothyroidism, autoimmune disorders

• The prognosis has improved with better medical management. Many now survive to middle age, when intellectual decline due to Alzheimer's disease is common. The association between the two disorders was crucial in the discovery of the latter's genetic basis (p. 140).

Fragile X syndrome

Fragile X syndrome is so called because of a fragile site on the long arm of the X chromosome seen when cells are grown in a folate-deficient medium. It occurs in about 1/1500 births and is the second commonest cause of learning disability (approximately 10% of cases). Its exact prevalence is uncertain because its phenotype (Table 17.7) is variable and accurate genetic testing has only recently become possible.

Most fragile X syndrome is due to a trinucleotide (triplet) repeat mutation in the FMR1 gene, impairing the gene's normal role in regulating expression of other genes. Being on the X chromosome, the syndrome is commoner in boys than girls. Along with several other X-linked disorders, it explains much of the higher rate of learning disability in males. However, the unusual nature of the FMR1

Table 17.7 Features of fragile X syndrome.

Commoner in males (>2 : 1)
All features are particularly variable
Learning disability
   May be mild, moderate, severe or profound
   Gets worse late in childhood
   Performance IQ affected more than verbal IQ
   Litany speech—repetitive, lacking in themes or
     content
   Poor attention and concentration
   Autistic features common
Physical features
   Large, protruding ears
   Long face with high-arched palate
   Flat feet
   Lax joints
   Soft skin
   Large testes (after puberty)
   Mitral valve prolapse

mutation means that some males who have the mutation are normal, and more females are affected than would be expected. Female carriers also have an increased risk of psychiatric disorders. The disorder gets worse in succeeding generations (*anticipation*).
• Genetic detection of affected individuals and carriers is feasible.
• There is no specific treatment. *Methylphenidate* and *folic acid* may improve the attentional deficits.
• FMR1 regulates the expression of other genes involved in the formation of synapses, and this function is impaired in fragile X syndrome because of the mutation.

Other chromosomal abnormalities

Severe learning disability is common with other abnormalities of the autosomes, but less frequent in sex chromosome aneuploidies.
• *Prader–Willi syndrome* is learning disability together with compulsive eating, obesity, disruptive behaviour, hypogonadism and psychosis. It is due to deletion of part of chromosome 15. *Angelman syndrome* (severe learning disability, puppet-like movements, laughter and a big tongue) is caused by the same abnormality when inherited from the mother rather than from the father.

Single gene disorders

There are over 1000 different genes known to cause learning disability, often via effects on metabolism or brain development. Most are very rare.

Phenylketonuria

Phenylketonuria (PKU) is the classic inborn error of metabolism (Table 17.8). The amino acid phenylalanine cannot be converted into paratyrosine because of a defective converting enzyme. It is autosomal recessive and affects 1 in 10000 live births.
• PKU is one of the few treatable causes of severe learning disability. A rigorous low phenylalanine diet must be started in the first months of life to prevent deterioration—hence the neonatal screen-

Table 17.8 Features of untreated phenylketonuria.

Severe learning disability
Tantrums and unpredictable aggression
Abnormal movements and mannerisms
Fair skinned
Short stature
Associated medical problems
   Eczema
   Vomiting
   Seizures

Table 17.9 Examples of metabolic disorders associated with learning disability.

Metabolic category	Example
Aminoacids	Homocysteinuria
Lipids	Tay–Sachs disease
Mucopolysaccharides	Hurler's syndrome
Carbohydrates	Galactosaemia
Purines	Lesch–Nyhan syndrome

Table 17.10 Pre- and perinatal environmental causes of learning disability.

Category	Comment
Obstetric complications	
In utero infections	
Rubella	Greatest risk (50%) if infection is in first trimester
HIV	Retardation in 50% of infected children
Syphilis	
Cytomegalovirus	
Toxoplasmosis	
Foetal alcohol syndrome	In some offspring of mothers who drink heavily
Other drugs and toxins	e.g. methylmercury
Placental insufficiency	
Placental abruption	
Eclampsia/toxaemia	
Birth complications	May be a consequence of earlier foetal abnormality
Ventricular haemorrhage	
Perinatal factors	
Hypothyroidism (cretinism)	An important cause in areas with low iodine diets
Hyperbilirubinaemia	
Other factors	
Cerebral palsy	} Learning disability commoner than expected, though IQ often in normal range
Hydrocephalus	
Spina bifida	

ing for phenylalanine levels. Carriers can be detected.

Other inherited errors of metabolism

Learning disability can result from disorders of other metabolic pathways (Table 17.9). The frequency of each is low and varies between ethnic groups. Most are associated with failure to thrive and hepatic and/or renal dysfunction.

- In *Lesch–Nyhan syndrome*, self-mutilation by biting is characteristic.
- All the cited examples are autosomal recessive and most can be detected prenatally. A few can be ameliorated by diet.

Other genetic disorders

Neurofibromatosis and *tuberous sclerosis complex* are neurocutaneous syndromes. Both are autosomal

Table 17.11 Postnatal causes of learning disability.

Infections
Meningitis
Encephalitis
Brain tumours
Head injury
Accidental
Non-accidental
Hypoxia (e.g. anaesthetic accident)
Lead poisoning
Rare idiopathic syndromes
Disintegrative psychoses

dominant but spontaneous mutations are also common.

• *Neurofibromatosis* (von Recklinghausen's disease) affects 1 in 4000 births. Diagnostic features are *cafe au lait* spots on the skin and multiple neurofibromas. Mild learning disability occurs in about 50% of cases of type 1 neurofibromatosis, which is due to a mutation in the Nf1 gene on chromosome 17.

• *Tuberous sclerosis complex* occurs in 1 in 6000 births. There are several characteristic skin lesions and multiple tumours (hamartomas) in brain and elsewhere. Epilepsy and progressive mental retardation occur in 60%. Autistic features are often seen. It is caused by two genes, TSC1 (hamartin) on chromosome 9, and TSC2 (tuberin) on chromosome 16.

• *Autism* is covered in Chapter 16.

Environmental factors

Learning disability can be caused by a variety of environmental insults. Most act pre- or perinatally (Table 17.10) but postnatal factors are also recognized (Table 17.11).

Key points

• Learning disability (mental retardation) is defined as an IQ below 70, with functional impairments in several areas and a childhood onset. It affects about 2% of the population, boys more commonly than girls.
• Psychiatric and behavioural problems are common, especially in those who also have epilepsy.
• Severe learning disability is usually caused by genetic or chromosomal abnormalities (e.g. Down's syndrome, fragile X). Mild retardation is often idiopathic and multifactorial.
• Learning disability is rarely treatable. Management is aimed at maximizing potential and quality of life, and at treating concurrent psychiatric and behavioural problems.
• Most people with learning disability live in the community.

Chapter 18

Psychiatry in other settings

The most important message of this book is that psychiatry is an integral part of medicine—there is nothing unique about psychiatric patients or psychiatric disorders. Rather it is the traditional separation of psychiatric services from the rest of medicine that has made this appear to be the case (Chapters 1 and 8). We have also emphasized that the conventional view of psychiatry, often gained from attachments to psychiatric wards, is potentially misleading as most psychiatric disorder presents to, and is managed by, other doctors in other settings. All doctors therefore need to possess the basic skills of psychiatric assessment and management. This chapter discusses the implications of the following facts:

• Psychiatric disorders are common in the population, and thus in all areas of medical practice.

• Outside specialist psychiatric services, somatic symptoms are often the presenting feature of psychiatric disorder.

• Psychiatric disorders frequently coexist with or complicate medical illnesses.

Epidemiology of psychiatric disorder in different settings

In the population

Epidemiological surveys show that at least 20% of the adult population have a psychiatric disorder at any one time. Neuroses and substance misuse account for most of this morbidity and psychosis is relatively rare (Table 18.1).

• Total psychiatric morbidity is strongly associated with social deprivation. Rates are two-fold higher in low than high socioeconomic classes, and in urban than rural areas.

• The neuroses are twice as common in women as men; the reverse is true for substance dependence.

• The prevalence for personality disorder, childhood psychiatric disorder and learning disability are covered in Chapters 15, 16 and 17 respectively.

Population prevalence is not the same as demand on the services. Many of the individuals in Table 18.1 will never present to any service with their disorder. The difference between the population prevalence and the number who seek medical help is the first step on the pyramid whose peak is the tiny and unrepresentative percentage of cases that become psychiatric in-patients (Figure 18.1). Various 'filters' explain the steep slope of the pyramid.

General practice

We have emphasized throughout this book—and illustrated by the pyramid in Figure 18.1—that it is in general practice where the bulk of psychiatric disorder is managed.

• The most common psychiatric disorders in general practice are the somatoform disorders, depression, neurosis and substance misuse. Patients with

Table 18.1 Approximate population prevalence of psychiatric disorder.

Disorder	Prevalence (%)
Mixed anxiety–depression	8
Alcohol dependence	5
Generalized anxiety disorder	3
Specific anxiety disorders	3
Depressive disorder	2
Drug dependence	2
Dementia	1
Eating disorders	<1
Psychosis	0.4

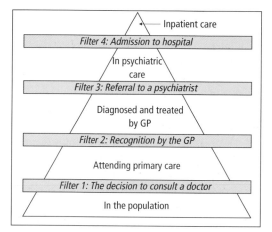

Figure 18.1 Psychiatric disorders in different settings and the filters to psychiatric care. Not everyone with a psychiatric disorder presents to a doctor. The decision to do so—the first filter to psychiatric care—depends on several factors: e.g. awareness that the symptoms may signify psychiatric disorder, their severity, choosing to see a practitioner of alternative medicine, stigma, etc. Of those who do see a doctor (in the UK, usually a GP), the psychiatric disorder is recognized and treated in about half. This filter is determined by the doctor's diagnostic and treatment decisions. About 10% of patients are referred to psychiatric services; this filter depends on the nature of the disorder, the doctor's characteristics and the availability of resources. A tiny minority at some stage have a psychiatric admission. This last filter is based mainly upon the diagnosis, the risk of harm (Chapter 4), and availability of psychiatric beds and alternative treatment options. This figure emphasizes that one's perspective on psychiatry depends largely on whereabouts on the pyramid you are standing.

psychosis are rare—most GPs have only a handful of patients on their books, and these are usually under specialist care.

Psychiatry as seen from general practice

Since psychiatrists and GPs see a different profile of psychiatric disorder, not surprisingly the two groups may have differing views about priorities. For example, a GP may wish to allocate resources to manage neurotic disorders—which fill her surgeries—whereas her local psychiatrist will probably argue that rarer, but more severe, disorders—which dominate his caseload—take priority. This difference may cause tensions when psychiatrists and GPs are jointly involved in planning services if resources are limited.

To try and improve co-ordination between primary care and psychiatric services, several recommendations have been made, though not always implemented:
- Psychiatric sector boundaries should reflect GP boundaries.
- Psychiatric and GP training should be closely integrated.
- Keeping of joint case records (though patients are not keen).
- Ensure consistent advice from GP and psychiatrist about diagnosis, treatment and prognosis.
- Responsibility for overall medical care held by GP.
- Local practice guidelines drawn up for the common psychiatric disorders.

Casualty departments

Deliberate self-harm is the major psychiatric problem in casualty departments (Chapter 4). Although only a minority of these patients have persistent psychiatric disorders, many have stress-related disorders and some have depressive disorders. Intoxication and delirium related to alcohol and drugs are also common, particularly in inner city hospitals and in people involved in accidents.
- Some patients with somatoform disorders and a few with factitious disorders (Chapter 10) are frequent users of casualty departments.

Medical and surgical out-patient clinics

Amongst patients attending medical and surgical out-patient clinics, a third have a psychiatric disorder. Half of these have depressive and anxiety disorders, and the remainder somatoform disorders.

• In both these groups, adequate recognition and treatment of their psychiatric disorder should be an integral part of management, since it has been shown to improve outcome.

• Depression is a common cause of apparent worsening of a medical condition.

• Panic disorder (Chapter 10) is an important cause of medically unexplained symptoms such as chest pain, dizziness and tingling.

Medical and surgical wards

About 20% of medical and surgical in-patients have a depressive or anxiety disorder coexisting with their medical disease, 10% have a significant alcohol misuse problem, and a quarter of elderly in-patients have an episode of delirium.

• Some patients with severe somatoform disorders get admitted and undergo multiple investigations and even surgery before the diagnosis is made.

• Remember alcohol withdrawal as a possible cause of delirium in in-patients.

Presentations of psychiatric disorder in medical settings

Many cases of psychiatric disorders that present in medical settings do so with psychological symptoms or behavioural disturbance. However, many others present in ways that are less obviously 'psychiatric', with:

• Somatic symptoms.
• A medical management problem.
• An apparent exacerbation of an established medical condition.

Psychiatric disorder and somatic symptoms

As mentioned above, a significant minority of patients seen in general practice and in hospital out-patient clinics have somatic symptoms which cannot be explained by medical disease, and many of these have a psychiatric disorder. The important diagnoses are depressive, anxiety and somatoform disorders.

• Figure 18.2 shows a simple diagnostic approach to medically unexplained somatic symptoms.

Somatic symptoms due to depressive and anxiety disorders

Depression is associated with bodily symptoms such as fatigue, weight loss and pain. As a result, a depressed person may be seen by any medical specialty. Similarly, anxiety produces the bodily symptoms of autonomic arousal, which include palpitations, breathlessness and sensory symptoms.

For any patient who presents with bodily symptoms that are not adequately explicable by a medical diagnosis, consider the possibility that the patient may have a depressive or anxiety disorder. This psychiatric diagnosis may be the only diagnosis or it may be complicating a medical condition, in which case two diagnoses must be made. When assessing a patient with somatic symptoms it is therefore necessary both to carry out the appropriate investigations to exclude physical disease and seek positive evidence of depression or anxiety.

• The converse situation—a misdiagnosis of depression or anxiety in a patient whose symptoms are caused by a medical disease—though much rarer, must not be overlooked (Chapter 13).

Ms M went to her doctor because of abdominal pain. She was upset, but both she and the doctor saw her distress as being a result of the pain. An urgent laparotomy was performed and a normal appendix removed. Only after she took an overdose the following month was a further history taken which revealed that she had been having problems with her mother and had developed symptoms of depressive disorder (low mood, anhedonia and poor sleep) prior to the pain starting. She was given an antidepressant drug, helped to tackle the family conflict and made a full recovery.

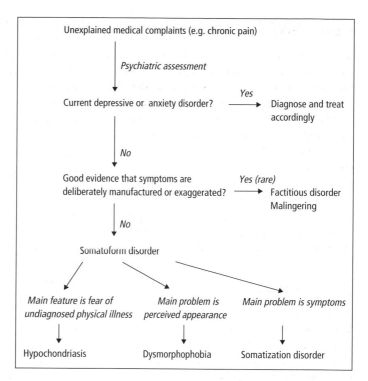

Figure 18.2 Psychiatric diagnoses in people with unexplained medical complaints.

Flowchart content:

Unexplained medical complaints (e.g. chronic pain)

↓ *Psychiatric assessment*

Current depressive or anxiety disorder? —— *Yes* → Diagnose and treat accordingly

↓ *No*

Good evidence that symptoms are deliberately manufactured or exaggerated? —— *Yes (rare)* → Factitious disorder / Malingering

↓ *No*

Somatoform disorder

- *Main feature is fear of undiagnosed physical illness* ↓ Hypochondriasis
- *Main problem is perceived appearance* ↓ Dysmorphophobia
- *Main problem is symptoms* ↓ Somatization disorder

Somatoform disorders

Of the patients with a functional somatic syndrome (Table 10.14) who do *not* have a depressive or anxiety disorder, most may be regarded as having a somatoform disorder (p. 108).

> *Mr H has attended a gastroenterology clinic intermittently for years with abdominal discomfort and flatulence. No significant abnormalities have been found despite numerous investigations throughout the length of his gastrointestinal tract. Trials of antispasmodics, laxatives and antiulcer drugs have not produced sustained effects. A new junior doctor reviews his case and sees a connection between stresses at home or work and the exacerbation of abdominal as well as anxiety symptoms. Mr H is unwilling to countenance a psychological basis for his problems but agrees to see a liaison psychiatrist who works closely with the clinic. Mr H embarks on a course of problem solving therapy and attends a stress management class. His irritable bowel syndrome improves markedly and he agrees (for the first time) that further medical interventions are not necessary.*

Psychiatric disorder presenting with a medical management problem

Psychiatric disorders may also present as a problem in medical management. For example:
- An old lady repeatedly pulls out her drip in the orthopaedic ward.
- A young woman is repeatedly admitted with an infected operative wound.
- A woman with diabetes refusing to take adequate insulin.
- A young man has thumped a doctor in surgical out-patients.

The diagnosis in these cases proved to be, respectively: delirium, factitious disorder, depression and no psychiatric diagnosis.
- The cases illustrate that any psychiatric disorder can present with a medical management problem, and that a psychiatric assessment, even if brief (Chapter 2), is essential.

• The final example makes the equally important point that people also behave badly for no psychiatric reason at all, and that the mental state must be assessed before diagnosing any psychiatric disorder—behaviour itself is rarely, if ever, sufficient as a basis for diagnosis.

Psychiatric disorder presenting as an apparent worsening of a medical disease

An exacerbation of symptoms or disability in a patient with a chronic medical condition may erroneously be attributed to a worsening of the disease process, when it is in fact due to the development of a comorbid psychiatric disorder. For example:

• A man with previously stable angina repeatedly presents with severe chest pain.

• A woman with previous hypothyroidism suffers a recurrence of severe lethargy.

• A woman with arthritis becomes housebound.

The diagnosis in these cases proved to be, respectively: panic disorder, depression and agoraphobia.

• The danger in these cases is that the patients are given unnecessary and potentially hazardous medical treatment instead of appropriate psychiatric management.

Psychiatric and medical comorbidity

Many patients with medical disease *also* have psychiatric disorder—the two occur together much more often than would be expected by chance. Chapter 13 covered the situations where a medical condition such as hyperthyroidism or Cushing's disease can produce psychiatric symptoms as part of its pathophysiology. However, there are several other reasons why medical and psychiatric disorders frequently coexist:

• Psychiatric symptoms may be a response to the diagnosis or limitations of a physical disease. For example, depression associated with cancer; sexual dysfunction after myocardial infarction; a body image disturbance after limb amputation.

• Psychiatric disorder may cause medical illness. For example, anorexia nervosa causing osteoporosis.

• There may be a shared cause, such as a major life event precipitating both a stroke and depression.

The coexistence of psychiatric disorder and medical disorder is clinically important because it:

• Magnifies suffering and disability.

• Worsens outcome. For example, mortality rates are increased in people with heart disease, cancer or stroke who have a comorbid depressive disorder.

• Prolongs medical care and increases overall health costs.

Management of psychiatric disorder in medicine

There are three main requirements for the effective management of psychiatric disorder in medical settings. These illustrate the knowledge, skills and attitudes which all doctors should have (Chapter 1):

• To be able to recognize it.

• To be able to treat it appropriately.

• To know how and when to refer to specialist psychiatric services.

Recognition

The diagnosis of psychiatric disorder in non-psychiatric settings is often missed. This error may be attributable to the doctor, the patient, or the circumstances (Table 18.2).

Doctors are better at the detection and assessment of psychiatric disorder if they:

• Realize that somatic symptoms are not always due to medical conditions.

• Always do a brief psychiatric assessment—even if just a few questions (Table 2.2).

• Ask the patient about their worries and concerns.

• Enable the patient to express emotion.

Treatment

The treatment of psychiatric disorder in medical settings follows the same principles as treatment in psychiatric settings. It requires that:

Table 18.2 Reasons psychiatric diagnoses are missed.

Doctor
Failure to consider the possibility
Failure to elicit psychiatric symptoms—through lack of effort or skill

Patient
Reports only somatic symptoms
Hides emotional distress and psychosocial stresses

Circumstances
Lack of time
Lack of privacy
Clinic geared solely toward detection of medical disease

- You can explain the psychiatric diagnosis to the patient in a way that they can accept. This is achieved by emphasizing that it is a real illness, that it is an understandable reaction and not a sign of weakness, and that it can be treated effectively.
- You are able to provide evidence-based treatments. Some doctors will regularly use simple psychological therapies themselves. Others will have ensured that they have members of the clinical team, such as specialist nurses or counsellors, who they can ask for assistance.
- You are confident in prescribing the main psychotropic drugs—especially antidepressants—and that you are up-to-date with their use, indications, interactions and side-effects.

Referral to specialist psychiatric services

A small but important minority of patients will require a referral to psychiatric services. The main indications for referral are:
- Request for second opinion.
- Failure of first-line management.
- Need for specialist treatment, such as ECT.
- Serious suicide risk.
- Presence of a condition, such as psychosis, requiring specialist services.

- Severe substance misuse.
- Need for compulsory treatment.

From primary care, referrals will usually be made to the local general psychiatric services, unless the problem falls into the remit of one of the subspecialties (Chapter 8). For patients in general hospitals there may be a hospital liaison psychiatry service that will assist both in management and in making appropriate referrals.

- Referrals, other than of exceptional emergencies, should only be made after the doctor has: (a) completed a basic assessment themselves; and (b) explained and agreed the referral with the patient.
- Following the referral, good communication between all the agencies involved is essential if problems and misunderstandings are to be avoided.

Key points

- Patients with psychiatric disorders are encountered in all medical settings. Neurotic symptoms, depression and anxiety disorders, substance misuse and organic mental disorders are all common in general practice and general hospitals. In these settings they often present with somatic symptoms.
- Medical disease is frequently accompanied by psychiatric disorder. The combination worsens prognosis if not effectively managed.
- Management of psychiatric disorder is based on the general principles described in this book, plus: (a) attention to the patient's medical condition and treatment; and (b) necessary adaptation to the medical setting.
- Because psychiatric disorders are so common in the general population, all doctors must be:
  – alert to the possibility of psychiatric disorder in all patients;
  – aware that psychiatric disorder often presents with bodily symptoms;
  – aware of the prevalence of psychiatric disorder in the physically ill;
  – able to screen for psychiatric disorder;
  – able to use simple psychological treatments;
  – able to use antidepressants;
  – aware when and how to refer to psychiatric services.

Multiple choice questions

1. **Hallucinations:**
   a. Can occur in severe depression.
   b. Are misperceptions of external stimuli.
   c. Which are visual suggest an organic disorder.
   d. Voices talking to the person are characteristic of schizophrenia.
   e. Which occur while waking from sleep are called 'hypnopompic'.

2. **Alzheimer's disease:**
   a. Usually presents in the seventh decade.
   b. Is usually inherited as an autosomal recessive disorder.
   c. Death occurs on average 2–3 years after diagnosis.
   d. Is associated with the apolipoprotein E4 genetic variant.
   e. Drug therapy is aimed at reducing excessive cholinergic neurotransmission.

3. **In dementia:**
   a. Incontinence and ataxic gait suggests normal pressure hydrocephalus.
   b. A fluctuating course and visual hallucinations suggests Pick's disease.
   c. Antipsychotics are first line treatment for behavioural symptoms (e.g. shouting, agitation).
   d. Myoclonic jerks are characteristic of Creutzfeldt–Jakob disease.
   e. About 90% of cases are caused by Alzheimer's disease.

4. **Compared to conventional antipsychotics, atypical antipsychotics:**
   a. Produce fewer extra-pyramidal side-effects.
   b. Cause less weight gain.
   c. Tend to be more selective for the dopamine D2 receptor.
   d. Are less sedative.
   e. Decrease suicide rates.

5. **When choosing an antidepressant:**
   a. Nausea is more common with SSRIs than tricyclics.
   b. SSRI-induced sexual dysfunction is usually transient.
   c. Avoid clomipramine in combination with other drugs.
   d. After recovery, halve the dose for maintenance therapy.
   e. Continuing antidepressants after recovery halves the risk of relapse.

6. **First rank symptoms:**
   a. Were described by Bleuler.
   b. If prominent are diagnostic of schizophrenia.
   c. Are a poor prognostic sign in schizophrenia.
   d. Can occur in mania.
   e. Are rare in developing countries.

7. **Cognitive behaviour therapy:**
   a. Is usually carried out by psychiatrists.
   b. Sometimes includes analysis of dreams.
   c. Usually involves homework and diary keeping.
   d. Is not effective in schizophrenia.
   e. In clinical trials is effective in 80–85% of cases of depression.

8. **In patients taking lithium:**
   a. Liver function tests are needed regularly.
   b. A fine tremor is a sign of lithium toxicity.
   c. She may experience a metallic taste.
   d. Hypothyroidism is a recognized side-effect.
   e. Plasma levels should be kept below 0.5 mmol/l.

9. **Electroconvulsive therapy:**
   a. Has fewer side-effects when given to the non-dominant hemisphere.
   b. Can only be given to patients under the Mental Health Act.
   c. Should not be given to those over 70 years old.
   d. Is only effective if a seizure is induced.
   e. Can be given to patients currently taking antidepressants.

10. **Sleep problems:**
    a. Initial insomnia is characteristic of depression.
    b. Are a recognized side-effect of SSRIs.
    c. Hypersomnia is characteristic of atypical depression.
    d. Sleep hygiene is an effective intervention.
    e. Narcolepsy usually presents before age 10.

11. **Eating disorders:**
    a. Anorexia nervosa is the commonest subtype.
    b. Many patients have features of both anorexia and bulimia nervosa.
    c. Cognitive behavioural therapy is the most effective treatment for bulimia.
    d. Are three times as common in women as men.
    e. Anorexia nervosa has approximately a ten-fold increased mortality rate.

12. **Causes of mood disorders:**
    a. Bipolar and unipolar mood disorders have similar heritabilities.
    b. Early life adversity and recent life events are interacting risk factors for depression.
    c. Depression is a common feature of Cushing's disease.
    d. Prolonged depression is associated with atrophy of the thalamus.
    e. Raised cortisol levels are present in 90% of subjects with moderate to severe depression.

13. **In post-traumatic stress disorder:**
    a. Debriefing is an effective preventative treatment.
    b. Hyperarousal is a principal feature.
    c. Alcohol misuse frequently occurs.
    d. Antidepressants are usually effective.
    e. Most cases resolve within a few months.

14. **In the treatment of mania:**
    a. Lithium carbonate is the standard monotherapy.
    b. Antipsychotics should be limited to those with delusions or hallucinations.
    c. Depressive symptoms often coexist.
    d. Delusions which occur are usually nihilistic.
    e. Afterwards, mood stabilizer medication is normally prescribed.

15. **Autism:**
    a. Has a similar incidence in boys and girls.
    b. About 25% suffer from epilepsy.
    c. Is associated with large ears and blonde hair in boys.
    d. Is an X-linked recessive disorder.
    e. About a third are mentally retarded.

16. **Which of the following are first rank symptoms of schizophrenia?**
    a. Thought disorder.
    b. Thought insertion.
    c. Thought block.
    d. Thought withdrawal.
    e. Thought broadcasting.

17. **Which of these drugs is a recognized cause of depressive symptoms?**
    a. Amphetamines.
    b. Digoxin.
    c. L-Dopa.
    d. Anticholinergics.
    e. Diuretics.

18. **Which of these medical disorders is a recognized cause of depressive symptoms?**
    a. Systemic lupus erythematosus.
    b. Addison's disease.

c. Hypothyroidism.

d. Cushing's disease.

e. Multiple sclerosis.

19. **Epidemiology of depression:**
    a. The lifetime risk of a depressive episode in men is 2–3%.
    b. Bipolar disorder has an equal sex incidence.
    c. 20% of medical in-patients meet criteria for a mood disorder.
    d. Suicide occurs in 1 in 20 patients with mood disorder.
    e. At least 50% of people with unexplained physical symptoms meet criteria for depression.

20. **Conduct disorder:**
    a. Is usually part of attention-deficit hyperactivity disorder.
    b. Is the commonest psychiatric disorder of childhood.
    c. The diagnosis is usually made around puberty.
    d. About half progress to dissocial personality disorder.
    e. Behavioural therapy is an effective intervention.

21. **Delirium:**
    a. Is usually associated with a disturbed sleep–wake cycle.
    b. Place disorientation usually occurs before time disorientation.
    c. Occurs in at least 10% of medical in-patients.
    d. Can be caused by urinary retention.
    e. Low dose antipsychotics are the first-line drug treatment.

22. **Which of the following are psychotic disorders?**
    a. Hypochondriasis.
    b. Paranoid personality disorder.
    c. Somatoform disorder.
    d. Korsakoff's syndrome.

e. De Clèrambault's syndrome (erotomania).

23. **Suicide:**
    a. Is commoner in married men than unmarried men.
    b. 70% of those who deliberately self-harm are suffering from major depression.
    c. Is commoner in retired than younger people.
    d. Occurs eventually in 20% of those who have previously self-harmed.
    e. About 50% of suicide victims have a history of alcohol abuse or dependence.

24. **Learning disability:**
    a. Is defined by an IQ of less than 60.
    b. Self-biting is characteristic of fragile X syndrome.
    c. Is caused by a chromosomal abnormality in the majority of cases.
    d. Is associated with an increased risk of developing dementia.
    e. Phenylketonuria can be treated by removing phenylalanine from the diet.

25. **In prophylaxis of bipolar disorder:**
    a. Lithium should not normally be prescribed for more than 2 years.
    b. Carbamazepine about as effective as sodium valproate.
    c. Elderly patients should not be prescribed lithium.
    d. Cognitive therapy reduces relapse rates.
    e. Thyroid function should be tested regularly in patients taking lithium.

26. **Heritability of psychiatric disorders:**
    a. Refers to the penetrance of a gene.
    b. Is measured using adoption studies.
    c. Heritability of schizophrenia is about 40%.
    d. Heritability of depression is about 40%.
    e. Heritability of anxiety disorders is less than 10%.

27. **Complex partial epilepsy:**
    a. Olfactory hallucinations are characteristic.
    b. Used to be called petit mal epilepsy.
    c. Schizophrenia is commoner than expected.
    d. Is associated with a several-fold increase in suicide.
    e. The seizure focus is usually in the thalamus.

28. **Personality disorder:**
    a. Cluster A is called 'Eccentric'.
    b. Dialectic behaviour therapy is effective in borderline personality disorder.
    c. Psychodynamic psychotherapy is effective in schizoid personality disorder.
    d. Anankastic personality disorder is also called avoidant personality disorder.
    e. Persecutory delusions are a feature of paranoid personality disorder.

29. **Substance misuse:**
    a. Phencyclidine (PCP) mainly blocks 5-HT receptors.
    b. Ecstasy may damage 5-HT fibres in the brain.
    c. LSD is addictive.
    d. Cannabis can be detected in the urine for several weeks.
    e. Chronic amphetamine use is associated with mood swings.

30. **A patient with borderline personality disorder:**
    a. Is unlikely to benefit from any treatments.
    b. May experience brief psychotic symptoms.
    c. Is at a lower risk of suicide compared to patients with other personality disorders.
    d. Usually first shows signs of the disorder in their 30s.
    e. Is likely to misuse alcohol and drugs.

31. **In ICD-10:**
    a. Hypochondriasis is classified as an anxiety disorder.
    b. Dysthymia is classified as a personality disorder.
    c. Dementia and delirium are forms of organic disorder.
    d. Depressive disorder is a form of neurosis.
    e. Symptoms must be present for at least 1 month to diagnose schizophrenia.

32. **Which of the following are used to treat attention deficit hyperactivity disorder?**
    a. Methylphenidate.
    b. Methylprednisolone.
    c. Atomoxetine.
    d. Zopiclone.
    e. Modafinil.

33. **Which of the following are features of dementia with Lewy bodies?**
    a. Parkinsonism.
    b. Visual hallucinations.
    c. Rapidly fluctuating mental state.
    d. Autosomal recessive inheritance.
    e. Can be transmitted by blood products.

34. **Medically unexplained somatic symptoms:**
    a. About 25% have a depressive disorder.
    b. Antidepressants are effective in treating chronic pain.
    c. Briquet's syndrome nearly always occurs in women.
    d. Mortality rate is significantly increased.
    e. Are rarely due to somatoform disorder.

35. **Which of the following are antidepressants?**
    a. Lofepramine.
    b. Loperamide.
    c. Sertraline.
    d. Aripiprazole.
    e. Venlafaxine.

Answers to multiple choice questions

1. **Hallucinations:**
   a. True
   b. False (True = false perception)
   c. True
   d. False (True = talking about the person)
   e. True

2. **Alzheimer's disease:**
   a. False (True = commoner in eighth and ninth decade)
   b. False (True = usually non-Mendelian (complex) inheritance)
   c. False (True = 5–8 years)
   d. True
   e. False (True = enhance cholinergic neurotransmission)

3. **In dementia:**
   a. True
   b. False (True = dementia with Lewy bodies)
   c. False (Avoid whenever possible)
   d. True
   e. False (True = 50–60%)

4. **Compared to conventional antipsychotics, atypical antipsychotics:**
   a. True
   b. False
   c. False
   d. False
   e. False (True = only for clozapine)

5. **When choosing an antidepressant:**
   a. True
   b. False
   c. True
   d. False (True = the dose that got you better keeps you better)
   e. True

6. **First rank symptoms:**
   a. False (True = Schneider)
   b. False (True = indicative but not pathognomonic)
   c. False (True = no prognostic value)
   d. True
   e. False (True = similar occurrence worldwide)

7. **Cognitive behaviour therapy:**
   a. False (True = psychologists or other health professionals)
   b. False
   c. True
   d. False (True = effective against residual delusions and hallucinations)
   e. False (True = 60–70%)

8. **In patients taking lithium:**
   a. False (True = renal function tests)
   b. False (True = coarse tremor)
   c. True
   d. True
   e. False (True = between 0.4 and 1.0 mmol/l)

9. **Electroconvulsive therapy:**
   a. True
   b. False
   c. False
   d. True
   e. True

10. **Sleep problems:**
    a. False (True = early morning waking)
    b. True
    c. True
    d. True
    e. True

11. **Eating disorders:**
    a. False (True = atypical eating disorder)
    b. True
    c. True
    d. False (True = ten-fold)
    e. True

12. **Causes of mood disorders:**
    a. False (True = bipolar disorder is much more heritable)
    b. True
    c. True
    d. False (True = atrophy of the hippocampus)
    e. False (True = less than 50%)

13. **In post-traumatic stress disorder:**
    a. False
    b. True
    c. True
    d. False
    e. True

14. **In the treatment of mania:**
    a. False (True = antipsychotic)
    b. False (True = effective in non-psychotic mania too)
    c. True
    d. False (True = grandiose)
    e. False (True = only after two manic episodes)

15. **Autism:**
    a. False (True = 80% are boys)
    b. True
    c. False (True = fragile X syndrome)
    d. False
    e. False (True = about 75%)

16. **Which of the following are first rank symptoms of schizophrenia?**
    a. False
    b. True
    c. False
    d. True
    e. True

17. **Which of these drugs is a recognized cause of depressive symptoms?**
    a. True
    b. True
    c. True
    d. False (True = delirium)
    e. True

18. **Which of these medical disorders is a recognized cause of depressive symptoms?**
    a. True
    b. True
    c. True
    d. True
    e. True

19. **Epidemiology of depression:**
    a. False (True = closer to 10%)
    b. True
    c. True
    d. False (True = 1 in 8)
    e. True

20. **Conduct disorder:**
    a. False (True = differential diagnosis)
    b. True
    c. False (True = usually by age 7)
    d. True
    e. False (True = no proven interventions known)

21. **Delirium:**
    a. True
    b. False (Time disorientation is characteristic)
    c. True
    d. True
    e. True (Except in delirium tremens)

22. **Which of the following are psychotic disorders?**
    a. False (True = neurotic disorder)
    b. False
    c. False
    d. True
    e. True

23. **Suicide:**
    a. False
    b. False (True = this figure applies to completed suicide)
    c. True
    d. False (True = about 5%)
    e. True

24. **Learning disability:**
    a. False (True = 70)
    b. False (True = Lesch–Nyhan syndrome)
    c. False (True = 5–35%)
    d. True
    e. True

25. **In prophylaxis of bipolar disorder:**
    a. False (True = aim for minimum of 2 years)
    b. False
    c. False
    d. True
    e. True

26. **Heritability of psychiatric disorders:**
    a. False (True = proportion of a disorder in the population due to genes)
    b. False (True = twin studies)
    c. False (True = 80%)
    d. True
    e. False (True = 30%)

27. **Complex partial epilepsy:**
    a. True
    b. False (True = psychomotor epilepsy)
    c. True
    d. True
    e. False (True = temporal lobe)

28. **Personality disorder:**
    a. True
    b. True
    c. False
    d. False (True = obsessional)
    e. False

29. **Substance misuse:**
    a. False (True = NMDA glutamate receptors)
    b. True
    c. False
    d. True
    e. True

30. **A patient with borderline personality disorder:**
    a. False
    b. True
    c. False
    d. False
    e. True

31. **In ICD-10:**
    a. True
    b. False
    c. True
    d. False
    e. True

32. **Which of the following are used to treat attention deficit hyperactivity disorder?**
    a. True
    b. False
    c. True
    d. False
    e. True

33. **Which of the following are features of dementia with Lewy bodies?**
    a. True
    b. True
    c. True
    d. False
    e. False

34. **Medically unexplained somatic symptoms:**
    a. True
    b. True
    c. True
    d. False
    e. False

35. **Which of the following are antidepressants?**
    a. True
    b. False (True = antidiarrhoeic)
    c. True
    d. False (True = atypical antipsychotic)
    e. True

Appendix 1

ICD-10 classification of psychiatric disorders

Category	Category	Example
F00–09	Organic disorders	F02.2 Huntington's disease
F10–19	Substance use disorders	F10.2 Alcohol dependence
F29–29	Schizophrenia and other psychoses	F20.0 Paranoid schizophrenia
F30–39	Mood disorders	F32.1 Moderate depressive episode
F40–49	Neurotic and stress-related disorders	F45.2 Hypochondriasis
F50–59	Eating, sleep and related syndromes	F50.2 Bulimia nervosa
F60–69	Disorders of personality and behaviour	F60.2 Dissocial personality disorder
F70–79	Mental retardation (Learning disability)	F72.0 Severe mental retardation
F80–89	Developmental disorders	F84.0 Autism
F90–99	Childhood disorders	F94.0 Elective mutism

Keeping up-to-date and evidence-based

Textbooks and articles can be biased and rapidly outdated. The following are sources of up to date, good quality evidence in psychiatry.

● To hone your skills in evidence-based medicine (EBM) we recommend an EBM textbook such as *Evidence-based Medicine. How to Practice and Teach EBM*, Sackett D, Straus S, Richardson S, Rosenberg W, Haynes RB (2000), 2nd edition, Churchill Livingstone.

Finding the evidence

Access to high quality evidence in psychiatry is improving all the time.

● The *National Electronic Library for Health* (www.nelh.nhs.uk) is a website that brings together many good resources including the Cochrane Database of Systematic Reviews, the British National Formulary, Clinical Evidence, and Medline. Access to these resources is free to all users living in the UK. People from elsewhere will have to pay for access to some of the restricted resources.

● The *National Electronic Library for Health Mental Health Specialist Library* (http://www.nelmh.org/) contains much more detailed information and evidence about psychiatric treatments. It also has a lot of evidence-based information for patients.

● Emerging new evidence in psychiatry is summarized in *Evidence-based Mental Health*—a quarterly journal from the BMJ Publishing Group. The content of the journal is also available on line (http://ebmh.bmjjournals.com/).

Clinical practice guidelines

Clinical practice guidelines (CPG) are recommendations on the appropriate treatment and care of people with specific disorders. CPG can be a useful help, but should augment rather than replace clinical expertise and experience. Before using a CPG, make sure that it is properly evidence-based, and relevant to your patients.

● In the UK, the *National Institute for Clinical Excellence (NICE)* prepares national evidence-based guidelines. As of December 2004, mental health guidelines have been published on schizophrenia, eating disorders, self harm and depression, with others to come. All NICE CPGs are available at www.nice.nhs.uk.

Further reading

For more detailed general reading about psychiatry we recommend the *Shorter Oxford Textbook of Psychiatry*, Gelder M, Mayou R, Cowen P (2001) 4th edition, Oxford University Press.

Chapter 1

Lieberman JA, Rush JA (1996). Re-defining the role of psychiatry in medicine. *Am J Psychiatry* **153**, 1388–1397.

Core psychiatry for tomorrow's doctors (1997). *Psychiatr Bull* **21**, 522–524.

Geddes JR, Harrison PJ (1997). Evidence-based psychiatry: Closing the gap between research and practice. *Br J Psychiatry* **171**, 220–225

Crisp AH, Gelder MG, Rix S, *et al.* (2000). Stigmatisation of people with mental illness. *Br J Psychiatry* **177**, 4–7.

Chapters 2 and 3

Kopelman MD (1994). Structured psychiatric interview. *Br J Hosp Med* **52**, 93–98 and 277–281.

Davies T (1997). Mental health assessment. *BMJ* **314**, 1536–1539.

Sims AP (2003). *Symptoms in the Mind. An Introduction to Descriptive Psychopathology*, 3rd edition. London, Saunders.

Chapter 4

Maden A (1996). Risk assessment in psychiatry. *Br J Hosp Med* **56**, 78–82.

Atakan Z, Davies T (1997). Mental health emergencies. *BMJ* **314**, 1740–1742.

Hirschfeld RMA, Russell JM (1997). Assessment and treatment of suicidal patients. *New Engl J Med* **337**, 910–915.

Szmukler G (2001). Violence risk prediction in practice. *Br J Psychiatry* **178**, 84–85.

Chapter 5

Kendell RE (1975). *The role of diagnosis in psychiatry.* Oxford, Blackwell Scientific.

Sharpe M (1990). The use of graphical life charts in psychiatry. *Br J Hosp Med* **44**, 44–47.

Maguire P, Pitceathly C (2002). Key communication skills and how to acquire them. *BMJ* **325**, 697–700.

Chapter 6

Lazare A (1973). Hidden conceptual models in psychiatry. *New Engl J Med* **288**, 345–351.

Cawley RH (1993). Psychiatry is more than a science. *Br J Psychiatry* **162**, 154–160.

Andreasen NC (1996). Linking mind and brain in the study of mental illnesses: a project for a scientific psychopathology. *Science* **275**, 1586–1593.

Chapter 7

Andrews G (1993). The essential psychotherapies. *Br J Psychiatry* **162**, 447–451.

Tillett R (1996). Psychotherapy assessment and treatment selection. *Br J Psychiatry* **168**, 10–15.

Holmes J (2002). All you need is cognitive behaviour therapy? *BMJ* **324**, 288–294.

Stahl SM (2002). *Essential Psychopharmacology*, 2nd edition. Cambridge, CUP.

Chapter 8

White K, Roy D, Hamilton I (1997). Community mental health services. *BMJ* **314**, 1817–1820.

Burns T (1997). Case management, care management and care programming. *Br J Psychiatry* **170**, 393–395.

Chapter 9

Piccinelli M, Wilkinson G (1994). Outcome of depression in psychiatric settings. *Br J Psychiatry* **164**, 297–304.

Harris TO, Brown GW (1996). Social causes of depression. *Curr Opinion Psychiatry* **9**, 3–10.

Hale AS (1997). Depression. *BMJ* **315**, 43–46.

Muller-Oerlinghausen B, Berghofer A, Bauer M (2002). Bipolar disorder. *Lancet* **359**, 241–247.

Chapter 10

Gelder MG (1986). Neurosis: another tough old word. *BMJ* **292**, 972–973.

Sharpe M, Wilks D (2002). Fatigue. *BMJ* **325**, 480–483.

Tonks A (2003). Treating generalized anxiety disorder. *BMJ* **326**, 700–702.

Sharpe M, Mayou R (2004). Somatoform disorders: a help or a hindrance to good patient care? *Br J Psychiatry* **184**, 465–467.

Jenicke MA (2004). Obsessive–compulsive disorder. *N Engl J Med* **350**, 259–265.

Chapter 11

Margison FR (1997). Abnormalities of sexual function and interest: origins and interventions. *Curr Opinion Psychiatry* **10**, 127–131.

Fairburn CG, Harrison PJ (2003). Eating disorders. *Lancet* **361**, 407–416.

Seteia MJ, Nowell PD (2004). Insomnia. *Lancet* **364**, 1959–1973.

Chapter 12

Andreasen NC (1995). Symptoms, signs and diagnosis of schizophrenia. *Lancet* **346**, 477–481.

Harrison PJ, Owen MJ (2003). Genes for schizophrenia? *Lancet* **361**, 417–419.

Mueser KT, McGurk SR (2004). Schizophrenia. *Lancet* **363**, 2063–2072.

Chapter 13

Crimlisk H, Taylor M (1996). How to cope with a neuropsychiatric case. *Br J Hosp Med* **56**, 103–107.

Geldmacher DS, Whitehouse PJ (1996). Evaluation of dementia. *New Engl J Med* **335**, 330–336.

Lishman WA (1997). *Organic Psychiatry*, 3rd edition. Oxford, Blackwells.

Burns A, Gallagley A, Byrne J (2004). Delirium. *J Neurol Neurosurg Psychiatry* **75**, 362–367.

Chapter 14

Hall W, Zador D (1997). The alcohol withdrawal syndrome. *Lancet* **349**, 1897–1900.

Schuckit MA (1997). Substance use disorders. *BMJ* **314**, 1605–1608.

Lingford-Hughes A, Nutt D (2003). Neurobiology of addiction and implications for treatment. *Br J Psychiatry* **182**, 97–100.

Chapter 15

Marlowe M, Sugarman P (1997). Disorders of personality. *BMJ* **315**, 176–179.

Tyrer P (2001). Personality disorder. *Br J Psychiatry* **179**, 81–84.

Lieb K, Zanarini MC, Schmahl C, *et al.* (2004). Borderline personality disorder. *Lancet* **364**, 453–461.

Chapter 16

Bassarath L (2001). Conduct disorder: a biopsychosocial review. *Can J Psychiatry* **46**, 609–616.

Wilens TE, Biederman J, Spencer TJ (2002). Attention deficit/hyperactivity disorder across the lifespan. *Annu Rev Med* **53**, 113–131.

Volkmar FR, Lord C, Bailey A, *et al.* (2004). Autism and pervasive developmental disorders. *J Child Psychol Psychiatry* **45**, 135–170.

Chapter 17

King BH, DeAntonio C, McCracken JT, *et al.* (1994). Psychiatric consultation in severe and profound mental retardation. *Am J Psychiatry* **151**, 1802–1808.

Battaglia A, Carey JC (2003). Diagnostic evaluation of developmental delay/mental retardation: An overview. *Am J Med Genet* **117C**, 3–14.

Fraser W, Kerr M (2003). *Seminars in the Psychiatry of Learning Disabilities*, 2nd edition, Gaskell Press, London.

Chapter 18

Craig TK, Boardman AP (1997). Common mental health problems in primary care. *BMJ* **314**, 1609–1612.

Ramirez A, House A (1997). Common mental-health problems in hospital. *BMJ* **314**, 1679–1681.

Wessely S, Nimnuan C, Sharpe M (1999). Functional somatic syndromes: one or many? *Lancet* **354**, 936–939.

WHO World Mental Health Consortium (2004). Prevalence, severity, and unmet need for treatment of mental disorders in the World Health Organization World Mental Health surveys. *JAMA* **291**, 2581–2590.

Index

Page numbers in *italics* represent figures, those in **bold** represent tables

absence seizures 147
absent grief 99
abstinence 151
  alcohol 156
  nicotine 159
  opioids 157
acute brain syndrome *see*
    delerium
addiction *see* dependence
adherence *see* compliance
adjustment disorders 50,
    106–7, *106*
  children 172
adjustment reactions *see*
    adjustment disorders
administration, community
    care 82
adolescents 84, *178*, 178
  in detention facilities 179
adult psychiatry, general **80–3**
advanced directives 139
aetiology **49–56**, *50*
  behavioural model 52
  biochemical factors 55
  biological factors 42, *43*, 54–5
  biopsychosocial model 42
  cognitive model *52*, 52–3
  epidemiology 49
  family theories 51
  genetics *54*, 54–5
  life events 50
  personality factors 53–4
  psychodynamic theories 53
  psychological models 51
  social models 49–50
  vulnerability factors 50
affect 87
  flattened 19
  incongruous 19
affective disorders *see* mood
    disorders
affective instability 165
aggression 34, 40, 164
agitation 22
agoraphobia *104*, 104, 192
akathisia 19, 66
alcohol 14, **152–6**
  abstinence 156
  assessment 9, **32**, 150
  casualty department 189

cirrhosis 150
clinical features 153–4
community psychiatric
    services 84–5
consumption *152*, 152, *153*
  at risk 150, 151, 154
contextual history 33
delerium tremens 153, *155*
dementia 143
dependence 32, 153
  treatment **68**, 155–6
detoxification 155
hallucinosis 154
harmful effects 33, 152, *154*,
    155
  on children 179
harmful use 154
Korsakov's syndrome 154
management 154–5
medical disorders 33, 154, 156
psychiatric disorders 154
psychosis 21
recommended limits 9, 152
Wernicke's syndrome 153–4,
    155
withdrawal 32, 153, 189
Alcoholics Anonymous 156
alprazolam 64
Alzheimer's disease *137*, *139*,
    140–2
  aetiology 54, 55, 56, 140, *142*
  cholinergic defects 55
  clinical features 140
  Down's syndrome 185
  drug treatment **67–8**, 142
  genetic aspects 54, 56, 141
  management 142
  risk factors *141*
ambitendency 19
amenorrhoea 23, 31
  anorexia nervosa 113
amisulpride 67
amitriptyline *61*, 61, 64, 69
amnesia, psychogenic 107
amnesic syndrome 17, *137*, 146
amok 101
amphetamines 118, 150, 157
amyloid precursor protein
    mutations 54, 56, 141
anabolic steroids 159

anankastic personality disorder
    106, *162*, 163
anergia 22, 87, 88
Angelman syndrome 185
anhedonia 10, 22, 87, 88
animal models 56
anorexia nervosa 11, 30,
    113–16, 121, 192
  aetiology 114–15
  clinical features 113–14
  differential diagnosis 115
  epidemiology 114–15
  in-patient treatment 115–16
  management 115
  prognosis 116
anterograde amnesia 148
anticholinergics **67**
anticipation 185
anticipatory grief 99
anticonvulsants, epilepsy 62,
    63, 148
antidepressants **57**, **59–62**
  bipolar disorder 95
  borderline personality
      disorder 164
  bulimia nervosa 117
  childhood depressive disorder
      173
  depression 93, 95
  duration of treatment 57, 59
  elderly patients 69
  hypochondriasis 109
  mode of action 59
  neurosis 102
  obsessive-compulsive disorder
      106
  panic disorder 105
  phobic anxiety 104
  post-traumatic stress disorder
      107
  prescribing 2, *93*, 193
  schizophrenia 127
  somatoform disorder 109
  withdrawal 32
  see also monoamine oxidase
      inhibitors (MAOIs);
      selective serotonin
      reuptake inhibitors
      (SSRIs); tricyclic
      antidepressants (TCAs)

antipsychiatry 51
antipsychotics **64–7**
  atypical *64*, 64, **66–7**, *66*, 95
    disadvantages 67
  breastfeeding 69
  chemical structure *64*, 64
  conventional *64*, 64, *66*
  delerium 145
  delusional disorders 135
  dementia 138
  depot 66
  depression 94
  elderly patients 69
  mania 95
  mode of action 64–5
  personality disorders 164
  pregnancy 69
  schizoaffective disorders 133
  schizophrenia 125, 126
  side effects 18–19, *65*, 65, *66*
    anticholinergics treatment
      65, 67
anxiety 2, 26, 101
  benzodiazepines 63
  coping strategies 28
  generalized/free floating 27
  insomnia 117
  neurosis module 27
  paroxysmal 103, 105
  phobic 27, 103–4, *104*
  separation 170–1, 172
  situational 27
  symptoms 10, 27, **103**
anxiety disorders **103–5**
  behaviour therapy 73
  childhood 170–1, *171*
  generalized 103, *104*, *105*, 105
  head injury 149
  hospital in-patients 190
  out-patient clinic patients
    190
  panic disorder 103, 105
  phobic 103–4, *104*
  somatic symptoms 190
anxiolytics **63–4**
  contraindications in
    pregnancy/breastfeeding
    69
  neurosis 102
  phobic anxiety 104
  tricyclic antidepressants
    (TCAs) 61, 64
anxious personality disorder
  162
apolipoprotein E (aopE) gene
  140
appearance 10, 14, 18, 22, 23,
  24, 27, 28
  unresponsive patient 34

appetite 23, 25, 29
approved social workers (ASWs)
  76, 77, 82
aripiprazole 67
Asperger's syndrome (autistic
    psychopathy) 176
assertive outreach 83
assertiveness training 73
assessment *see* psychiatric
    assessment
ataxia 10
atomoxetine 175
attention deficit hyperactivity
    disorder 173, **174–5**,
    174, 178
  specific reading disorder 176
attitudes 2–3
atypical eating disorder 113
autism 51, **175–6**, *175*
  tuberous sclerosis 187
autistic psychopathy (Asperger's
    syndrome) 176
autistic spectrum disorders 175
avoidance behaviour 103, 104

behaviour therapy 52, 70, *71*,
    72, **73**
  dialectical 74, 164
  obsessive-compulsive disorder
    106
  phobic anxiety 104
behavioural conditioning in
    neurosis 103
behavioural disorders of
    children 173
behavioural theories **52**
la belle indifférence 108
benzodiazepines **63–4**, 69, 118
  acute stress reactions 106
  alcohol detoxification 155
  mania 95
  misuse 159
  mode of action 63
  overdose 64
  schizophrenia 125
  withdrawal 32, 63, 64
bereavement counselling 99
bereavement response 99
β-amyloid and Alzheimer's
    disease 54, 55, 141
  treatment strategies 142
binge eating 30, 116
  disorder 117
biochemical theories 55
biofeedback 73
biological factors 42, *43*, 54–5
biological models 54–5
biological treatments 57
biopsychosocial model 2, 42

bipolar disorder 11, 90, **91–2**
  adolescents 178
  aetiology 96, 97
  children 172
  chronic 91
  cognitive behaviour therapy
    95
  depressive episode treatment
    95
  lithium treatment 62
  management 95
  prognosis 96
  rapid cycling 92
  relapse prevention 95
body dysmorphic disorder *see*
    dysmorphophobia
body image distortion 30
body mass index 30, 31
borderline personality disorder
    162, 164–5
  sexual abuse history 179
bouffée dilirante 134
bovine spongiform
    encephalopathy (BSE)
    143
brain
  abnormalities 1
  biochemical studies 55
  functional imaging 55
  minimal dysfunction 164
  schizophrenia 131–2
    development 132
  structural imaging 55–6
breastfeeding 69, 98
  drug prescribing **69**
brief psychodynamic
    psychotherapy 72–3
brief reactive psychosis 134
Briquet's syndrome
    (somatization disorder)
    110
bulimia nervosa 30, 113,
    116–17, 121, 165
  aetiology 117
  clinical features 116
  cognitive behaviour therapy
    74
  epidemiology 117
  management 117
  sexual abuse history 179
buprenorphine 68, 156
buspirone 64

caffeine 159
CAGE questionnaire **9**, 32
candidate genes 54
cannabis 150, 158
Capgras' delusion 135
carbamazepine **63**, 69, 138

care plan 83
care programme approach
    (CPA) **82–3**, 86
    schizophrenia management
        125, 128
case control studies 49
case management, key worker
    82
case summary *46*, 46
casualty departments 189
catalepsy (posturing) 19
cataplexy 118
catatonia 19
    unresponsive patient 34, 35
causative factors **41–2**
    see also aetiology
challenging behaviour 182
child abuse 76, 164, **179**
    duty of care 168, 179
    somatoform disorder 108
child psychiatry 80, **84**
childhood disorders **168–80**
    adolescents *178*, 178
    aetiology 169, *170*
    anxiety 170–1, *171*
    attention deficit hyperactivity
        disorder 173, *174*, 174–5
    autism *175*, 175–6
    behavioural 173
    classification 168
    conduct disorder 169, *173*,
        173–4, *174*
    developmental 175
        pervasive 175–6
        specific 176–7
    emotional 169, 171–2
    encopresis 177
    enuresis 177
    epidemiology 168–9
    family factors 51
    learning disability 181, 182,
        183
    management 169
    mood 172–3
    physical illness 179
    prognosis 170, *171*
    psychosis 178
    school refusal 172
    selective (elective) mutism
        178
    somatoform disorder 171
    tics 177–8
childhood events
    depression 50
    personality disorders 163
    somatoform disorder 108
childhood history 13, 42
children
    in institutional care 178

interviewing 168, *169*
    legal issues 78
    prescribing 69
    psychiatrically ill parents 179
Children Act (1989) 78
chloral hydrate 64
chlordiazepoxide 155
chlorpromazine 65, 159
cholinesterase inhibitors **68**,
    142
chromosomal abnormalities 54,
    184, 185
    sex chromosomes 164
chronic brain syndrome/failure
    see dementia
chronic fatigue syndrome 27
    children 172
    see also neurasthenia
citalopram 59
classical conditioning 52
classification *see* psychiatric
    classification
clinical psychologist 82
clomipramine *61*, 61, 118, 172
clonidine 157
closed questions 8
clouding of consciousness 12,
    17, 144
    delerium 144
    unresponsive patient 34
clozapine 65, 67, 127, 143
cocaine 150, 157–8
codeine 156
cognitive analytical therapy 74
cognitive behaviour therapy **74**
    alcohol misuse 156
    anorexia nervosa 115
    bipolar disorder 95
    bulimia nervosa 117
    childhood obsessive-
        compulsive disorder 172
    depression 94, 95
    hypochondriasis 109
    neurasthenia 111
    neurosis 102
    panic disorder 105
    phobic anxiety 104
    post-traumatic stress disorder
        107
    premenstrual syndrome 98
    schizophrenia 127
    somatoform disorder 109
cognitive function 7
    assessment **16–18**
cognitive impairment 10
    assessment **12**, 17
    depression 17, 23–4
    head injury 149
cognitive theories **52–3**, *52*

cognitive therapy 53, 70, *71*,
    72, **73–4**
cohort studies 49
common law 76
communication skills 2
community addiction services
    84
community care 2, 14, 80,
    81–2
    care programme approach
        (CPA) 82–3
    crisis teams 81
    learning disability teams 184
community learning disability
    teams 184
community mental health
    teams (CMHTs) 82, 86
community psychiatric nurses
    (CPNs) 82
comorbidity 4, 86, 192
    hospital in-patients 190
competence, psychiatric
    opinion 78
compliance (adherence/
    concordance) 57, *59*
compulsion 11, 27
    dependence 32
compulsory treatment 57, **76**
    see also Mental Health Act
        (1983)
computerized tomography (CT)
    55
concentration 23, 24, 89
concordance *see* compliance
conditioning 52
conduct disorder 169, *173*,
    173–4, *174*, 179
    children in institutional care
        178
    specific reading disorder 176
confabulation 17, 146
confidentiality 8, 40, 78, 179
confusional state, acute *see*
    delerium
consciousness
    unresponsive patient 34
    see also clouding of
        consciousness
consent
    community care 82
    informed 76
    parental in child assessment
        168
constipation 23, 83
contextual factors 3, 7, 41
    assessment **12–13**
    risk assessment 36
contracts 78
conversion disorder **107–8**

coping strategies 24, 28
coprolalia 178
core assessment **8–14**, *9*
    contextual information
        12–13
    history 8–9
    investigations 14
    mental state examination
        10–12
    physical examination 13–14
    shrinking the core ('one
        minute screen') *14*, 14
Cotard's syndrome 88
counselling 75
countertransference 53, *72*
court diversion schemes 85
court reports 45, 78, 85
crack 157
Creutzfeldt–Jakob disease 143
crisis intervention services 81
critical psychiatry 51
cross-dressing 121
cyclothymia 91, 165
cyproterone acetate 121

danazol 98
dangerous and severe
        personality disorder 40,
        166–7
dangerousness assessment 85
day hospitals 81
De Clèrambault's syndrome
        135
deafness 16, 176
defence mechanisms *53*, 53
delayed grief 99
delerium 12, 14, 16, 17, 18, 34,
        83, 136, **144–5**, 191
    aetiology *144*, 144, *145*
    clinical features 144
    management 145
    prognosis 145
    tremens 32, 63, 153, *155*
delusion 11, **19–20**, 65, 122
    content 19
    grandiose 20, 25, 90
    mania 25
    nihilistic 20
    partial 11
    perceptions 19
    persecutory (paranoid) 19–20
    primary 19
    of reference 19
    secondary 19
delusional disorders 18, 129,
        132
    acute 134
    management 135
    morbid jealousy 134

persistent 134
    prognosis 135
    somatic 134
delusional mood 19
dementia 12, 14, 16, 17, 18, 81,
        83, **136–43**
    aetiology 137, *138*
    alcoholic 143
    assessment 138
    clinical features 136–7, *139*
    cortical 137, *139*
    depression differentiation
        137
    differential diagnosis 137–8,
        139
    driving 78
    drug treatment **67–8**
    familial disorders 49
    head injury 49
    investigations 138, *140*
    management 138–9
    neuropathology 56
    praecox 12
    presenile 137
    prognosis 139–40
    screening test 17
    subcortical 137, *139*
dependence 150
    alcohol 153, 155–6
    amphetamines 157
    nicotine 159
    opioids 156
    substance misuse 32
    treatment 155–6
dependent personality disorder
        162
depersonalization 12, 27–8
depersonalization-derealization
        syndrome **112**
depression 2, 18, **87–9**, 192
    aetiology 96
    agitated 92
    amphetamines 157
    antipsychotics 94
    assessment 22
    atypical 61, 92
    bipolar 95
    children 173
    classification 90
    clinical presentation *89*, 89
    cognitive behaviour therapy
        94, 95
    cognitive impairment 17,
        23–4
    cognitive model 53
    coping strategies 24
    dementia 138
        differential diagnosis 137
    double 92

drug therapy **57**, **59–62**, *93*,
        93–5
electroconvulsive therapy
        69–70, 94
endogenous 92
general practice 188
grief comparison *99*, 99
with learning disability 182
lithium 94
MAOIs 94
maternal 179
melancholia 23
mild 87, 93
moderate 87–8
module 21, **22–4**
mood 87
neurosis 101
non-response to first-line
        treatment 94
out-patient clinic patients
        190
postnatal 98
postschizophrenic 125
psychiatric referral 94
psychological treatment 94
psychotic 18, 19, 23, 88
reactive 92
relapse prevention 95
screening questions 10
severe 80, 88
social origins 50
somatic symptoms *88*, 190
steroid hypothesis 55
substance misuse 150
suicide 38
depressive disorder 22, 87,
        90–1
    aetiological factors 96–7, *97*
    childhood 173
    classification 90
    cognitive behaviour therapy
        74
    cognitive theories 53
    epidemiology *92*, 92
    hospital in-patients 190
    insomnia 117
    management 92–5, *93*
    prognosis 96
    psychosurgery 70
    recurrent 90, 95
depressive episode 87, 90
    bipolar disorder 92, 95
    management 95
depressive personality disorder
        90
depressive stupor 24, 88
deprivation dwarfism 179
derealization 12, 27–8, 112
desensitization 73

desipramine 61
detoxification 151, 155
  opioids 157
developmental disorders 175
  pervasive 175–6
  specific 176–7
dexamethasone suppression test
  55
dhat 101
diagnosis 3–4, **41**, 192, *193*
  hierarchical principles 4
  hypotheses 15
Diagnostic and Statistical
  Manual of Mental
  Disorders (DSM-IV) 4
  personality disorders 161,
  166
dialectical behaviour therapy
  74, 164
diazepam 64
dieting 30
differential diagnosis 4
discharge summary 45, 46
disinhibited gestures 24
disorganization 124
dissocial (psychopathic)
  personality disorder
  162, 163, 164, **165**, 174,
  175
dissociative disorders 27, 34,
  51, 101, **107–8**, *107*
disulfiram 68, 156
diurnal variation of mood 22
doctor–patient relationship 2, 3
  transference 72
domestic violence 76
donepezil 68, 142
dopamine hypothesis of
  schizophrenia 131
dopamine receptors 55, 129
  antagonism 64–5
Down's syndrome 54, 182,
  184–5, *184*
driving, fitness 78
drug treatment **57–69**, *58*, 193
  compliance (adherence/
  concordance) 57, *59*
  elderly patients **69**
  pregnancy/breastfeeding **69**
  prescribing principles 57, *59*
drug-induced psychosis 18
dysarthria 11
dysmorphophobia (body
  dysmorphic disorder) 29,
  108, **109**
dyspareunia **119**
dysphasia 11, 137
dysthymia 90
dystonia 19, 65, 67

early morning waking 23
eating disorder 7, **113–17**, 121
  assessment 30
  attitudes to weight/shape 30
  atypical 113
  body weight 30, 31
  differential diagnosis 31
  maternal 179
  module **30–1**
  physical examination 31
  risk factors 114–15, *115*
  see also anorexia nervosa;
  bulimia nervosa
echopraxia/echolalia 19
ecstasy (methylenedioxy-
  methamphetamine;
  MMDA) 158
ejaculatory failure 118
elderly patients **83–4**
  drug prescribing **69**
electroconvulsive therapy (ECT)
  69–70, 94
  childhood depressive disorder
  173
  depression 94
  depressive stupor 88
  informed consent 78
  mania 95
emergency assessment 14
emotional abuse 179
emotional disorder, childhood
  169, 171–2
employment 76
  history 13
encephalitis lethargica 123
encopresis 177
enuresis 177
environmental factors 50
  learning disability *186*, *187*,
  187
  schizophrenia *130*, 130–1
epidemiology 49, 188–90, *189*
epilepsy **146–8**, *147*
  anticonvulsants 62, **63**, 148
  childhood disorders 179
  complex partial
  (psychomotor) siezures
  146, *148*
  psychological problems
  147–8
  seizures 146–7, *147*
erectile dysfunction **119**
erotomania 135
ethnic minorities 85
euphoria 25
euthymia 87
evidence-based treatment 2, 57,
  193
  psychotherapy 71

excessive grief 99
exhibitionism 121
expressed emotion (EE) 127
extrapyramidal side effects
  65–6
eye contact 10, 22
eye movement desensitization
  and reprocessing 74,
  107

factitious disorder 29, 108,
  111–12, 189, 191
  by proxy 179
failure to thrive 179
family 50
  disorder clusters 54
  education 75
  history 13, 24, 42
  role in child psychiatry 169
  support 75, 125
  theories 51
family therapy 75
  schizophrenia 127
fetishism 121
first rank symptoms *21*, 21,
  122, *123*
flight of ideas 25, 90
flooding 73
flumazenil 64
fluoxetine 59, 69, 117, 172, 173
folic acid 185
folie à deux 135
forensic history 13, 85
forensic psychiatry 80, **85**, 121
  learning disability assessment
  182
formal thought disorder 11
formulation, psychiatric 45, 46,
  47
fragile X syndrome 54, 176,
  185, *185*
Fregoli's delusion 135
frontotemporal dementia *139*,
  143
fugue 107
functional magnetic resonance
  imaging (fMRI) 55

galantamine 68
gender identity disorders 121
general hospital psychiatry 80
general practitioneer (GP) 2, 14,
  82, 188–9
  communicating care 45
  writing to 45, 46–7
genetic factors 50, 51, 54–5
  heritability *54*, 54
  heterogeneity 55
  polymorphisms 54

Gilles de la Tourette syndrome
see Tourette syndrome
gonadotrophin agonists 98
graded exposure 73, 104, 120
grief 22, 98–9
  abnormal (pathological) 99
  depression comparison 99,
    99
  normal 99
  reactions 106
group homes
  learning disabled adults 183
  schizophrenia 128
group therapy 74

hallucinations 12, 18, 20, 23,
    65, 122
  alcoholic 154
  auditory 20, 88, 154
    mood congruent 20
  hypnogogic 12, 118
  hypnopompic 12
  LSD 158
  mania 25–6
  olfactory 20
  partial 12
  somatic 20
  third person 20
  visual 20
hallucinogens 158
haloperidol 65, 145
harm reduction approaches 157
harmful substance use 150, 151
  alcohol 154
head injury 49, 138, **148–9**
health care workers 86
heritability *54*, 54
heroin 150, 156
heterocyclic antidepressants 60
histrionic personality disorder
    162
homelessness 85
homicide 85
homosexuality 121
housing 13, 75, 76
5-HT system 55, 59, 60, 114, 176
  anxiety symptoms 103
  ecstasy 158
  hypofunction 97
Huntington's disease 54, 137,
    139, **143**
hyperkinetic disorder 174
  see also attention deficit
    hyperactivity disorder
hypersomnia *118*, 118
hypnogogic hallucinations 12,
    118
hypnopompic hallucinations
    12

hypnotics 118
  see also anxiolytics
hypochondriacal psychosis,
    monosymptomatic
    134–5
hypochondriasis 11, 29, 108,
    109
hypofrontality 131
hypomania 89
  bipolar disorder II 91
hypothalamic-pituitary-adrenal
    (HPA) axis 50, 55, 97
hysteria 107

ideas of reference 19
idiot savants 175
illness behaviour 51
illusion 12
  des soisies 135
imipramine 69, 177
impulsivity 165
in-patient care 80–1
  admissions 14
  child psychiatry 84
incidence 49
informants 8, 13, 34, 161
inherited errors of metabolism
    186, 186
insight 10, 21
  assessment **12**
  mania 26
insomnia **117–18**
  depression 23
  initial 23
  primary 117
  treatment 63, 118
International Classification of
    Diseases (ICD-10) 4
  depressive disorders 90
  personality disorders 161
interpersonal psychotherapy
    74, 94
  bulimia nervosa 117
interview setting 8
interviewing 8
  motivational 156
  skills 2, 3, 8, 15
intoxication 150, 157, 189
irritable bowel syndrome 110
isolation 23, 75

jealousy, morbid 40, 134, 150

ketamine 131, 158
key worker 82, 83
  schizophrenia 128
knight's move thinking 20
koro 101
Korsakov's syndrome 146, 154

lamotrigine **63**, 69, 95
language impairment 17
lanugo hair 31
lavender oil aromatherapy 138
learned behaviour 52
learned helplessness 52
learning disability 80, **181–7**
  assessment 181, *183*
  associated conditions 184–7
  behaviour therapy 73
  childhood disorders 181,
    182, *183*
  chromosomal abnormalities
    184, 185
  clinical features 181, *182*
  community teams 184
  definition 181
  environmental factors *186*,
    187, 187
  essential lifestyle planning
    184
  in-patient/residential care 81,
    184
  inherited errors of
    metabolism *186*, 186
  management 183–4
  mild/moderate/severe *182*
  psychiatric disorder 182,
    183
  risk assessment 182
  single gene defects 185–7
legal issues 78
Lesch-Nyhan syndrome 186
Lewy body dementia 138, *139*,
    142–3
liason psychiatry 80, **84**
libido 23, 53
  loss 118
  mania 25
  suppression 121
life charts 43, *44*
life events 24, 42, 50, 108, 192
likelihood ratio 9, 12
lithium **62**, 69
  bipolar disorder 26, 95
  breastfeeding 69
  depression 94
  mania 95
  pregnancy 69
  side effects 62
  toxicity 62
lofepramine *61*, 61
loosening of association 20
lysergic acid diethylamide (LSD)
    150

magic mushrooms 158
magnetic resonance imaging
    (MRI) 55, 56

major tranquilizers *see* antipsychotics
malingering 29, 34, 108, 111
management 43, **44**
  plan 5
mania 18, 80, 87, **89–90**
  aetiology 97
  antipsychotics 95
  assessment 24
  bipolar disorder I 91
  drug-induced 97
  electroconvulsive therapy 95
  lithium 95
  mild (hypomania) 89, 95
  moderate 90
  module 21, **24–6**
  physical examination 26
  psychosis 18, 19
  severe 90
  symptoms *89*, 89
  treatment 95
  violence risk 40
manic depression *see* bipolar disorder
manic episode 87, 91
  clinical features 89
mannerism 19
maternity blues 97–8
Meadows' syndrome 179
medical complaints, psychiatric disorder 190, *191*, 191
  worsening of symptoms 192
medical disorders
  in-patient psychiatric comorbidity 190
  organic psychiatric disorder *148*
  psychiatric manifestations *148*
  substance misuse 33
medical history 9, 14
melancholia 23
memantine 68, 142
memory impairment 17
menopause 98
menstrual disorders 23
menstrual history 30–1
Mental Health Act (1983) 70, **76–8**, *76*, 82
  dissocial (psychopathic) personality disorder 165
  sections *77*, 77–8
Mental Health Act (Scotland) **78**, *78*
Mental Health Care and Treatment Act (Scotland) (2003) *78*, 78
mental retardation *see* learning disability

mental state examination (MSE) 3, 6, 15
  core **10–12**
methadone 68, 156, 157
methylenedioxymethamphetamine (MMDA) 158
methylphenidate 175, 185
mini-mental state examination (MMSE) *17*, 17
minor emotional disorder 101
mirtazapine 62
mixed affective states 90, 92
mixed anxiety–depression 101
moclobemide 61–2
modafinil 118, 175
monoamine oxidase inhibitors (MAOIs) **61–2**
  breastfeeding 60
  cautions/contraindications 61
  depression 94
  mode of action 61
  side effects 61
mood
  assessment 10, 19, **21–6**
  congruity 88
  delusional 19
  depression 22
  diurnal variation 22
  mania 25
  objective 10
  reactivity 22
  somatoform disorder 29
  subjective 10
mood disorders 7, **87–100**, *88*
  aetiology 96
  children 172–3
  classification *90*, 90
  course *91*
  epidemiology *92*, 92
  management 92–5
  organic 90, *96*, 96
  prognosis 96
  rapid cycling 92
  suicide risk 96
  terminology *92*
mood stabilizers **62–3**
  borderline personality disorder 164
  elderly patients 69
  mania 95
  pregnancy 69
  schizoaffective disorders 133
morbid jealousy 40, 134, 150
morphine 156
motivation for change 151
motivational interviewing 156
motor abnormalities 18–19

movement
  assessment 18–19
  unresponsive patient 35
multi-infarct dementia 142
multidisciplinary teams 82
Munchausen's syndrome 111, 112
  by proxy 179
mutism
  akinetic 34
  selective (elective) 35, 178
myalgic encephalomyelitis (ME) 111

N-methyl-D-aspartate (NMDA) receptors
  antagonists **68**, 131, 142
  schizophrenia 131
naltrexone 68, 157
narcissistic personality disorder *162*
narcolepsy 118
needs assessment 13
negative reinforcement 52
negative symptoms 122, 123, 127
negativism 19
neglect 179
neologism 19
neurasthenia 27, **111**
  symptoms *111*
neurobiological developments 2
neuroendocrine challenge test 55
neurofibrillary tangles 141
neurofibromatosis 186, 187
neuroleptic malignant syndrome 35, 66
neuroleptics *see* antipsychotics
neuropathology 56
neurosis 7, 53, **101–12**
  aetiology 103
  assessment 26
  classification *102*
  cultural variants 101
  depersonalization-derealization syndrome 112
  diagnosis 102
  dissociative disorder 107–8
  epidemiology 102, 188
  general practice 188, 189
  management 102–3
  module **27–8**
  personality disorder 101
  prognosis 103
  somatic symptoms 27
  somatoform disorders 108–9
  stress reactions 106
  undifferentiated 101
  see also anxiety disorders

neurotic disorders 101
classification 102
neurotic symptoms 101
neuroticism 97, 103
nicotine 159
night terrors 178
nightmares 178
children 170
non-psychiatric setting **188–93**
epidemiology 188–90, 189
management of psychiatric
disorder 192–3
prevalence of psychiatric
disorder 188, 189
non-verbal cues 8
noradrenaline system 59, 60
anxiety symptoms 103
hypofunction 97
normal pressure hydrocephalus
139, **143**
nurse practitioners 82

obedience, automatic 19
obsession 11, 23
neurosis module 27
obsessive-compulsive disorder
11, 23, **105–6**, 106, 178
childhood 171–2
cognitive behaviour therapy 74
neurosis module 27
psychosurgery 70
Tourette syndrome 178
treatment 106
oestrogens 98
olanzapine 67, 95
open questions 8
operant conditioning 52
opioids **156–7**
dependence treatment **68**
harm reduction approaches
157
maintenance therapy 157
withdrawal 156, 156–7
oppositional defiant disorder 173
organic psychiatric disorder 4,
136–49, 145–9, 146
amnesic syndrome 146
childhood disorders 179
epilepsy 146–8
head injury 148–9
medical disorders 148
psychosis 18
see also delerium; dementia
out-patient clinics 190
overvalued ideas 11

paedophilia 121
panic attack 27, 105, 105, 147
cognitive model 52, 52

panic disorder 63, 103, 104,
105, 190, 192
with agoraphobia 104
cognitive behaviour therapy
74
cognitive model 52, 52–3
paralysis 107
paranoid (persecutory) delusion
19–20
paranoid personality disorder
162, 164
paranoid psychosis 134
amphetamines 157
chronic (paranoia) 134
paraphilias 121
paraphrenia 122, 137
parasomnias 118
parasuicide 38
parental training 174
parents, psychiatrically ill 179
parkinsonism 19, 65–6
Parkinson's disease dementia
143
paroxetine 107
passivity 20
perceptions 23, 25
assessment 10, **11–12**
delusional 19
perpetuating factors 41, 43, 43,
50
persistent somatoform pain
disorder 108, **110**
personal history 13
personality 13, 24
as aetiological factor 53–4
head injury-related change
149
personality disorders 28, **160–7**
aetiology 163–16
anankastic 27, 106, 162, 163
assessment 161
borderline 162, 164–5, 179
classification 161, 162
clinical features 160, 162
cluster A 162, 164
cluster B 162, 164–5
cluster C 162, 165
conceptual problems 166–7
dangerous and severe 40,
166–7
dependent 162
depressive 90
diagnosis 160–1
dissocial (psychopathic) 162,
163, 164, **165**, 165, 174,
175
epidemiology 163, 163
histrionic 162
immature 163

management 163
mature 163
multiaxial classification 166,
166
narcissistic 162
paranoid 162, 164
prognosis 163
psychiatric disorder
relationship 165–6, 166
violence risk 40
personality traits 160, 163
phencyclidine 131, 158–9
phenelzine 61
phenobarbitone 148
phenylketonuria 185–6, 186
phenytoin 148
phobias, childhood 172
phobic anxiety 63, 103–4, 104
cognitive behaviour therapy
74
physical examination **13–14**
physical therapies 58
Pick's disease 143
pimozide 135
population surveys 49
positive reinforcement 52
positive symptoms 65, 122, 123
positron emission tomography
(PET) 55
postconcussional syndrome
149
postnatal depression 98
post-traumatic stress disorder
27, 74, 106, **107**, 107,
165
posturing (catalepsy) 19
Prader-Willi syndrome 185
precipitating factors 9, 41, 42,
43, 43, 50
predisposing factors 41, 42, 43,
43, 50
pregnancy, drug prescribing **69**
premature ejaculation 120
premenstrual dysphoric
disorder 98
premenstrual syndrome 98
prescribing
elderly patients **69**
pregnancy/breastfeeding **69**
principles 57, 59
substitute 157
presenilin mutations 141
pressure of speech 25, 90
prevalence of psychiatric
disorders 49, 188, 189
primary care 188
primary gain 107
prion disease 56, 139, 140, **143**
problem lists 46, 47

problem-solving skills training 75, 174
procyclidine 67
prognosis 43, **44**
prolonged grief 99
propranolol 64
pseudodementia 12, 24, 137
pseudohallucinations 12, 20
pseudoseizures 107, 147
psychiatric assessment 2, 3, 6–8, *7*, *42*
  causative factors 41–2
  communication 3, 4–5, **45–7**
  completing 4, **41–4**
  contextual information 41
  core 3, 6, **8–14**, *9*
  diagnostic process 41
  information for patient 45–6, 47
  management decisions 43, 44
  modules 3, 6, 7–8, **16–35**
  in non-psychiatric setting 192
  prognosis 44
  summarizing cases **45–7**
psychiatric assessment modules **16–35**
  cognitive function 16–18
  depression 22–4
  eating disorders 30–1
  mania 24–6
  mood assessment 21–6
  neurosis 27–8
  psychosis 18–21
  somatoform disorders 28–9
  substance misuse 32–3
  unresponsive patient 34–5
  use 16
psychiatric care, filters to 188, *189*
psychiatric classification *4*, 4
  children 168
  multiaxial *166*, 166, 168, *169*, 183
psychiatric history 3, 9
psychiatric interview 3, 6, **8**, 15
psychiatric services **80–6**, *81*
psychiatric specialties 80
psychoanalysis 53
psychodynamic theories 53
psychodynamic therapy 70, **71–3**, *71*, *72*
psychogenic psychosis 134
psychogeriatrics 80, **83–4**
psychological disorders 1
psychological factors 3, 42, *43*
psychological medicine *see* liason psychiatry
psychological models 51

psychological treatment 57, **70–5**, 193
  depression 94
  neurosis 102
  phobic anxiety 104
  schizophrenia 127–8
psychomotor poverty 124
psychomotor retardation 22, 88
psychopathic disorder *see* dissocial personality disorder
psychopharmacology *see* drug treatment
psychosis 7
  acohol 21
  acute in substance misuse 150
  assessment 18
  benzodiazepines 63
  brief reactive 134
  children 178
  cognition 21
  delusions 11
  depressive (psychotic depression) 88
  general practice 189
  module **18–21**
  monosymptomatic hypochondriacal 134–5
  mood 19
  motor abnormalities 18–19
  organic disorders 18, 21
  paranoid 134, 157
  perceptions 20
  psychogenic 134
  puerperal 98
  therapy 64
  thoughts 19–20
  see also bipolar disorder; delusional disorder; organic psychiatric disorder; schizophrenia
psychosurgery **70**
psychotherapeutic skills 2, 3
psychotherapy *58*, **70–5**, *74*
  adjustment disorder 107
  adverse effects 71
  behavioural 70, *71*, *72*, **73**
  cognitive 70, *71*, *72*, **73–4**
  cognitive behavioural 74
  depression 94
  evidence-based therapy 71
  principles 70–1, *71*
  psychodynamic 70, **71–3**, *71*, *72*
  simple therapies 75
  supportive 75
public education 76
puerperal disorders **97–8**

puerperal psychosis 98
  electroconvulsive therapy 70
punishment 52

reading disorder, specific 176–7
reality distortion 21, 124
reality orientation 138
reboxetine 62
referral 8–9, 94, 193
Regional Secure Units 85
rehabilitation 76, 151
reinforcement 52
relationships 13
relaxation therapy 73, 118
retrograde amnesia 148
Rett's syndrome 176
risk **36–40**
  formulation 36–7
  management 36, 37–8
    immediate interventions 37
    risk of violence 40
  to others 40
risk assessment **36–7**, 40
  learning disability 182
  substance misuse module 32
risk factors 49
  genetic predisposition 54
  of poor outcome 44
risperidone 66, 95
rivastigmine 68
running commentary 20

St. John's Wort 62
schizoaffective disorder 132, **133**
schizoid personality disorder *162*
schizophrenia 11, 12, 18, 67, **122–35**
  acute 122, 124, 125
  adolescents 178
  aetiology 129
  brain imaging studies 55, 56
  cannabis use 158
  catatonic 19, 34, 35, 123
  chronic 123–4, *124*, *126*, 126–7
    relapse prevention 126–7
  clinical features 122, 123–4
  cognitive behaviour therapy 74
  cognitive impairment 21, 124
  depression 125
  differential diagnosis 124, *125*
  disorganization 124
  dopamine hypothesis 55, 131

schizophrenia (cont'd)
  environmental risk factors
      130, 130–1
  epidemiology 128–9
  family theories 51
  first rank symptoms *21*, 21,
      122, *123*
  genetic factors 129–30, *130*
  hallucinations 20
  head injury 149
  hebephrenic 123
  in-patient care 80, 81
  investigations 124–5
  late onset (paraphrenia) 122,
      137
  with learning disability 182
  management 64, 125–8, *126*
      admission for assessment
          125
      early intervention
          programmes 125–6
      medical review 127
  mood abnormalities 19
  N-methyl-D-aspartate
      (NMDA) receptors 131
  negative symptoms 122, 123,
      127
  neurodevelopmental model
      132, *133*
  neuropathology 131–2
  positive symptoms 65, 122,
      123
  prognosis 128, *129*
  psychological theories 132
  psychomotor poverty 124
  reality distortion 124
  related disorders 132–3
  residual 123
  social theories 132
  spectrum disorders 129
  subtypes *123*, 123
  susceptibility genes *130*
  though disorder 20
  violence risk 40
schizophreniform disorder
    122
schizotypal disorder 129, 132,
    135
Schneiderian symptoms 21
school refulsal *172*, 172
seasonal affective disorder 92
secondary gain 51, 107
sedatives *see* anxiolytics
selective (elective) mutism 35,
    178
selective serotonin and
      noradrenaline reuptake
      inhibitors (SNRIs) **62**

selective serotonin reuptake
      inhibitors (SSRIs) 57,
      59–60, 98
  breastfeeding 69
  depression 93
  mode of action 59, *60*
  pregnancy 69
  prescribing in childhood
      173
  side effects 60
  suicide risk 60
  tricyclic antidepressants
      comparison *60*
self-esteem 179
  social phobia 104
self-harm (deliberate self-harm)
      38, 40, 76, 186
  adolescents 173
  assessment 39
  borderline personality
      disorder 164
  casualty departments 189
  children in institutional care
      178
  eating disorders 31
  liason psychiatry 84
  repeated 39
  risk 36
      management 39
self-help groups 82
  alcohol misuse 156
self-monitoring 73
separation anxiety 170–1,
    172
serotonin system *see* 5-HT
    system
sertraline 59, 107
seven-minute screen 17
sex chromosome abnormalities
    164
sex offenders 121
sex therapy 119–20
sexual abuse 164, 165, 179
sexual desire 23, 25
  loss 118, 120
  objects of 121
sexual dysfunction **118–20**
  assessment 119, *120*
  psychological treatment
      119–20
  types *119*
sexual history 13
sexual preference disorders
    121
sick role 51
sildenafil 119
single photon emission
    tomography (SPET) 55

sleep 23, 29
  disorders **117–18**, 121
  disturbance in children 170,
      178
  hygiene 118
  mania 25
  paralysis 118
social deprivation
  attention deficit
      hyperactivity disorder
      174
  conduct disorder 173
social factors 3, 42, *43*, 49–50,
    75
social interventions 57, **75–6**,
    82
  acute 75
  dementia 139
  during psychiatric admission
      75
  during psychiatric care
      75–6
  neurosis 102
  personality disorders 164
  schizophrenia 128
social phobia 104–5
social policy 76
social skills 75
  training 73, 156
social workers 77, 78, 82
solvent misuse 159
somatic functional syndromes
    110–11, *110*
somatic symptom disorders
    110
somatic symptoms 7, 14, 26,
    29, 188, 190
  assessment 28
  neurosis 27, 101
  somatization 108
  disorder 29, 110
somatoform autonomic
      dysfunction 108, **110**
somatoform disorders 26, 27,
    51, 101–2, **108–9**
  assessment 28, 109
  casualty department 189
  childhood 171
  cognitive behaviour therapy
      74
  general practice 188
  hospital in-patients 190
  management 109
  module **28–9**
  out-patient clinic patients 190
  relation to functional somatic
      syndromes 110–11
  symptoms *108*, 190, 191

Special Hospitals 85
speech 10, 19, 22
  assessment **11**
  depression module 22
  mania 25
  psychosis 19
speed *see* amphetamines
stages of change model *151*, 151
stereotyped movement 19, 35
stereotypy 19
steroid hypothesis of depression 55
steroids, anabolic 159
stigma 2, 3, 51, 76
stimulants
  attention deficity hyperactivity disorder 175
  conduct disorder 174
  misuse 157-8
stimulus control 118
stress reactions 50
  acute 28, **106**, *106*
  adjustment disorders *106*, 106-7
  personality trait decompensation 160
  see also post-traumatic stress disorder
stress-related disorders 26, 27, 101-2, **106**
  assessment 26
  classification *102*
stressors 24
  current circumstances assessment 13
  life events 50
  social interventions 75-6
  specific to women 98
stupor 34
  depressive 24, 88
  unresponsive patient 34
substance misuse 7, 80, **150-9**, *151*, 188
  aetiology 151-2
  anabolic steroids 159
  assessment 31-2, 150-1
  benzodiazepines 159
  caffeine 159
  cannabis 158
  children in institutional care 178
  community psychiatric services 84-5
  complications 151
  conduct disorder 173, 174

drug treatment **68**
epidemiology 150
general practice 188
hallucinogens 158
harmful effects 33
management 151
maternal 179
medical disorders 33
module **32-3**
motivation for change 151
nicotine 159
psychiatric assessment 9
psychosis 21
solvents 159
stimulants 157-8
types 150
violence risk 40
substitute prescribing 157
suicide **38-9**
  attempted 38
  incidence 38
  intent 10, 23, 36, 38, 88, 164
  prevention *40*, 40
  risk 10, 40, 80, 88
    alcohol dependence 154
    assessment 38-9
    factors *37*, 38
    management 39, 40
    mood disorder 96
    postpubertal children 173
    SSRIs 60
  schizophrenia 128
supportive psychotherapy 75

tardive dyskinesia 14, 19, 66
tau protein 141, 143
temazepam 64
temper tantrums 147, 178
temporal lobe epilepsy 146
therapeutic community 75, 163, 164
thiamine deficiency, alcohol-induced 146
thought
  block 20
  broadcasting 20
  control 20
  echo 20
  insertion 20
  withdrawal 20
thought disorder 11, 20, 65, 122
  flight of ideas 25
  knight's move thinking 20
thoughts 10, **11**

assessment 10, **11**
content 11, 19-20, 23, 25, 29
depression 88
flow 11, 20
mania 25, 90
nature 11, 23, 25
possession 20
psychosis 19-20
thyroid function 14
tics 177-8
tolerance 32
torsade de pointes 66
Tourette syndrome 171, 177-8
transcultural differences 50, 85, 101
transference 53, *72*, 72
transgenic animal models 56
transsexualism 121
transvestism 121
trazodone 59, 62, 64
tremor 10
tricyclic antidepressants (TCAs) 57, **60-1**, *61*
  breastfeeding 69
  contraindications 61
  depression 93, 94
  elderly patients 69
  enuresis 177
  mode of action 60-1
    receptors blocked *61*
  overdose 61
  pregnancy 69
  side effects *61*, 61
  SSRIs comparison *60*
tri-iodothyronine 94
truancy *172*, 172
tuberous sclerosis 54, 176, 186-7

undifferentiated somatoform disorder 108, 110
unipolar disorder 90
unresponsive patient 7
  assessment 34
  module **34-5**
unsocialized conduct disorder 173
urine drug screen 14

vaginismus 120
valproic acid **63**, 69, 95
vascular dementia 138, *139*, **142**
velocardiofacial syndrome 129-30

venlafaxine 62, 94
violence risk 40
voluntary organizations 82
von Recklinghausen's disease 187
vulnerability factors 50

waxy flexibility 19
weight 30, 31
Wernicke's syndrome 153–4, 155
will making 78
withdrawal 150
   alcohol 153
   opioids *156*, 156–7

substance misuse 32
thought 20
word salad 20

zaleplon 64
zolpidem 64
zopiclone 64